WASHOE COUNTY LIBRARY

D0828292

ACSM's Guide to Exercise and Cancer Survivorship

ACSM's Guide to Exercise and Cancer Survivorship

American College of Sports Medicine

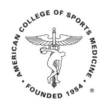

Melinda L. Irwin, PhD, MPH

Yale School of Medicine

— *Editor* —

Human Kinetics

Library of Congress Cataloging-in-Publication Data

ACSM's guide to exercise and cancer survivorship / American College of Sports Medicine ; Melinda L. Irwin, editor.
   p. ; cm.
  American College of Sports Medicine's guide to exercise and cancer survivorship
  Guide to exercise and cancer survivorship
Includes bibliographical references and index.
ISBN-13: 978-0-7360-9564-8 (print)
ISBN-10: 0-7360-9564-0 (print)
I. Irwin, Melinda L. II. American College of Sports Medicine. III. Title: American College of Sports Medicine's guide to exercise and cancer survivorship. IV. Title: Guide to exercise and cancer survivorship.
  [DNLM: 1. Neoplasms--therapy. 2. Exercise Therapy. QZ 266]
  LC-classification not assigned
  616.99'4062--dc23

                              2011029666

ISBN-10: 0-7360-9564-0 (print)
ISBN-13: 978-0-7360-9564-8 (print)

Copyright © 2012 by American College of Sports Medicine

All rights reserved. Except for use in a review, the reproduction or utilization of this work in any form or by any electronic, mechanical, or other means, now known or hereafter invented, including xerography, photocopying, and recording, and in any information storage and retrieval system, is forbidden without the written permission of the publisher.

Notice: Permission to reproduce the following material is granted to instructors and agencies who have purchased *ACSM's Guide to Exercise and Cancer Survivorship:* pp. 17-18, 52-54, 57-58, 76, 77-78, 98, 107-108, 120-121, 149, 155, 159, 167, 168-169, 175. The reproduction of other parts of this book is expressly forbidden by the above copyright notice. Persons or agencies who have not purchased *ACSM's Guide to Exercise and Cancer Survivorship* may not reproduce any material.

The web addresses cited in this text were current as of July 2011, unless otherwise noted.

Acquisitions Editor: Myles Schrag; **Developmental Editor:** Amanda S. Ewing; **Assistant Editor:** Anne Cole; **Copyeditor:** Patsy Fortney; **Indexer:** Nancy Ball; **Permissions Manager:** Dalene Reeder; **Graphic Designer:** Keri Evans; **Graphic Artist:** Denise Lowry; **Cover Designer:** Keith Blomberg; **Photographer (cover):** Neil Bernstein; **Photo Asset Manager:** Laura Fitch; **Photo Production Manager:** Jason Allen; **Art Manager:** Kelly Hendren; **Associate Art Manager:** Alan L. Wilborn; **Illustrations:** © Human Kinetics, unless otherwise noted; **Printer:** Sheridan Books

Printed in the United States of America   10 9 8 7 6 5 4 3 2 1

The paper in this book is certified under a sustainable forestry program.

Human Kinetics
Website: www.HumanKinetics.com

United States: Human Kinetics, P.O. Box 5076, Champaign, IL 61825-5076
800-747-4457
e-mail: humank@hkusa.com

Canada: Human Kinetics, 475 Devonshire Road Unit 100, Windsor, ON N8Y 2L5
800-465-7301 (in Canada only)
e-mail: info@hkcanada.com

Europe: Human Kinetics, 107 Bradford Road, Stanningley, Leeds LS28 6AT, United Kingdom
+44 (0) 113 255 5665
e-mail: hk@hkeurope.com

Australia: Human Kinetics, 57A Price Avenue, Lower Mitcham, South Australia 5062
08 8372 0999
e-mail: info@hkaustralia.com

New Zealand: Human Kinetics, P.O. Box 80, Torrens Park, South Australia 5062
0800 222 062
e-mail: info@hknewzealand.com

E5187

Contents

Contributors

Karen Basen-Engquist, PhD, MPH
Professor
Department of Behavioral Science, Cancer
  Prevention, and Population Sciences
The University of Texas MD Anderson Cancer
  Center

Claudio Battaglini, PhD
Assistant Professor
Department of Exercise and Sport Science
University of North Carolina at Chapel Hill

Kristin L. Campbell, BSc PT, PhD
Assistant Professor
Department of Physical Therapy
Faculty of Medicine
University of British Columbia

Wendy Demark-Wahnefried, PhD, RD
Professor and Webb Endowed Chair of Nutrition
  Sciences
Associate Director
University of Alabama at Birmingham
  Comprehensive Cancer Center

Christine M. Friedenreich, PhD
Senior Research Scientist/Epidemiologist
AHFMR Health Senior Scholar
Alberta Health Services—Cancer Care

Daniel C. Hughes, PhD
Institute for Health Promotion Research
University of Texas Health Science Center—
  San Antonio

Lee W. Jones, PhD
Associate Professor
Research Director, Duke Center for Cancer
  Survivorship
Department of Radiation Oncology
Duke University Medical Center

Larissa A. Korde, MD, MPH
Fred Hutchinson Cancer Research Center
Seattle, Washington

Stephanie Martch, MS, RD, LD
Project Director
The University of Texas MD Anderson Cancer
  Center

Heather K. Neilson, MSc
Epidemiology Research Associate
Alberta Health Services—Cancer Care

Heidi Perkins, PhD
Lecturer
Department of Kinesiology
Rice University

Tara Sanft, MD
Assistant Professor
Yale School of Medicine
Director of the Adult Survivorship Clinic
Yale Cancer Center

Kathryn Schmitz, PhD, MPH
Associate Professor
Department of Biostatistics and Epidemiology
University of Pennsylvania School of Medicine

Carole M. Schneider, PhD
Director, Rocky Mountain Cancer Rehabilitation
  Institute
Professor, School of Sport and Exercise Science
University of Northern Colorado

Anna L. Schwartz, PhD, FNP, FAAN
Affiliate Professor
School of Nursing
University of Washington

ACSM Reviewers

James R. Churilla, PhD, MPH, MS, RCEP
ACSM Program Director Certified
Assistant Professor
Clinical and Applied Movement Sciences
Brooks College of Health
University of North Florida

Ildiko Nyikos, MA, ACSM RCEP
Research Specialist
Lakeshore Foundation

William F. Simpson, PhD, CES, FACSM
Associate Professor
University of Wisconsin–Superior
    Department of Health and Human Performance
Associate Professor
Director, Exercise Physiology Laboratory

Mark A. Patterson, MEd, RCEP
Registered Clinical Exercise Physiologist
Department of Cardiovascular Services
    and Department of Vascular Therapy
Kaiser Permanente—Colorado Region

Madeline Paternostro Bayles, PhD, FACSM
Professor
Health and Physical Education
Indiana University of PA

S.A.E. Headley, PhD, FACSM, RCEP, CSCS
Professor
Exercise Science and Sport Studies
Springfield College

Sherry Barkley, PhD, CES, RCEP
Assistant Professor and Chair
HPER Department
Augustana College

Nikki Carosone, MS, CPT
Long Island University
School of Health Sciences
Adjunct Professor of Exercise Physiology
General Manager
Plus One Health Management

Paul Sorace, MS, RCEP
Clinical Exercise Physiologist
Hackensack University Medical Center

Peter Ronai, MS, FACSM, RCEP, CES, CSCS-D
Clinical Assistant Professor
Exercise Science
Sacred Heart University

Preface

In the last couple of decades, we have made considerable progress in diagnosing certain cancers earlier and treating many cancers more effectively. During this time physical activity has emerged as an important modifiable health behavior that also plays a key role in both the prevention and treatment of certain cancers. Although we have known since the 1980s that being physically active is associated with reductions in the risk of being diagnosed with many cancers,[1] it was not until 2005 that the first paper was published examining the importance on survival of being physically active *after* a diagnosis of cancer.[2] Since 2005, many more studies have been published that consistently show a benefit of being physically active and a reduced risk of developing a recurrence or dying of cancer or other related causes.[3-6]

A common question people ask after a diagnosis of cancer is, "What can I do to improve my chances of survival?" Because physical activity has been shown to have a multitude of health benefits including fewer side effects of chemotherapy and radiation and improved quality of life and survival, and because it is safe and easy to implement,[7, 8] more clinicians and oncologists than ever before are recommending that their patients exercise. Patients are seeking opportunities to learn how to exercise safely given the side effects of their surgeries and treatments or their prediagnosis lifestyles.

As a result of the growing research showing that exercise ameliorates the side effects of treatment and improves survival rates, and the increase in inquiries about physical activity to cancer foundations across the country, the American Cancer Society (ACS) and the American College of Sports Medicine (ACSM) decided to issue physical activity guidelines for cancer survivors.[7, 8] The ACS first published its physical activity guidelines for cancer survivors in 2006;[7] the ACSM followed with its own guidelines in 2010.[8] Both sets of guidelines were created in roundtable discussions that occurred over many days in meetings and telephone and e-mail conversations among internationally recognized scientists studying the effects of exercise on cancer survivorship and oncologists treating cancer patients.

The ACS and ACSM physical activity guidelines are very important for motivating more clinicians to recommend exercise and refer their patients to qualified fitness professionals, which in turn may encourage health insurance companies to cover exercise programs for cancer survivors, as they do cardiac rehabilitation programs. Equally important, however, is ensuring that fitness professionals are educated in how to work with cancer survivors. They must understand what a cancer diagnosis entails, the types of surgeries and treatments commonly prescribed, how these treatments affect the body, and how exercise may facilitate a faster recovery from surgery and treatment and ultimately improve survival rates.

To meet this need for fitness professional training, in late 2006 the ACS, under the direction of Colleen Doyle, the ACS Director of Nutrition and Physical Activity Division, reached out to the ACSM to discuss the development of a certification exam for fitness professionals. The purpose of this exam would be to test fitness professionals' knowledge about the benefits of exercise for cancer survivors, and their ability to adapt and tailor exercise programs for this population.

Although some courses on how to develop exercise programs for cancer survivors were being offered around the country, none were based on evidence-based medicine, and none were developed with the input of scientists and oncologists. Thus, the ACS and ACSM invited 10 scientists and oncologists to develop a specialty certification for fitness professionals working with cancer survivors. The scientists and oncologists first met in early 2007 to discuss the qualifications needed for becoming certified and the scope of practice for fitness professionals with this certification. The first draft of the certification exam was beta-tested in 2007, and it went live in December 2008. The certification was titled ACSM/ACS Certified Cancer Exercise Trainer (CET).

Fitness professionals can now take this computer-based exam at various testing locations around the country (visit www.acsm.org for more information). Although a number of organizations offer workshops, books, or information on how to modify exercise programs for cancer survivors, the ACSM CET is the only evidence-based certification exam that underwent a rigorous development process that included experts in the field—both researchers and clinicians— treating cancer patients.

In early 2009, the ACSM, with its educational partner Fitness Resource Associates, developed a webinar series for those wanting to take the CET exam as well as for those wanting to learn about exercise and cancer patients to earn CECs or simply for their own edification. Dr. Kathryn Schmitz, associate professor at the University of Pennsylvania and an international leader in the field of exercise and cancer survivorship research, developed and presents the webinar curriculum.

Although the webinars have been extremely beneficial for increasing knowledge regarding how to modify exercise programs for cancer survivors, the ACSM thought it was also important to offer a textbook to use both to prepare for the exam and to refer to when working with cancer survivors. *ACSM's Guide to Exercise and Cancer Survivorship* includes 10 comprehensive, yet concise chapters that present the science behind the benefits of exercise to cancer survival, as well as the application of that science to the development or adaptation of exercise programs for those diagnosed with cancer. The intention of each chapter is to train the trainer in developing and adapting exercise programs for cancer survivors. Although this textbook was written primarily for the fitness professional, it is very relevant to any professional working with cancer survivors—physical therapists, occupational therapists, nurses, oncologists, general practitioners, and nutritionists—as well as to people diagnosed with cancer or caring for cancer survivors.

The chapters focus on all the knowledge and skills (which are listed at the beginning of each chapter) that are the source for the content of the CET exam while also offering examples of exercise adaptations for cancer survivors. Topics include the incidence and prevalence of the most common cancers; common cancer treatments and side effects; the benefits of exercise after a diagnosis of cancer; exercise testing, prescription, and programming;

nutrition and weight management; health behavior change counseling; injury prevention; and program administration. Each chapter was written by an expert in the field of treating cancer survivors or researching the effects of exercise on cancer survivorship. Each chapter also includes a handful of take-home messages to offer practical applications of the topics discussed. The take-home messages highlight issues such as safety and how to deal with certain situations. Each chapter also includes forms and questionnaires, such as sample letters to the client, medical and cancer treatment history forms, and exercise questionnaires, to help fitness professionals begin an exercise program with a new client. This book is a resource manual for studying for the ACSM/ACS Certified Cancer Exercise Trainer exam, while also offering comprehensive information on how to develop and adapt exercise programs for cancer survivors.

Today, with this textbook, along with the ACSM webinars, the ACS and ACSM physical activity guidelines, and the ACSM/ACS Cancer Exercise Trainer certification, there are more resources than ever before to help one specialize and excel in developing safe and effective exercise programs for cancer survivors. Research tells us that exercise after a cancer diagnosis decreases the risk of a recurrence, improves survival rates, and decreases the side effects of treatment.[2-8]

Those who were physically active before a cancer diagnosis often wonder whether exercising was protective. Research shows that exercise delays tumor growth so that a person may be diagnosed later (e.g., at age 70 rather than 50) or at an earlier disease stage (e.g., stage I rather than stage III). Research also shows exercise benefits those who were not physically active before diagnosis. It is never too late to start an exercise program. Becoming physically active can have clinically meaningful effects such as better recovery from surgery, fewer negative side effects of treatment, and increased survival rates.

We hope this textbook will increase fitness professionals' knowledge of the importance of exercise after a cancer diagnosis, as well as their skills at developing and adapting exercise programs. The more certified exercise trainers there are, the more exercise opportunities there will be in our communities for those diagnosed with cancer. Our hope is that this textbook is not just a tool for educating the fitness professional, but is also a means toward increasing the physical activity levels of, and in turn improving the quality and quantity of years for, people diagnosed with cancer.

References

1. Thune I, Ferberg A. Physical activity and cancer risk: Dose-response and cancer, all sites and site specific. *Med Sci Sports Exerc.* 2001; 33(6): S530-S550.

2. Holmes MD, Chen WY, Feskanich D, et al. Physical activity and survival after breast cancer diagnosis. *JAMA.* 2005; 293(20): 2479-2486.

3. Irwin ML, Smith A, McTiernan A, et al. Association between pre- and post-diagnosis physical activity on mortality in breast cancer survivors: The Health, Eating, Activity, and Lifestyle (HEAL) Study. *J Clin Oncol.* 2008; 26(24): 3958-3964.

4. Holick CN, Newcomb PA, Trentham-Dietz A, et al. Physical activity and survival after diagnosis of invasive breast cancer. *Cancer Epidemiol Biomarkers Prev.* 2008; 17(2): 379-386.

5. Pierce JP, Stefanick ML, Flatt SW, et al. Greater survival after breast cancer in physically active women with high vegetable-fruit intake regardless of obesity. *J Clin Oncol.* 2007; 25: 2345-2351.

6. Sternfeld B, Weltzien E, Quesenberry CP Jr., et al. Physical activity and risk of recurrence and mortality in breast cancer survivors: Findings from the LACE study. *Cancer Epidemiol Biomarkers Prev.* 2009 Jan; 18(1): 87-95.

7. Doyle C, Kushi LH, Byers T, Courneya KS, Demark-Wahnefried W, Grant B, McTiernan A, Rock CL, Thompson C, Gansler T, Andrews KS. Nutrition, Physical Activity and Cancer Survivorship Advisory Committee; American Cancer Society. Nutrition and physical activity during and after cancer treatment: An American Cancer Society guide for informed choices. *CA Cancer J Clin.* 2006; 56(6): 323-353.

8. Schmitz KH, Courneya KS, Matthews C, Demark-Wahnefried W, Galvão DA, Pinto BM, Irwin ML, Wolin KY, Segal RJ, Lucia A, Schneider CM, von Gruenigen VE, Schwartz AL, American College of Sports Medicine. American College of Sports Medicine roundtable on exercise guidelines for cancer survivors. *Med Sci Sports Exerc.* 2010; 42(7): 1409-1426.

Acknowledgments

This textbook, although primarily focused on the development and adaptation of exercise programs for cancer survivors, also covers many additional topics including cancer prevention, cancer diagnosis, surgical and treatment options, side effects of surgery and treatment, nutrition, injury prevention, program development, and many other cancer survivorship topics. I am extremely grateful to all the scientists and clinicians who contributed their expertise and knowledge to this book. These prominent experts volunteered their time so that this book would be made available, primarily for the fitness professional, but also for the cancer survivor wanting to make healthy lifestyle changes.

Although a growing number of exercise programs for cancer survivors are becoming available throughout the United States and abroad, and this is indeed a good thing, many of these programs are not evidence based or led by certified fitness professionals. Fortunately, the American Cancer Society (ACS) and the American College of Sports Medicine (ACSM) had the foresight to bring together the clinicians and scientists who are conducting and leading research studies of exercise and cancer survivorship to develop an evidence-based certification exam for fitness professionals. Thus, I want to thank ACS, specifically Colleen Doyle, and ACSM, including Mike Niederpruem, Hope Wood, Kerry O'Rourke, Kela Thomas, and Richard Cotton, for moving this field forward and being the only organizations to offer such a certification exam. I have never been prouder of being a member and fellow of ACSM than I am now.

I also want to thank the editors and staff at Human Kinetics for publishing this textbook. From my initial telephone calls and e-mail exchanges with Myles Schrag, senior acquisitions editor, to the final stages of editing with Amanda Ewing, everything went very smoothly. Although I would have loved this book to have been published one, two, or even five years ago because of the growing number of cancer survivors and the urgent desire of many professionals to educate and counsel them on the benefits of exercise, the research on this topic was still in its infancy. Thanks to the cutting-edge research that has been conducted in the past five years, there is no better time than now to publish this book.

On that note, I am extremely grateful to the U.S. National Cancer Institute, ACS, Susan G. Komen for the Cure, the Lance Armstrong Foundation, and other organizations that sponsor and fund research studies focused on exercise and cancer survivorship. In addition, ACSM and ACS have sponsored the development of consensus statements and recommendations for physical activity for cancer survivors. This book is based on those evidence-based recommendations.

I also want to acknowledge the many fitness professionals eager to safely train cancer survivors. These fitness professionals are seeking out opportunities, such as the ACSM/ACS Cancer Exercise Trainer certification exam as well as this textbook, to increase their knowledge of how to appropriately develop and adapt exercise programs.

Last, and most important, I dedicate this book to the many cancer survivors I have encountered over the years at meetings and conferences and in my role as a researcher. Thank you for pushing the field forward, for participating in research, and for making sure opportunities exist beyond surgery and treatment that focus on the whole person.

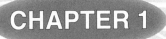

Diagnosis and Treatment of Cancer

Larissa A. Korde, MD, MPH

Content in this chapter covered in the CET exam outline includes the following:

- General knowledge of the descriptive epidemiology of cancer, including the prevalence, incidence, and survival statistics for the major cancer types.

- General knowledge of cancer biology (e.g., initiation, promotion/progression, and metastases), particularly for the four most common cancers: lung, breast, colon, and prostate.

- Knowledge of currently accepted screening practices for surveillance of recurrence for common cancers (e.g., mammography, colonoscopy, prostate specific antigen, pap smears).

- Knowledge of the pathology tests used to diagnose common cancers (e.g., biopsy, imaging technologies, and blood tests for tumor markers).

- General knowledge of current cancer treatment strategies, including surgery, systemic therapies (e.g., chemotherapy) and targeted therapies (e.g., anti-angiogenesis inhibitors).

- Understand typical durations of cancer therapy for the major cancers (breast, prostate, melanoma, ovary, lung, colon), and that therapies are continually evolving/changing.

- Knowledge of the most common warning signs of recurrence for common cancers, and when to recommend that clients seek additional medical evaluation.

Cancer is an important cause of morbidity and mortality in the United States. It is estimated that more than 12 million Americans have a current or past diagnosis of cancer. Knowledge of cancer incidence, risk factors, treatment, and treatment side effects is important for health care practitioners and fitness professionals working with cancer survivors. This chapter provides an overview of basic cancer biology and addresses incidence, screening, and risk factors for common malignancies. In addition, this chapter briefly reviews cancer treatment and side effects.

Cancer Incidence and Survival

In the United States, cancer is currently the leading cause of death among women 40 to 79 years of age and men 60 to 79 years of age, and is second to heart disease as the most common cause of death in adults of all ages. Of note is the fact that death from heart disease has steadily decreased over the past three decades, whereas cancer mortality has declined only slightly among people younger than 85 in the past decade. Among those 85 and older, cancer mortality has been basically stable from 1975 to 2005. Lung cancer is the most common cause of cancer death in men, accounting for 29% of cancer deaths; prostate and colorectal cancer account for 11% and 9% of cancer deaths in men. Lung cancer is also the most common cause of cancer mortality in women, accounting for 26% of cancer deaths; breast cancer is responsible for about 15% of cancer mortality and colorectal cancer for approximately 9%.[1]

Although lung cancer is the most common cause of cancer mortality in both men and women, it is not the most commonly diagnosed cancer in either gender. Prostate cancer is the most prevalent malignancy among men. It is estimated that prostate cancer will account for 28% of all cancer diagnoses in men, whereas lung cancer will be responsible for approximately 15% of cancer diagnoses. In women, breast cancer is the most prevalent form of cancer, accounting for approximately 28% of diagnoses, with lung cancer making up about 14% of malignant cases. In both men and women, colorectal cancer is estimated to be responsible for about 10% of cancer diagnoses in 2011.[1] Estimates of the number of new cancer cases and deaths for 2010 are shown in figure 1.1.

Take-Home Message
Cancer is a major health problem in the United States and is an important cause of morbidity and mortality among American adults. As cancer treatment and screening improve, the number of cancer survivors increases. A working knowledge of cancer risk factors, incidence, and treatment, as well as the long-term sequelae of cancer, are important for professionals working with cancer survivors.

Cancer Biology

Cancer occurs when cells in the body escape normal mechanisms of control, leading to abnormal cell division and proliferation. Cancer cells can also invade surrounding tissues (i.e., metastasis) and eventually can spread to distant sites through the blood and lymph systems. Cancer can arise in virtually any part of the body, and cancer types are grouped into broad categories. *Carcinoma* is cancer that begins in the skin or in tissues that line or cover internal organs. *Sarcoma* refers to cancer that begins in supportive or connective tissue, such as muscle, bone, fat, and blood vessels. *Leukemia* begins in blood-forming tissues and results in abnormal blood cells that circulate throughout the body in the blood. *Lymphoma* and *myeloma* are cancers that originate in cells of the immune system.

Cancer develops and progresses through the accumulation of genetic abnormalities, or mutations, within cells. Mutations can occur in genes that induce increased activity (oncogenes) or can cause inactivations of genes that generally control cellular activity (tumor suppressor genes). Through the accumulation of mutations, cancer cells become resistant to the normal cellular signaling processes, leading to uncontrolled growth and resistance to apoptosis (cell death). Tumors develop the ability to form new blood vessels (angiogenesis), which allows them to be self-sufficient and to spread. Cancers spread by two basic mechanisms: *invasion* (direct penetration into neighboring tissues) and *metastasis* (penetration into lymphatic and blood vessels leading to distant spread and eventual seeding in distant sites).

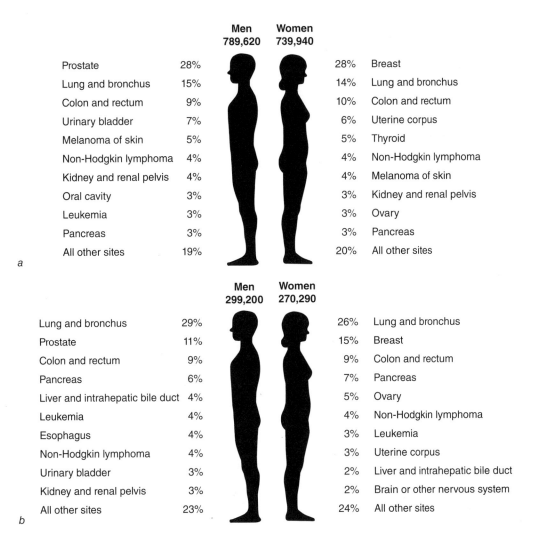

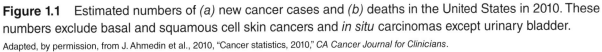

Figure 1.1   Estimated numbers of *(a)* new cancer cases and *(b)* deaths in the United States in 2010. These numbers exclude basal and squamous cell skin cancers and *in situ* carcinomas except urinary bladder.

Adapted, by permission, from J. Ahmedin et al., 2010, "Cancer statistics, 2010," *CA Cancer Journal for Clinicians*.

Most gene mutations that lead to the occurrence of cancer are somatic, meaning that they occur within individual cells. However, a small number of cancers are associated with inherited cancer syndromes, in which particular gene mutations that predispose people to cancer are passed down from parent to child. Families that experience multiple cancers or cancers that occur at earlier-than-usual ages (e.g., younger than 50 for breast cancer) may warrant referral to a cancer genetics professional.

Cancer Staging

A staging system is a standardized way to describe the extent to which a cancer has spread. The process of staging cancer arose from the observation that survival rates were generally higher for cancers that were localized compared with those that had spread beyond the organ or site of origin. Staging can be based on clinical information (e.g., the size of the tumor on physical examination or imaging) or pathologic information (measurements taken by the pathologist after surgical removal of a tumor).

For solid tumors, the American Joint Committee on Cancer (AJCC) generally uses a classification system that takes into account the size of a tumor (T), the degree of lymph node involvement (N), and the presence or absence of distant metastases (M). Depending on the TNM classification, a tumor is assigned a stage grouping, from stage 0 to stage

IV. Stage 0 refers to *in situ*, or noninvasive, cancer. This is also sometimes referred to as intraepithelial neoplasia. Stages I and II generally represent disease that is confined to the site of origin and locoregional area. Stages III and IV refer to disease that has spread to distant sites (metastatic disease).[2] In general, solid tumors that are diagnosed at an early stage (I and II) are less likely to result in mortality than advanced-stage disease (III and IV).

The U.S. Surveillance, Epidemiology and End Results (SEER) program monitors cancer incidence and mortality in the United States and presents five-year relative survival figures for various types of cancer. The five-year relative survival rate compares the observed survival among people with a given stage of cancer to what is expected for people without cancer. This database does not currently report using the AJCC classification system (staging), but rather, groups cancers into local, regional, and distant stage disease. Five-year relative survival rates for the most common solid tumors in men and women are shown in figure 1.2.[3]

Lymphoid neoplasms arise from cells of the immune system, including B-cells, T-cells, plasma cells, and NK (natural killer)-cells. A number of systems are used for classifying lymphoid neoplasms. Traditionally, classification systems have distinguished between *lymphomas*, which generally present with an obvious tumor in either lymph nodes or an extranodal site, and *leukemias*, which

typically involve the bone marrow and peripheral blood. However, in some cases both manifestations of lymphoid malignancies may be present.

Tumors that arise from plasma cells, which are part of the B-cell lineage, include multiple myeloma and plasmacytoma, and are also considered to fall into the spectrum of lymphoid neoplasms. The current standard used in clinical trials is the Revised European-American Classification of Lymphoid Neoplasms (REAL) and World Health Organization (WHO) classification, which uses clinical, morphologic, immunophenotypic, and genetic features over 25 categories of lymphoid neoplasms.[2] The REAL/WHO classification system includes all lymphoid neoplasms: Hodgkin's lymphoma, non-Hodgkin's lymphoma, lymphoid leukemias, and plasma cell neoplasms. The staging

Take-Home Message
Cancer staging is based generally on the size of the primary tumor, the presence or absence of the involvement of local or regional lymph nodes, and the presence or absence of distant metastases. Stage at diagnosis is directly related to the prognosis and guides the choice of treatment.

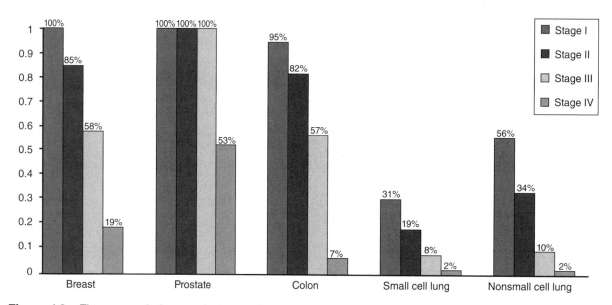

Figure 1.2 Five-year relative survival rates for common cancers by stage at diagnosis.
Data from Gloeckler Ries et al. 2003.[3]

TABLE 1.1   Summary of Ann Arbor Classification of Staging of Lymphoma

Stage	Disease involvement
I	Involvement of a single lymph node region
IE	Involvement of a single extralymphatic organ or site
II	Involvement of two lymph node regions on the same side of the diaphragm (II) or with involvement of contiguous extralymphatic organ or tissue (IIE)
III	Involvement of lymph node regions on both sides of the diaphragm (III) and/or limited contiguous extralymphatic organ or site (IIIE)
IIIS	As III with involvement of the spleen, or spleen + extranodal organ or site (IIIES)
IV	Diffuse or disseminated involvement of one or more extralymphatic organs, with or without associated nodal involvement, including disease present in the bone marrow or liver, or nodular involvement of the lung(s); OR isolated extralymphatic organ involvement in the absence of adjacent regional lymph node involvement, but in conjunction with disease in distant sites

All stages are further divided on the basis of the absence (A) or presence (B) of systemic symptoms, including fever, night sweats, and/or unexplained weight loss of greater than 10% of normal body weight.

Adapted from Greene et al. 2002.[2]

system used for defining the extent of disease for Hodgkin's and non-Hodgkin's lymphoma is based on the Ann Arbor classification, and is summarized in table 1.1.

Cancer Screening and Diagnosis

The purpose of cancer screening is to detect a cancer at an asymptomatic stage. Because stage of disease is generally associated with prognosis, the detection of cancer at an early stage can lead to a reduction in mortality.[4,5] In addition, cancer screening can reduce morbidity, because treatment for earlier-stage cancers or premalignant disease is often less aggressive than that for more advanced disease.[5] For screening for a particular disease to be effective, two general criteria must be met:

1. A test or procedure exists that can detect the disease earlier than if it were detected by symptoms.
2. There must be evidence that earlier treatment of the disease results in improved survival.

In addition to the potential survival benefits of a screening test, a number of potential harms must also be considered. Although most screening examinations are noninvasive or minimally invasive, the test itself may pose a risk of complications (e.g., perforation during a colonoscopy). In addition, screening tests can result in either false positive results, leading to an additional workup for an abnormality that does not represent true disease, or false negative results, leading to false reassurance in a person who has the disease. An ideal screening test has both a low false negative rate and a low false positive rate, usually referred to as specificity and sensitivity, respectively.

Current ACS screening guidelines are presented in table 1.2. Note that although lung cancer is the second most common malignancy in adults, routine screening is not recommended because, to date, no screening examinations have been shown to lead to an earlier diagnosis or improvement in survival rates. Similarly, although screening for ovarian cancer has been studied extensively, current data do not support a benefit for routine screening.

It is important to note that an abnormal screening result, such as an elevated prostate-specific antigen (PSA), the presence of abnormal cytology on a Pap smear, or an abnormal finding on mammography, may not necessarily result in a diagnosis of cancer. Rather, an abnormality on screening leads to additional workup aimed at diagnosing or ruling out a malignancy. This may include additional imaging (specific imaging studies that assist in the diagnosis of particular cancers are discussed later), but the definitive diagnosis of cancer is generally made by

TABLE 1.2 American Cancer Society Screening Recommendations for Average-Risk, Asymptomatic People

Cancer site	Population	Screening test	Frequency
Breast	Women aged ≥20 years	Breast self-examination (BSE)	Providers should discuss BSE with women beginning in their early 20s, emphasizing the importance of reporting any changes or symptoms. Women who choose to practice BSE should be instructed in proper technique.
		Clinical breast examination (CBE)	For women in their 20s and 30s, CBE as part of a routine physical examination at least every three years is recommended. Asymptomatic women 40 years or older should continue to have CBE, preferably on an annual basis.
	Women aged ≥40 years	Mammography	Women should begin annual mammography at 40.*
Colorectal	Men and women aged ≥50 years	Fecal occult blood testing (FOBT) or fecal immunochemical test (FIT); OR	Annually
		stool DNA test; OR	Interval uncertain
		flexible sigmoidoscopy; OR	Every five years
		FOBT or FIT and flexible sigmoidoscopy; OR	Annual FOBT or FIT and flexible sigmoidoscopy every five years
		double contrast barium enema; OR	Every five years
		colonoscopy; OR	Every 10 years
		computed tomography colonography	Every five years
Prostate	Men aged ≥50 years	Digital rectal exam (DRE) and prostate-specific antigen test (PSA)	Men with at least a 10-year life expectancy should have the opportunity to make an informed decision with a health care provider about whether to be screened for prostate cancer, after receiving information about the benefits, risks, and uncertainties associated with prostate cancer screening.
Cervix	Women aged ≥18 years	Pap test	Cervical cancer screening should begin approximately three years after a woman begins to have sexual intercourse, but no later than 21 years of age. Screening should initially be performed with either a conventional Pap test (yearly) or a liquid-based Pap test (every two years). At or after age 30, women who have had three normal consecutive Pap tests may be screened every two to three years with a Pap test, +/– an HPV (human papillomavirus) DNA test. Women who are >70 years of age who have had three normal consecutive Pap tests and no abnormal tests in the past 10 years, and those who have had a hysterectomy, may elect to stop cervical cancer screening.
Endometrium	Women at menopause		Women should be informed about the risks and symptoms of endometrial cancer and strongly encouraged to report any unexpected bleeding or spotting to their physician.
Cancer-related checkup	Men and women aged ≥20 years		Periodic health examination should include examination for cancers of the thyroid, testes, ovaries, lymph nodes, oral cavity, and skin. All patients should be counseled on health practices related to sun exposure, tobacco, diet, nutrition, risk factors, sexual practices, and environmental and occupational exposures.

* The U.S. Preventive Services Task Force recommends biennial mammographic screening for women between the ages of 50 and 74.[6]

Adapted, by permission, from R.A. Smith et al., 2010, "Cancer screening in the United States, 2010: A review of current American Cancer Society guidelines and issues in cancer screening," CA Cancer Journal for Clinicians 60(2): 99-119.

direct examination of tissue, usually by way of a needle or excisional biopsy. The workup and treatment for the most common cancers are described in their respective sections (i.e., breast cancer, prostate cancer, and so on) that follow.

Take-Home Message
To be effective, a cancer screening test must result in diagnosis at an early stage, which must result in a decrease in the chance of dying from the disease. Currently, screening is recommended for breast and cervical cancer in women, prostate cancer in men, and colorectal cancer in men and women.

Breast Cancer

The majority of breast cancers are detected either by an abnormal screening mammogram or a lump palpated by either the patient or her physician. A small percentage of patients present with local symptoms such as breast pain, breast enlargement, nipple retraction, or nipple discharge.[7] Abnormal findings on screening mammography include calcifications, architectural distortions, and frank masses. Areas of abnormality can be further evaluated with ultrasound, which helps to determine whether a mass is present and whether the lesion is solid or cystic. If a malignancy is suspected by imaging or physical examination, a biopsy should be performed; this can be done either with radiologic guidance or via a surgical excision. Breast magnetic resonance imaging (MRI) is also useful in select cases, either for screening in women with a very high risk of breast cancer, such as those with a genetic predisposition, or to provide additional information regarding the extent of disease present in the breast.

Local therapy for breast cancer includes surgical removal of the tumor, evaluation of the axillary lymph nodes, and if indicated, radiation therapy. When a primary tumor is present, surgical options include mastectomy (removal of all breast tissue) and breast-conserving treatment with a lumpectomy (removal of the tumor with a wide margin of normal tissue) followed by radiation. For women with large tumors or multifocal disease, lumpectomy may not be an option. Numerous studies

have shown that, for appropriate candidates and when followed by radiation, lumpectomy has the same overall survival rates as mastectomy, although breast-conserving therapy is associated with a slightly higher risk of local recurrence.[8, 9]

Surgical management of invasive breast cancer should also include evaluation of the axillary lymph nodes. This can take the form of either an axillary lymph node dissection or a sentinel lymph node biopsy, in which the lymph node or nodes that directly drain the area of the tumor are identified and removed. If these initial nodes contain cancer cells, the standard of care is to perform an axillary dissection. However, if the sentinel node is free of disease, the patient can be spared a full nodal dissection.[10] This is particularly important because a full nodal dissection is associated with a higher risk of lymphedema than is a sentinel node procedure.[11] Studies suggest that 3 to 5% of patients who undergo sentinel lymph node biopsy develop lymphedema, versus 16 to 19% of those who undergo axillary lymph node dissection.[12, 13] For patients with known lymph node involvement based on biopsy or clinical findings, an axillary dissection is the standard of care.

For women who choose breast conservation, and for some women who undergo mastectomy (e.g., those with positive surgical margins or numerous involved lymph nodes), radiation is generally recommended. For women with stage 0 breast cancer (ductal carcinoma *in situ*; DCIS) who undergo lumpectomy, radiation is also generally recommended. Standard whole breast radiation is typically given five days per week for five to six weeks.

The term *adjuvant treatment* refers to treatment that occurs after the surgical removal of a cancer; it is aimed at preventing recurrence of disease. Adjuvant treatment may include radiation, as described earlier, or systemic treatments such as hormonal therapy, chemotherapy, and targeted biologic therapy. The necessity of and options for systemic treatment are based on a number of characteristics of the tumor, including size, grade, the presence or absence of lymph node involvement, and the expression of certain receptors that can guide the use of specific therapies.

Women with DCIS (stage 0 breast cancer) who express hormone receptors may benefit from adjuvant hormonal treatment. Estrogen receptor is expressed in 50 to 60% of DCIS cases.[14] In women treated with lumpectomy and radiation, additional treatment with tamoxifen for five years reduces the risk of local recurrence and contralateral breast cancer.[15, 16]

In patients with invasive breast cancer whose tumors express estrogen or progesterone receptors, or both (about 70 to 75% of breast cancers), studies have shown that treatment with hormonally directed medications such as tamoxifen or aromatase inhibitors (anastrozole [brand name Arimidex]; letrozole [Femara]; exemestane [Aromasin]) can reduce the risk of recurrence by 40% or greater, and may also have an effect on overall survival.[17] These medications are pills that are taken once daily, usually for at least five years.

About 20 to 30% of breast tumors express HER2/neu, a protein that is associated with a more aggressive subtype of breast cancer.[18] Trastuzumab (Herceptin), a monoclonal antibody to HER2/neu is commonly used in combination with chemotherapy for treatment of metastatic, HER2-positive breast cancer.[19] Recently, trastuzumab has also been shown to reduce recurrence risk and improve survival in early-stage breast cancer patients.[20, 21] In this setting, trastuzumab is generally given in combination with chemotherapy initially, and then continued for one year. Trastuzumab is administered intravenously, either weekly or every three weeks. The major side effect of trastuzumab is an increased risk of cardiotoxicity, and thus cardiac function should be monitored by echocardiogram or nuclear scan periodically.

The need for chemotherapy in early-stage breast cancer is also based on tumor characteristics. The National Comprehensive Cancer Network (NCCN) recommends chemotherapy for women with tumors that are node positive, and for those with node-negative disease with certain unfavorable features (large tumor size, high tumor grade or other high-risk histologic features, hormone receptor negativity). There are numerous accepted chemotherapy regimens for breast cancer; most include two or three drugs given concurrently or in sequence.

Chemotherapy drugs commonly used in the treatment of early-stage breast cancer include adriamycin, cyclophosphamide, paclitaxel, docetaxel, methotrexate, and 5-fluorouracil. Chemotherapy for breast cancer is generally given in two- to four-week cycles for four to six cycles, for a total duration of 12 to 24 weeks of treatment. For many standard breast cancer regimens, treatment is given intravenously on the first day of each cycle; in other treatments, different drugs may be administered on different days of the cycle (e.g., weekly or every two weeks). After completion of treatment, patients should initially have a physician visit with clinical breast examination every three to six months, and should also continue annual mammography. Currently, additional imaging evaluation for recurrent or distant disease is not routinely recommended in the absence of specific symptoms.

In patients with stage IV, or metastatic, disease, the complete eradication of disease is very unlikely, and thus treatment is aimed at palliation of symptoms and shrinkage of disease burden. In this setting, multiple modalities of therapy can be considered, including radiation therapy, hormonal therapy (for estrogen or progesterone receptor–positive disease), chemotherapy and targeted therapy, and supportive management such as pain medication and bone-targeted agents such as zoledronic acid (Zometa). Treatment plans should be individualized based on the location of disease, tumor burden and aggressiveness, and symptoms.

Prostate Cancer

Prostate cancer primarily affects older men, with a mean age at diagnosis of 68.[22] Many men with prostate cancer, particularly those with localized disease, die of other illnesses before their prostate cancer causes significant disability. Consequently, choice of treatment is often driven by the age at diagnosis, the presence of intercurrent illness, and possible side effects of therapy.

There is controversy regarding the value of screening for prostate cancer and the optimal treatment for each stage of disease.[23] For a man with an abnormal screening result, additional workup generally involves a transrectal biopsy of the prostate gland, which is usually performed under local anesthesia with ultrasound guidance. Additional information that may aid in determining the prognosis of the tumor and making therapeutic decisions include the level of PSA elevation, Gleason score (a histologic grading score on a scale of 2 to 10, with higher scores indicating high-grade tumors with poorer prognoses), patient age and comorbid conditions, and clinical stage.[24]

Localized prostate cancer can be treated with radical prostatectomy or radiation. In selected cases with favorable prognostic factors, watchful waiting with treatment only at evidence of tumor progression is also an option.[25] Surgical management is usually reserved for patients in good health with tumors confined to the prostate gland (stage I or II).[26] Full surgical staging in patients undergoing radical prostatectomy includes an evaluation of the extent of disease (whether the tumor is confined to the capsule of the prostate gland) and resection margins, and an evaluation of the pelvic lymph nodes in higher-risk patients.[27] If intraoperative evaluation reveals pelvic nodal metastases, radical prostatectomy is not usually performed, because risk of recurrence is much greater with extraprostatic disease.

Patients with disease confined to the prostate and surrounding tissue (stages I through III) are candidates for definitive external beam radiation therapy. Long-term results of radiation therapy depend on the initial stage of disease; more than 75% of patients with T1 disease (incidentally discovered or screen detected) are alive without recurrence of prostate cancer at 10 years, whereas those with T4 disease (invading into adjacent organs or pelvic wall) have less than 25% recurrence-free survival at 10 years.[28] Interstitial brachytherapy (permanently placed radioactive iodine implants in the prostate gland) is used at certain centers for patients with favorable tumor characteristics, such as a low Gleason score and T1 or T2 tumors, and may be associated with a lower risk of impotence and other radiation-related side effects.[29] For more advanced tumors, both brachytherapy and external beam radiation may be used. After prostatectomy or radiation, patients should be followed with PSA testing and DRE every three to six months; abnormal test results should prompt a further workup with imaging.

The growth of prostate cancers can be driven by androgens, primarily testosterone. Treatments that reduce androgen levels in the body, referred to as androgen deprivation therapy, are commonly used in the treatment of locally advanced and metastatic prostate cancer, although the timing of the initiation of therapy has been the issue of some debate.[30] These include orchiectomy (surgical removal of the testes), LHRH agonists (medications such as leuprolide [Lupron] or goserelin [Zoladex] usually given by subcutaneous injection, either monthly or every three months), and antiandrogens (flutamide [Eulexin], bicalutamide [Casodex], and nilutamide

[Nilandron], taken orally on a daily basis). These treatments lower testosterone levels, leading to a desired effect on tumor recurrence and progression, but have side effects including loss of libido, osteoporosis, and impotence.[31] For this reason, decisions for treatment should be individualized. Metastatic prostate cancer is generally treated initially with androgen deprivation, but it eventually becomes resistant to endocrine maneuvers, at which time chemotherapy may be initiated.

Lung Cancer

Lung cancer is the leading cause of cancer mortality in the United States in both men and women.[1] Approximately 90% of all lung cancers are related to smoking, with a strong dose–response relationship. Risk decreases with smoking cessation, but former smokers are still at higher risk of lung cancer than those who have never smoked.[32] People exposed to secondhand smoke are also at increased risk of developing lung cancer compared with nonsmokers without exposure to cigarette smoke.[33] To date, screening of asymptomatic people with an elevated risk of lung cancer because of smoking or other exposures is not recommended, because this strategy has not been shown to decrease mortality.[34]

Presenting symptoms of lung cancer relate to the location and extent of the tumor. Symptoms related to localized obstruction of major airways and the infiltration of lung tissue or surrounding blood vessels include cough, shortness of breath, and hemoptysis (coughing up blood). Tumors that invade locally into adjacent structures can cause chest pain, pleural effusion (accumulation of fluid in the space around the lungs), or shoulder and arm pain in the case of tumors in the lung apices. Metastatic disease can present with symptoms of distant organ involvement, such as bone pain, neurologic symptoms, or mental status changes.[35]

In those with new or progressive symptoms, an imaging workup, initially with a chest X-ray or computed tomography (CT) scan of the chest, is recommended. The next step is to obtain a tissue diagnosis. This can often be done via bronchoscopy (a minimally invasive technique for visualizing the inside of the airways) for central lesions, but may require a CT-guided needle biopsy or surgery in patients with peripheral lesions or pleural disease. Additional imaging, such as a CT scan, a positron emission tomography (PET apices) scan, or a brain MRI may be required to evaluate for distant disease. In addition, in patients who appear to be candidates for surgical resection, a pulmonary function evaluation should be performed to determine whether they are at risk of pulmonary compromise or postoperative complications.[36]

For treatment and prognosis, lung cancer is divided into two histologic categories: small cell lung cancer (SCLC) and non–small cell lung cancer (NSCLC). The majority of patients with SCLC present with advanced-stage disease, and thus thorough staging with imaging, evaluation of the mediastinum, and bone marrow biopsy are recommended. For patients with disease limited to the thorax, lobectomy (removal of one lobe of the lung) or pneumonectomy (removal of the entire lung), followed by adjuvant chemotherapy and thoracic irradiation is the treatment of choice. In addition, patients with SCLC are at very high risk for the development of brain metastases, and thus prophylactic cranial irradiation should be considered. For patients whose disease is metastatic at presentation, combination chemotherapy has been shown to improve their chances of survival.[35] The most common chemotherapy regimen used for treatment of SCLC is cisplatin and etoposide. When given without concurrent radiation, these drugs are usually administered intravenously on a daily basis for the first three days of a 21- to 28-day cycle, for four to six cycles.

Non–small cell lung cancer accounts for about 80% of all lung cancers and includes squamous cell carcinoma, large cell carcinoma, and adenocarcinoma. For patients with operable NSCLC (smaller lesions with limited or no nodal involvement), the treatment of choice is lobectomy, although in some cases bilobectomy or pneumonectomy is required. In patients with high-risk histological features, positive surgical margins, or more extensive disease noted at surgery, postoperative chemotherapy or chemoradiation is often recommended. Because of the high risk of recurrence, surveillance with chest CT every four to six months is recommended after completion of therapy.

For patients with extensive local disease at the time of diagnosis and those with tumors in certain locations that are difficult to resect, treatment options may include surgery, chemotherapy, or radiation, or a combination of modalities. Decisions

about resectability should be made by a multidisciplinary team of thoracic specialists. In some cases, preoperative chemotherapy, with or without concurrent radiation, can render tumors operable when they initially presented as inoperable.

In general, metastatic disease is not considered operable. Local treatment options for such patients include localized radiation to decrease tumor burden, and, in some cases, surgical resection of solitary metastases. Systemic chemotherapy with single agent or doublets should be considered for patients with a good performance status. Chemotherapy agents commonly used to treat NSCLC include cisplatin, carboplatin, paclitaxel, docetaxel, gemcitabine, and etoposide. The addition of targeted therapies, such as bevacizumab (a monoclonal antibody that blocks vascular endothelial growth factor) or erlotinib (a small molecule inhibitor of the enzyme tyrosine kinase, which is involved in numerous cell cycling and survival pathways), has been shown to improve survival rates, and should also be considered for patients without a contraindication to these agents.[37, 38] Side effects from these targeted therapies include an increased risk of bleeding, hypertension, and renal toxicity.

With the advent of targeted therapies, the management of many cancers, including NSCLC, is rapidly evolving. As knowledge about both tumor biology and treatment response improves, we are increasingly able to recognize which tumors are most likely to respond to a given therapy, thus enabling the more individualized management of cancer patients. As an example, numerous studies have recently shown that patients whose tumors do not contain a mutation in the gene k-ras, which is

Take-Home Message
The most common cancer among men in the United States is prostate cancer, accounting for more than 25% of cancer cases. In women, breast cancer is the most common malignancy, accounting for roughly 28% of cancer diagnoses. However, the most common cause of cancer death among both men and women in the United States is lung cancer.

known to be involved in cancer development and progression, are more likely to respond to treatment with targeted therapy drugs such as erlotinib and cetuximab.[39] As more information of this sort becomes available, we will be increasingly able to provide certain treatments to patients who are most likely to respond, and to spare those who are not likely to benefit from those therapies because of their toxicities.

Colorectal Cancer

Colorectal cancer is highly treatable and often curable when confined to the bowel; thus, screening for this disease is routinely recommended for people over the age of 50. Colon cancers may be asymptomatic or may present with vague abdominal complaints such as pain or bloating. Minor changes in bowel habits or blood in the stool may also be seen; with right-sided lesions, chronic blood loss may lead to symptomatic anemia. Left-sided lesions may cause obstructive symptoms such as nausea or vomiting. Very distal or rectal lesions can present with feelings of rectal fullness and urgency.[40]

An initial workup for colorectal cancer should include a digital rectal examination (DRE) and a colonoscopy with a biopsy of any suspicious lesions. As with other cancers, tissue examination is required to confirm the diagnosis of malignancy. Staging depends on the degree of invasion into the bowel wall, whether tumor is present in the regional lymph nodes, and whether there is evidence of distant spread of disease. A CT scan may aid in determining the extent of disease. Carcinoembryonic antigen (CEA) is a blood marker that may be elevated in patients with colorectal cancer. CEA should be checked at baseline; if elevated, it can be monitored postoperatively for evidence of disease recurrence.[40]

Primary treatment for colorectal cancer involves surgical excision of the tumor and the evaluation of adjacent draining lymph nodes and surrounding connective tissue. The surgical procedure of choice is usually a hemicolectomy; in some cases, this procedure can be performed laparoscopically.[41] Resection of rectal tumors generally requires a surgical margin free of tumor. In some cases, a sphincter-sparing approach may be possible.

For patients with nodal involvement or tumors invading the muscle, postoperative chemotherapy may be considered. Prior to this decade, the main-stay of chemotherapy for colorectal cancer was 5-fluorouracil (5-FU). Newer regimens combine either intravenous 5-FU or capecitabine, an oral form of 5-FU, with newer chemotherapy agents such as oxaliplatin or irinotecan or targeted therapy such as cetuximab or bevacizumab. As with lung cancer, emerging data suggest that cetuximab is particularly effective for patients in whom tumors do not have mutations of the k-ras gene.[42]

Postoperative radiation therapy should be considered for patients with tumors that have invaded into the muscle in the bowel wall or have perforated the bowel wall, and in those with positive surgical resection margins. In patients with rectal cancer, chemotherapy and radiation are often given concurrently and may be prescribed prior to or after completion of surgical resection.[42]

Local recurrences of colon cancer usually happen at the surgical site or in adjacent lymph nodes. The most common sites of distant spread are the lung and liver. For patients with a single or few metastatic lesions, resection of metastatic lesions may result in cure. Chemotherapy for advanced disease is an evolving field, but generally involves sequential or concurrent use of the agents described previously for treatment in the adjuvant setting.

Patients with a diagnosis of colon cancer that have completed therapy should be carefully monitored with physician visits and CEA testing (if indicated) every three months initially, and then every six months. A follow-up colonoscopy should be performed within a year of diagnosis, and then every one to five years depending on whether additional premalignant lesions are present. In patients at high risk of recurrence, surveillance may also include a CT scan of the abdomen.[43]

Take-Home Message
Treatment for cancer can involve local therapy (usually surgery, radiation, or both) or systemic therapy (chemotherapy, hormonal treatment, or targeted therapy). Newer targeted therapies exploit certain known abnormalities present in tumors to give the most effective treatment with the fewest side effects.

Cancer Recurrence Warning Signs

Signs of cancer recurrence are generally related to the site and the extent of the disease. For example, metastatic disease in the lung may present with symptoms of obstruction, similar to those for primary lung cancer; bony metastases generally present with pain at the site of the lesion. Thus, any new or progressive symptoms in cancer survivors, particularly those whose initial presentation was associated with a high risk of recurrence, should be evaluated by a physician and by blood work and imaging as appropriate. It is also important to note that, although the risk of recurrence for most cancers is highest within the first several years following diagnosis and treatment, for cancers that are more indolent, such as prostate cancer or hormone receptor–positive breast cancer, recurrence can occur many years or even decades after the initial diagnosis. In addition, survivors of most cancers are also at risk for a second primary tumor of the same type, or for certain cancers that can occur as complications of chemotherapy or radiation.

Summary

It is estimated that there are over 12 million cancer survivors in the United States, representing about 4% of the U.S population.[44] Breast is the most common cancer in women, and prostate is the most common cancer in men; lung cancer is the leading cause of cancer death in both men and women. Risk of cancer recurrence, and ultimately, survival, are related to the extent of disease present at the time of diagnosis and the effectiveness of treatment. Screening is recommended for cancers for which early detection can lead to decreases in morbidity and mortality. Overall, about 67% of people diagnosed with cancer survive their disease, and a significant portion of these are long-term survivors. Cancer treatments include surgery, radiation, and systemic treatments such as chemotherapy, hormonal therapy, and targeted therapy, all of which can have both short- and long-term side effects. Thus, a thorough understanding of the progression of disease, treatment

modalities, and follow-up are important for professionals involved in the care of cancer patients and survivors.

References

1. Jemal A, Siegel R, Ward E, Hao Y, Xu J, Thun MJ. Cancer statistics, 2009. *CA Cancer J Clin.* 2009 Jul-Aug; 59(4): 225-249.

2. Greene FL, Fleming ID, Fritz AG, Balch CM, Haller DG, Morrow M, eds. *AJCC Cancer Staging Manual.* 6th ed. Chicago: American Joint Committee on Cancer; 2002.

3. Gloeckler Ries LA, Reichman ME, Lewis DR, Hankey BF, Edwards BK. Cancer survival and incidence from the Surveillance, Epidemiology, and End Results (SEER) program. *Oncologist.* 2003; 8(6): 541-552.

4. Mandel JS, Bond JH, Church TR, et al. Reducing mortality from colorectal cancer by screening for fecal occult blood. Minnesota Colon Cancer Control Study. *N Engl J Med.* 1993 May 13; 328(19): 1365-1371.

5. Smith RA, Cokkinides V, Brooks D, Saslow D, Brawley OW. Cancer screening in the United States, 2010: A review of current American Cancer Society guidelines and issues in cancer screening. *CA Cancer J Clin.* 2010 Mar-Apr; 60(2): 99-119.

6. Screening for breast cancer: U.S. Preventive Services Task Force recommendation statement. *Ann Intern Med.* 2009 Nov 17; 151(10): 716-726, W-236.

7. Jardines HB, Doroshow JH, Fisher P, Weitzel J. Breast cancer overview: Risk factors, screening, genetic testing and prevention. In: Pazdur R CL, Hoskins WJ, Wagman LD, eds. *Cancer Management: A Multidisciplinary Overview.* Manhasset, NY: CMP Healthcare Media; 2004: 165-190.

8. Fisher B, Anderson S, Bryant J, et al. Twenty-year follow-up of a randomized trial comparing total mastectomy, lumpectomy, and lumpectomy plus irradiation for the treatment of invasive breast cancer. *N Engl J Med.* 2002 Oct 17; 347(16): 1233-1241.

9. Fisher B, Jeong JH, Anderson S, Bryant J, Fisher ER, Wolmark N. Twenty-five-year follow-up of a randomized trial comparing radical mastectomy, total mastectomy, and total mastectomy followed by irradiation. *N Engl J Med.* 2002 Aug 22; 347(8): 567-575.

10. McMasters KM, Tuttle TM, Carlson DJ, et al. Sentinel lymph node biopsy for breast cancer: A suitable alternative to routine axillary dissection in multi-institutional practice when optimal technique is used. *J Clin Oncol.* 2000 Jul; 18(13): 2560-2566.

11. Tsai RJ, Dennis LK, Lynch CF, Snetselaar LG, Zamba GK, Scott-Conner C. The risk of developing arm lymphedema among breast cancer survivors: A meta-analysis of treatment factors. *Ann Surg Oncol.* 2009 Jul; 16(7): 1959-1972.

12. Langer I, Guller U, Berclaz G, et al. Morbidity of sentinel lymph node biopsy (SLN) alone versus SLN and completion axillary lymph node dissection after breast cancer surgery: A prospective Swiss multicenter study on 659 patients. *Ann Surg.* 2007 Mar; 245(3): 452-461.

13. McLaughlin SA, Wright MJ, Morris KT, et al. Prevalence of lymphedema in women with breast cancer 5 years after sentinel lymph node biopsy or axillary dissection: Objective measurements. *J Clin Oncol.* 2008 Nov 10; 26(32): 5213-5219.

14. Leonard GD, Swain SM. Ductal carcinoma in situ, complexities and challenges. *J Natl Cancer Inst.* 2004 Jun 16; 96(12): 906-920.

15. Fisher B, Dignam J, Wolmark N, et al. Tamoxifen in treatment of intraductal breast cancer: National Surgical Adjuvant Breast and Bowel Project B-24 randomised controlled trial. *Lancet.* 1999 Jun 12; 353(9169): 1993-2000.

16. Houghton J, George WD, Cuzick J, Duggan C, Fentiman IS, Spittle M. Radiotherapy and tamoxifen in women with completely excised ductal carcinoma in situ of the breast in the UK, Australia, and New Zealand: Randomised controlled trial. *Lancet.* 2003 Jul 12; 362(9378): 95-102.

17. Herold CI, Blackwell KL. Aromatase inhibitors for breast cancer: Proven efficacy across the spectrum of disease. *Clin Breast Cancer.* 2008 Feb; 8(1): 50-64.

18. Slamon DJ, Press MF, Souza LM, et al. Studies of the putative transforming protein of the type I human T-cell leukemia virus. *Science.* 1985 Jun 21; 228(4706): 1427-1430.

19. Slamon DJ, Leyland-Jones B, Shak S, et al. Use of chemotherapy plus a monoclonal antibody against HER2 for metastatic breast cancer that overexpresses HER2. *N Engl J Med.* 2001 Mar 15; 344(11): 783-792.

20. Piccart-Gebhart MJ, Procter M, Leyland-Jones B, et al. Trastuzumab after adjuvant chemotherapy in HER2-positive breast cancer. *N Engl J Med.* 2005 Oct 20; 353(16): 1659-1672.

21. Romond EH, Perez EA, Bryant J, et al. Trastuzumab plus adjuvant chemotherapy for operable HER2-positive breast cancer. *N Engl J Med.* 2005 Oct 20; 353(16): 1673-1684.

22. American Cancer Society. *Cancer Facts and Figures: 2010.* Atlanta: American Cancer Society; 2010.

23. Garnick MB. Prostate cancer: Screening, diagnosis, and management. *Ann Intern Med.* 1993 May 15; 118(10): 804-818.

24. Gittes RF. Carcinoma of the prostate. *N Engl J Med.* 1991 Jan 24; 324(4): 236-245.

25. van den Bergh RC, Roemeling S, Roobol MJ, et al. Outcomes of men with screen-detected prostate cancer eligible for active surveillance who were managed expectantly. *Eur Urol.* 2008 Sep 17: 28-35.

26. Zincke H, Bergstralh EJ, Blute ML, et al. Radical prostatectomy for clinically localized prostate cancer: Long-term results of 1,143 patients from a single institution. *J Clin Oncol.* 1994 Nov; 12(11): 2254-2263.

27. Fournier GR, Jr., Narayan P. Re-evaluation of the need for pelvic lymphadenectomy in low grade prostate cancer. *Br J Urol.* 1993 Oct; 72(4): 484-488.

28. Duncan W, Warde P, Catton CN, et al. Carcinoma of the prostate: Results of radical radiotherapy (1970-1985). *Int J Radiat Oncol Biol Phys.* 1993 May 20; 26(2): 203-210.

29. Koukourakis G, Kelekis N, Armonis V, Kouloulias V. Brachytherapy for prostate cancer: A systematic review. *Adv Urol.* 2009: 327945.

30. Schroder FH. Early versus delayed endocrine therapy for prostate cancer. *Endocr Relat Cancer.* 2007 Mar; 14(1): 1-11.

31. Sanda MG, Dunn RL, Michalski J, et al. Quality of life and satisfaction with outcome among prostate-cancer survivors. *N Engl J Med.* 2008 Mar 20; 358(12): 1250-1261.

32. Peto R, Darby S, Deo H, Silcocks P, Whitley E, Doll R. Smoking, smoking cessation, and lung cancer in the UK since 1950: Combination of national statistics with two case-control studies. *BMJ.* 2000 Aug 5; 321(7257): 323-329.

33. Asomaning K, Miller DP, Liu G, et al. Secondhand smoke, age of exposure and lung cancer risk. *Lung Cancer.* 2008 Jul; 61(1): 13-20.

34. Bach PB, Kelley MJ, Tate RC, McCrory DC. Screening for lung cancer: A review of the current literature. *Chest.* 2003 Jan; 123(1 Suppl): 72S-82S.

35. Glisson BS, Movsas B. Small-cell lung cancer. In: Pazdur R, Hoskins WJ, Wagman LD, eds. *Cancer Management: A Multidisciplinary Approach.* 8th ed. Manhasset, NY: CMP Healthcare Media; 2004: 105-121.

36. McKenna RJ, Shin DM, Khuri FR. Non-small-cell lung cancer, mesothelioma and thymoma. In: Pazdur R, Hoskins WJ, Wagman LD, eds. *Cancer Management: A Multidisciplinary Approach.* 8th ed. Manhasset, NY: CMP Healthcare Media; 2004: 123-64.

37. Sandler A, Gray R, Perry MC, et al. Paclitaxel-carboplatin alone or with bevacizumab for non-small-cell lung cancer. *N Engl J Med.* 2006 Dec 14; 355(24): 2542-2550.

38. Shepherd FA, Rodrigues Pereira J, Ciuleanu T, et al. Erlotinib in previously treated non-small-cell lung cancer. *N Engl J Med.* 2005 Jul 14; 353(2): 123-132.

39. Linardou H, Dahabreh IJ, Kanaloupiti D, et al. Assessment of somatic k-RAS mutations as a mechanism associated with resistance to EGFR-targeted agents:

A systematic review and meta-analysis of studies in advanced non-small-cell lung cancer and metastatic colorectal cancer. *Lancet Oncol.* 2008 Oct; 9(10): 962-972.

40. Ellenhorn JD, Coia LR, Alberts SR. Colorectal and anal cancers. In: Pazdur R, Hoskins WJ, Wagman LD, eds. *Cancer Management: A Multidisciplinary Approach.* Manhasset, NY: CMP Healthcare Media; 2004: 323-355.

41. Lacy AM, Garcia-Valdecasas JC, Delgado S, et al. Laparoscopy-assisted colectomy versus open colectomy for treatment of non-metastatic colon cancer: A randomised trial. *Lancet.* 2002 Jun 29; 359(9325): 2224-2229.

42. Van Cutsem E, Kohne CH, Hitre E, et al. Cetuximab and chemotherapy as initial treatment for metastatic colorectal cancer. *N Engl J Med.* 2009 Apr 2; 360(14): 1408-1417.

43. Desch CE, Benson AB, 3rd, Somerfield MR, et al. Colorectal cancer surveillance: 2005 update of an American Society of Clinical Oncology practice guideline. *J Clin Oncol.* 2005 Nov 20; 23(33): 8512-8519.

44. Horner MJ, Krapcho M, Neyman N, Aminou R, Howlader N, Altekruse SF, Feuer EJ, Huang L, Mariotto A, Miller BA, Lewis DR, Eisner MP, Stinchcomb DG, Edwards BK, eds. *SEER Cancer Statistics Review, 1975-2006.* Bethesda, MD [updated based on November 2008 SEER data submission, posted to the SEER Web site, November 12, 2009]; Available from: http://seer.cancer.gov/csr/1975_2006.

CHAPTER 2

Side Effects and Persistent Effects of Cancer Surgery and Treatment

Tara Sanft, MD, and Melinda L. Irwin, PhD, MPH

Content in this chapter covered in the CET exam outline includes the following:

- Knowledge of the common side effects and symptoms of typical cancer treatments (surgeries, chemotherapy, radiation, hormone manipulations, other drugs).

- Knowledge of the major long-term effects of treatment among childhood cancer survivors that may require careful screening and program adaptation for these individuals.

- Knowledge of the common sites of metastases and ability to design and implement appropriate exercise programs consistent with this knowledge.

- Knowledge of the signs and symptoms associated with new-onset lymphedema, and the major cancer types associated with increased lymphedema risk (e.g., breast, head, and neck cancer).

- Knowledge of how cancer treatment may alter cardiovascular risk factors, and inappropriate cardiovascular responses to exercise testing or training.

- Knowledge of the effect of cancer treatment on balance and mobility and the ability to develop an appropriate exercise program that minimizes fall/injury risk.

- Knowledge of cancer diagnosis and treatment effects on physiological response to acute and chronic exercise, particularly with regard to physical deconditioning, body composition changes, and range of motion.

Despite advances in cancer therapy, approximately 500,000 adults die each year from cancer in the United States.[1] Recent research efforts have been directed toward tailoring cancer therapy based on patient and tumor characteristics, to optimize efficacy and minimize toxicity. Given that many existing cancer therapies are costly and have significant side effects that can result in long-term morbidity and even mortality, nonpharmacologic methods of preventing cancer recurrence may offer an attractive addition to the currently available treatment options. This may be especially true in patients for whom current therapies are less effective, such as those with so-called triple-negative (estrogen, progesterone, and HER2/neu negative) breast cancer, or those with early-stage colon cancer who have completed chemotherapy but have a high risk of recurrence. Interventions directed toward improving quality of life and lessening feelings of depression, insomnia, and fatigue are particularly important because many cancer survivors suffer these problems and are unaware of nonpharmacologic practices that may help. Additionally, because people who have survived cancer have an increased risk for developing cardiovascular disease, physical activity programs may have a positive effect on this outcome as well.[2]

When designing an exercise program for those who have completed treatment for cancer, fitness professionals must be familiar with the side effects associated with cancer surgery and treatment, as well as late effects (i.e., side effects that occur years after completing treatment). This chapter addresses the common side and late effects associated with cancer surgery and treatment.

Side Effects of Cancer Surgery and Treatment

Side effects of surgery and treatment differ depending on the type of surgery (e.g., sentinel node biopsy vs. axillary node dissection; lumpectomy vs. mastectomy) and treatment (e.g., radiation therapy, chemotherapy, hormonal therapy). Before we discuss the common side effects, we briefly discuss common surgeries and treatments offered to people diagnosed with cancer.

Most cancer patients receive surgery. This surgery could be minor (e.g., removal of a mole) or major (e.g., removal of a large section of the colon). About half of cancer patients undergo ionizing radiation treatments. Radiotherapy may be delivered pre- or postoperatively, alone or with concomitant chemotherapy. The mode of delivery, schedule, and frequency are unique to the form of cancer; a common schedule involves frequent appointments over a defined time period (e.g., radiation therapy five days per week for six weeks).

The majority of cancer patients also receive chemotherapy, which is prescribed orally or delivered intravenously on cyclical schedules. The type and duration of treatment are individualized, lasting from a few months to much longer depending on the type and severity of both the cancer and the chemotherapeutic agents used (e.g., one day, or cycle, of chemotherapy followed by two weeks of recovery; then one day, or cycle, of chemotherapy, and so on, for eight cycles).

Hormonal therapies, used most notably to treat certain types of breast and prostate cancer, are in the form of drug therapy or surgery (e.g., removal of the ovaries [oophorectomy] or testicles [orchiectomy]). Patients taking oral drugs commonly take them daily, sometimes for many years. Finally, a growing number of targeted therapies are being developed for cancers that are tumor specific (e.g., trastuzumab [Herceptin], a monoclonal antibody given to breast cancer survivors who overexpress the HER2/neu receptor or exhibit gene amplification).[3]

Fitness professionals need to remember that cancer therapies are constantly changing. To best evaluate a cancer survivor's exercise tolerance and prescribe a safe and effective exercise program, the fitness professional needs to understand the specifics of the client's diagnosis and the treatments received. A new client treatment form can be helpful in this regard (see figure 2.1). Further, this information will need to be understood in the context of the person's health (premorbid conditions) and fitness levels prior to cancer diagnosis. Knowledge of the treatments received and the associated side effects can help the fitness professional review the body systems adversely affected, which may have positive or negative implications for exercise tolerance and training.

Figure 2.1 **New Client Treatment Form**

Name: _____

Cancer type: _____   Stage of diagnosis: ☐ 0 ☐ I ☐ II ☐ III ☐ IV

Date of diagnosis: _____   Oncologist and date of last visit: _____

Treatment

1. Did you have surgery?   ☐ Yes   ☐ No

   Date of surgery:_____   Site of surgery: _____

   Impairments from surgery (if any): _____

   _____

   _____

2. Did you have chemotherapy?   ☐ Yes   ☐ No

   Date of completion: _____   Name of chemotherapy: _____

   Are you currently receiving chemotherapy?   ☐ Yes   ☐ No

   Name of chemotherapy you are currently receiving:_____

   Do you have persistent side effects from chemotherapy?   ☐ Yes   ☐ No

   Please list any symptom(s) that is bothering you now that you believe could be related to your prior
   chemotherapy (e.g., numbness in fingers and toes, pain, depression): _____

   _____

   _____

3. Did you have radiation therapy?   ☐ Yes   ☐ No

   Site of radiation: _____   Date of radiation completion:_____

   Impairments or symptoms from radiation (if any):_____

   _____

   _____

4. Are you taking any medication currently related to your cancer treatment (e.g., antihormonal therapy
   for breast cancer [tamoxifen])?   ☐ Yes   ☐ No

   Name of medication: _____

   Please list any symptom you have now that you believe is related to your medication: _____

   _____

   _____

(continued)

New Client Treatment Form *(continued)*

5. Please indicate if you have any of the following, and describe, as necessary.

☐ Fatigue: _____

☐ Depression: _____

☐ Anxiety: _____

☐ Difficulty sleeping: _____

☐ Weight gain or loss: _____

☐ Change in appetite: _____

☐ Pain: _____

☐ Shortness of breath: _____

☐ Edema: _____

☐ Joint stiffness or pain: _____

☐ Fractures: _____

☐ Myalgias: _____

☐ Muscle weakness: _____

☐ Lymphedema: _____

☐ Neuropathy: _____

☐ Other: _____

From ACSM, 2012, *ACSM's guide to exercise and cancer survivorship* (Champaign, IL: Human Kinetics).

Take-Home Message
The Institute of Medicine (IOM) recommends that all cancer survivors receive a survivorship care plan, a document detailing treatments received, potential side effects, and surveillance guidelines.[4] Currently, research is being done to ensure that more survivors receive survivorship care plans. Survivors may complete their own survivorship care plan, assuming they remember the therapies they have received, at the LiveStrong website (www.livestrongcareplan.org). Once the person has filled in the types and names of treatments, this online program generates a document detailing potential long-term and late effects, which may be useful when planning exercise and rehabilitation programs.

The adverse side effects of cancer treatments may be acute, resolving over a period of days or weeks, or they may be persistent, lasting years after treatment is completed. For the purpose of this chapter, we use the term *persistent effects*, an umbrella term that includes both long-term and late effects. Long-term effects are side effects or complications that begin during or very shortly after treatment and persist afterward, and for which the cancer survivor must compensate. Late effects are distinct from long-term effects in that they appear months or years after treatment completion (e.g., cardiomyopathies after exposure to cardiotoxic agents).

Table 2.1 lists persistent effects of cancer treatments, including effects on body systems relevant to exercise training: cardiovascular, musculoskeletal, nervous, endocrine, and immune. It should be noted that for persistent adverse effects of cancer treatment, there may be predisposing host factors, including age, gender, and other comorbid health

TABLE 2.1   Persistent Changes Resulting From the Most Commonly Used Curative Therapies

Changes	Surgery	Chemotherapy	Radiation	Hormonal therapy, oophorectomy, or orchiectomy	Targeted therapies
Second cancers		✓	✓	✓	
Fatigue	✓	✓	✓	✓	✓
Pain	✓	✓	✓	✓	✓
Cardiovascular changes: damage or increased CVD risk		✓	✓	✓	✓
Pulmonary changes	✓	✓	✓		
Neurological changes: peripheral neuropathy		✓			
Cognitive changes	✓	✓	✓	✓	✓
Endocrine changes: reproductive changes (e.g., infertility, early menopause, impaired sexual function)	✓	✓	✓	✓	✓
Body weight changes (increases or decreases)	✓	✓		✓	
Fat mass increases	✓	✓		✓	
Lean mass losses	✓	✓		✓	
Worsened bone health		✓	✓	✓	
Musculoskeletal soft tissues: changes or damage	✓	✓	✓	✓	
Immune system: impaired immune function or anemia		✓	✓	✓	✓
Lymphedema	✓		✓		
Gastrointestinal system: changes or impaired function	✓	✓	✓	✓	✓
Organ function changes	✓	✓	✓		✓
Skin changes	✓	✓	✓	✓	✓

conditions, that synergize to influence the incidence and severity of adverse treatment effects. A recent IOM report on adult cancer survivorship offers an in-depth review of the persistent effects of treatment.[4]

Fatigue

Cancer-related fatigue is defined as a distressing, persistent sense of tiredness or exhaustion that is related to the cancer or its treatment.[5] It is out of proportion to the level of recent activity and interferes with functioning. Cancer-related fatigue is reported in 70 to 100% of patients undergoing treatment, and survivors report persistent fatigue lasting months to years after finishing therapy.[6]

The National Comprehensive Cancer Network (NCCN) published guidelines to evaluate cancer-related fatigue. The initial assessment includes evaluating factors known to contribute to fatigue: emotional distress, pain, sleep disturbance, medication side effects, hypothyroidism, and anemia. If these or other potentially reversible causes exist, they should be treated with the intent of lessening feelings of fatigue. If none of these factors are present or fatigue persists despite adequate therapy, then nonpharmacologic interventions are recommended. Nonpharmacologic interventions include activity enhancement with exercise programs, psychosocial interventions for stress and anxiety management, attention-restoring therapy, nutrition counseling, and sleep therapy. Pharmacologic interventions include the treatment of anemia and the use of psychostimulants such as methylphenidate (Ritalin).

Sleep Disturbance

Sleep disturbance is common among cancer survivors, and data are emerging on the prevalence of insomnia syndrome in this population.[7] Insomnia is defined as difficulty falling asleep, difficulty staying asleep (episodes of wakefulness lasting more than 30 minutes), early-morning awakening, and nonrestorative sleep. In one large study of more than 900 cancer survivors, 30% of survivors reported insomnia. About 20% of participants reported using sleeping pills or tranquilizers, and 60% reported taking naps at least "some of the time."[8] Recent data have shown that a yoga program may improve sleep quality.[9]

Take-Home Message

A study of patients with lymphoma randomly assigned participants to Tibetan yoga or a waitlist control group. The patients in the yoga group reported less sleep disturbance, better sleep quality, and less use of sleep medications.[9] Yoga is a safe, nonpharmacologic intervention that may benefit many survivors with sleep disturbance.

Pain

Although the data vary, most literature suggests that a significant percentage of cancer survivors experience pain attributed to their cancer or its treatment.[10-12] Within this literature, several groups of survivors at highest risk have been identified, including those within five years of treatment, those who have undergone more intensive treatment, and those with a lower socioeconomic status.[10, 13] The etiology of pain in survivors can be attributed to a wide variety of factors. These include damage

to tissue and nerves from the original tumor, treatment-related injury from surgery, radiation or chemotherapy, and pain caused by noncancer conditions that may be a result of cancer treatment (e.g., osteoporotic fracture as a result of bone loss from androgen deprivation therapy in a prostate cancer patient).

Mechanisms of pain can be thought of as being mediated by two pathways: nociceptive and neuropathic.[14] Nociceptive pain is caused by damage to skin, muscles, connective tissue, and viscera. This often results in either sharp, localized pain (somatic) or vague, crampy pain (visceral). Neuropathic pain results from injury to the central and peripheral nervous systems and is often reported as a burning or shooting sensation. A thorough history and physical examination can elicit the etiology of a patient's pain and further characterize the pain as nociceptive or neuropathic or containing elements of both.

The approach to treatment of pain should be individualized to each patient and account for etiology, mechanism, and severity. The World Health Organization (WHO) guidelines for cancer pain is a widely accepted algorithm for treatment that categorizes pain by severity into mild, moderate, and severe pain.[15] Interventions include acetaminophen and nonsteroidal anti-inflammatory medication for mild pain and opioids, both weak and strong for moderate and severe pain, respectively. Additionally, the guidelines include a variety of adjuvant therapies aimed at decreasing pain by manipulating a different mechanism contributing to the pain syndrome, thereby enhancing overall control. Examples of adjuvant medications include anticonvulsant drugs, tricyclic antidepressants, and muscle relaxants. Nonpharmacologic interventions include massage, physical therapy, hypnosis, and relaxation.

Cardiovascular Changes

Cancer therapy for multiple malignancies results in both direct damage to the cardiovascular system and indirect damage via increasing risk factors associated with cardiovascular disease. Treatment-related effects can damage all parts of the heart including the muscle, electrical system, and valves. Symptoms of congestive heart failure include dyspnea on exertion, edema of the lower extremities, and weight gain. Specific chemotherapy agents that can damage heart muscle and lead to congestive heart failure include anthracyclines, taxanes, and trastuzumab. [4, 16] The association between anthracyclines and congestive heart failure is dose dependent, increases with age, and is more common when combined with other therapies such as radiation. Decreased ejection fraction, rhythm disturbance, and ventricular dysfunction are associated with these agents and can occur during treatment, within one year, or many years after the disease is treated.[17, 18] Trastuzumab (Herceptin) causes decreased ejection fraction and can lead to congestive heart failure, although the incidence is very low and symptoms often reverse once therapy is discontinued.[19]

Radiation to the chest can cause cardiac toxicity by increasing inflammation in the heart and surrounding tissues, which can lead to fibrosis and scarring. The ultimate effect of this is restrictive cardiomyopathy, or a decreased ability of the heart to expand. Symptoms of restrictive disease include shortness of breath and can be seen as late as 10 years after treatment.[20] Radiation can also damage cardiac vasculature, resulting in an increased risk of cardiac ischemia and myocardial infarction.[21] Patients who have received radiation to the chest for lymphoma, breast cancer, and lung cancer are at highest risk. Many studies examining radiation side effects involve large populations of patients treated decades ago with outdated radiation techniques. Newer, more focused, and targeted radiation techniques have reduced the incidence of this side effect.

Pulmonary Changes

Pulmonary symptoms related to surgery, radiation, and chemotherapy are not uncommon in cancer survivors; they are reported in 20 to 50% of certain patient populations, including survivors of germ cell tumors, Hodgkin's lymphoma, and breast cancer, as well as bone marrow transplant recipients.[2] Although some studies have identified abnormal pulmonary function tests in cancer survivors, it is unclear how significant these findings are in the asymptomatic patient.[22–25] Certain symptoms such as shortness of breath and decreased exercise tolerance may be seen, depending on the mode of treatment (e.g., surgical removal of a lung cancer that includes removing a lobe of the lung). Small studies in patients who had surgery for lung cancer found that inpatient pulmonary rehabilitation programs have positive effects on functional ability,

peak exercise capacity, and shortness of breath.[26, 27] Other studies in this population are ongoing.

Bleomycin is the most common chemotherapeutic agent to cause pulmonary toxicity, most often in the form of pneumonitis, or inflammation of the lung tissue. It is used to treat patients with germ cell tumors in combination with etoposide and cisplatin (commonly referred to as BEP) and also in Hodgkin's lymphoma in combination with doxorubicin, vinblastine, and dacarbazine (commonly referred to as ABVD). Pneumonitis is a rare complication, with an incidence of less than 10% in patients with germ cell tumor, but it can affect up to 30% of patients with Hodgkin's lymphoma who may also receive radiation to an area of the lungs. Multiple other chemotherapeutic agents have been associated with pulmonary toxicities.

Radiation pneumonitis can be seen in patients who have received radiation to the chest and lungs for various tumor types. The incidence of radiation pneumonitis is also rare; it usually occurs one to three months after completing therapy and resolves with no further clinical consequences.[28–30] A rare but devastating long-term side effect of radiation is pulmonary fibrosis, which can result in severely decreased lung capacity and eventual respiratory failure.

Neurological Changes

Numerous neuropathic syndromes are associated with cancer and its treatment. For instance, the tumor itself may encase nerves, causing burning, tingling, and electrical pain. After surgical resection of a malignancy, some patient experience phantom pain or the sensation of pain in a nonexistent limb. Other patients experience persistent pain at the site of a surgical incision such as a lumpectomy or thoracotomy scar.

Neuropathy is a loss of sensation (often described as numbness) or pain (radiating, burning, or tingling) associated with damage to peripheral nerves. Symptoms of neuropathy are often seen in association with cancer treatment, especially with taxanes, vinca alkaloids, platinum agents, and thalidomide. Symptoms usually start gradually and worsen with increasing doses and duration of therapy. The provider may ask if the patient has difficulty with specific tasks (e.g., picking up a coin from the counter or buttoning a shirt) to assess the severity of the neuropathy.

Neuropathy may or may not resolve after therapy, and further studies are needed to delineate the natural history depending on chemotherapeutic agent, dosing, and underlying comorbid conditions.[31] Multiple neuropathy prevention strategies have been studied without success.[32] Treatment includes anticonvulsants such as gabapentin and pregabalin, which have shown mixed evidence of effectiveness.[33, 34] Alternatives include tricyclic antidepressants, lidocaine patches, and opioid analgesics. Nonpharmacologic treatments include transcutaneous electrical nerve stimulation (TENS) and physical therapy.

Ototoxicity is a common side effect in patients treated with cisplatin chemotherapy. It may be characterized by high-frequency hearing loss or tinnitus, or a perception of sound with an absence of external sound. Researchers analyzing quality of life after adjuvant chemotherapy in patients with early-stage lung cancer found that hearing scores were significantly worse compared to those who did not receive chemotherapy. Poor hearing persisted even after nine months.[35] Long-term hearing loss has been reported in survivors of testicular cancer, with persistent symptoms reported in up to 20% of survivors.[36, 37]

Other neurological complications of cancer therapy include a phenomenon described as chemo-brain—a neurological decline after systemic chemotherapy. Subjectively, many cancer survivors report feeling more forgetful and experiencing an inability to concentrate and intermittent confusion. Objectively, patients who have received chemotherapy have scored lower on neuropsychological tests compared to healthy controls, although no overall statistically significant difference has been found.[38] The symptoms of chemo-brain correlate better with measures of depression and anxiety than they do with neuropsychological test results.[39] Studies are necessary for further describing the incidence, characteristics, risk factors, and treatment of this distressing symptom.

Endocrine Changes

Effects of cancer treatment on the endocrine system have been understood for decades. The pediatric survivorship population is the most commonly studied. Pediatric survivors are often the most severely affected because their growth and development can be compromised. Among adults, the majority of endocrine changes are specific to the location of the tumor and the specific modality used to treat it. For instance, patients with head and neck cancer often receive radiation as part of curative therapy. As a result, hypothyroidism is a common side effect and can be seen years after completion of therapy.[40, 41] Symptoms of hypothyroidism include fatigue, weight gain, constipation, depression, and weakness. Detection and treatment with thyroid hormone replacement can reverse these symptoms entirely.

Reproductive health can be threatened during cancer treatment, and chemotherapeutic agents such as alkylators (e.g., cyclophosphamide) can induce infertility in both men and women. Premature ovarian failure can cause hot flashes, vaginal dryness, and osteoporosis. Alkylating agents used to treat testicular cancer can also cause infertility, but this usually reverses two to three years after completion of therapy.

Many cancer survivors experience declines in bone health. Treatment of various malignancies includes steroids, either as part of the treatment plan or for symptomatic control of nausea and vomiting. Steroids are associated with osteoporosis and increased fracture risk. Additionally, premature menopause caused by surgery, radiation, or systemic therapy can lead to bone loss, osteopenia, and osteoporosis. Endocrine therapy used to treat breast and prostate cancer accelerates bone loss, and bone mineral density is monitored as part of routine care while the person is on these medications, sometimes for years. Osteopenia and osteoporosis puts survivors at risk for fracture, which can lead to debilitation, pain, and financial burden. Treatment includes dietary supplementation of vitamin D and calcium, weight-bearing exercises, and bisphosphonate therapy.

Musculoskeletal Changes

The musculoskeletal system can change in many ways after cancer treatment. For instance, treatment of breast cancer with endocrine therapy such as aromatase inhibitors can cause pain in the small joints in as many as 47% of patients, and joint stiffness occurs in as many as 44%.[42] In some patients, joint symptoms are so severe they cannot complete the recommended duration of treatment (usually five years of therapy). A recent study showed that acupuncture significantly reduced symptoms of aromatase inhibitor–related arthralgias.[43] A study led by Dr. Melinda Irwin at Yale University is currently examining the benefit of resistance and aerobic exercise on attenuating joint stiffness and other side effects of aromatase inhibitors in women with breast cancer.

Androgen deprivation therapy (ADT) as treatment for prostate cancer causes changes in the composition of lean body mass, with a decrease seen as early as 36 weeks after starting therapy.[44] ADT also increases fat mass, which predisposes men to cardiovascular disease, type 2 diabetes, and premature death.[44] Considering that one in six men will be diagnosed with prostate cancer in his lifetime, and that the five-year survival is nearly 100%,[1] the musculoskeletal changes that occur with treatment have implications regarding physical functioning, which can affect strength, productivity, and independence.

Immune Function Changes

Lymphedema refers to swelling in a limb as a result of lymphatic obstruction or destruction. This usually occurs after a surgical resection of a tumor, when there is damage to the lymphatic system draining the area around the tumor. Lymphedema is associated with limb heaviness, aching, and numbness, which results in chronic pain and can lead to a loss of function and an increased risk of infection.

The majority of patients who report lymphedema are breast cancer survivors, although patients with a history of ovarian, colon, prostate, and testicular cancer can experience lower-extremity lymphedema. The majority of patients develop lymphedema within the first couple of years of diagnosis, although late-onset swelling can occur many years after surgery.[45] Treatment includes manual lymphatic drainage, compression garments, exercise, and skin care. Historically, breast cancer survivors have been encouraged to avoid heavy lifting (greater than 5 lb, or 2.3 kg) with the affected arm, but recent evidence suggests that controlled, progressive resistance training does not adversely affect the limb with lymphedema.[46–49] An updated consensus on the approach to survivors with lymphedema is needed in light of this recent evidence.

Gastrointestinal Changes

The gastrointestinal system can be disrupted in various ways following cancer treatment. Management of pain with opioids can cause constipation; radiation to the head and neck can cause esophageal strictures, which impair eating; and radiation to the abdomen or pelvis can result in malabsorption, adhesions, and diarrhea. Although surgical techniques have improved, survivors with colorectal cancer who have had surgical resection can experience chronic diarrhea, fecal incontinence, urgency, and incomplete evacuation.[51–53] In a survey of colon cancer survivors at least five years from diagnosis, 49% of respondents reported chronic diarrhea, and 16% reported three or more bowel movements daily.[54] These findings have implications on a cancer survivor's mobility, productivity, and quality of life.

Organ Function Changes

In addition to changes in multiple anatomical systems, cancer treatment may permanently impair specific organs. Often, the functions of these organs are monitored before, during, and immediately after treatment. Long-term monitoring for organ damage is used on an individual basis.

Take-Home Message
A common misconception is that women who have had breast cancer surgery are restricted in terms of exercise with the arm of the affected side. This is not true, as highlighted by research that showed that slowly progressive weightlifting did not increase limb swelling in women at risk for breast cancer–related lymphedema. The women in the supervised exercise group received two sessions weekly for 13 weeks. Each session lasted 90 minutes and consisted of upper-body and lower-body resistant exercises. Three sets of each exercise were performed at each session, 10 repetitions per set. Weight was increased by the smallest possible increment after two sessions of completing three sets of 10 repetitions with no change in arm symptoms.[50]

Renal Damage

Platinum-based chemotherapy and regimens containing ifosfamide or methotrexate can cause significant renal damage, or nephrotoxicity. During the treatment phase, renal function and electrolytes are monitored closely, and dose adjustments are made based on changes in glomerular filtration rate (GFR). Long-term renal impairment is associated with hypertension and an increased risk of cardiovascular disease.

Multiple studies looking at the long-term effects of nephrotoxic chemotherapy in the pediatric cancer survivor population suggest that the majority of cancer survivors have normal renal function as distant as 10 years after treatment, with less than 5% of the population having abnormalities in electrolyte balance.[55,56] The Children's Oncology Group (COG) recommends yearly blood pressure and urinalysis monitoring to evaluate for hypertension and proteinuria, respectively. They also recommend a one-time check of renal function, which should include a check of blood urea nitrogen (BUN), creatinine, and electrolytes. If the levels of these elements are abnormal, ongoing management needs to be considered.[57]

Liver Damage

Acute liver damage can occur at any time during chemotherapy; however, the long-term side effects that anticancer treatment has on the hepatobiliary system are not well understood. The Children's Oncology Group (COG) performed a literature review on the late effects on the hepatobiliary system in children and adolescents with cancer.[58] The potential effects of therapy on the liver include the formation of fibrosis, which can lead to cirrhosis; portal hypertension; and the development of hepatocellular carcinoma. Additionally, patients requiring frequent blood transfusions are at risk for viral hepatitis and iron overload; and patients requiring total parenteral nutrition (TPN) may develop cholestasis. Those patients who have had stem cell transplantation are at risk for graft-versus-host disease, which can involve the liver. The follow-up care guidelines put forth by the COG apply to survivors of childhood cancers, but one-time monitoring of liver enzymes and bilirubin production is reasonable in adults who have received hepatotoxic chemotherapy. A physician should also consider screening for viral hepatitis, especially if the patient received multiple transfusions before 1993.

Skin and Hair Changes

Skin and hair changes after cancer treatment include generalized loss or thinning of hair and skin discoloration from radiation or chemotherapeutic agents. In patients who have had stem cell transplantation, graft-versus-host disease (GVHD) can affect all organs, including the skin. Changes seen in this disease include skin tightening, diffuse maculopapular rash, dryness, and ulcerations. The treatment of GVHD of the skin includes immunosuppressive agents, such as high-dose steroids. Topical steroids, high-dose long-wave ultraviolet radiation (UVA1), and photochemotherapy (PUVA) may be used to reduce the severity of skin problems.

Basal cell carcinoma is a skin problem that can be seen in survivors who have received radiation. In a survey of more than 2,000 survivors of childhood cancer, basal cell carcinoma was found in 11% of patients who remained in remission from their primary cancer.[59] Although basal cell and squamous cell carcinomas of the skin (collectively referred to as nonmelanomatous skin cancer) are thought to be nonaggressive and highly treatable, multiple recurrences are common,[60] requiring expensive excisions that can leave disfiguring scars.

Recurrence, New Primaries, and Second Cancers

Perhaps one of the most daunting concerns for cancer survivors is the possibility of recurrence. The National Comprehensive Cancer Network (NCCN) has guidelines on monitoring patients for recurrent disease. Outside of clinical history, physical examination, and certain screening tests such as mammography, colonoscopy, and prostate-specific antigen (PSA), there are not specific tests that can definitively demonstrate whether a patient has recurrent disease. Understandably, symptoms that may seem benign in the patient without a history of cancer can be very worrisome in a cancer survivor. For instance, low back pain is the fifth most common reason for a visit to a doctor in the United States, and most symptoms improve substantially within the first month.[61-63] In a patient with a history of breast or prostate cancer, however, back pain may be the first symptom of recurrence and could herald serious conditions such as malignant spinal cord compression. For these reasons, practitioners must take the cancer survivor's history into account when evaluating seemingly benign complaints.

In addition to recurrence, survivors may worry about the development of a new malignancy, either related to the environmental factors that put them at risk for the original cancer (e.g., smoking increases the risk of head and neck as well as lung cancer) or to the treatment for the original cancer (certain chemotherapies are associated with bone marrow damage that can lead to myelodysplasia and acute leukemias). Knowing the survivor's treatment history can help providers understand the risk of developing additional malignancies.

Summary

Cancer survivors are a unique medical population with a wide variety of treatment options (surgery, radiation, and chemotherapy) that put them at risk for both short- and long-term side effects. The actual risk to each person depends on the type of cancer, the treatments received, and other factors relating to genetics, lifestyle, and behavior. Awareness that a cancer survivor may have a variety of long-term effects after treatment will help providers tailor treatments to address these effects as well as work on modifying each survivor's risk with the goal of not only reducing the risks of morbidity, mortality, or recurrence, but also enhancing the quality of life.

References

1. Jemal A, et al. Cancer statistics, 2009. *CA Cancer J Clin.* 2009; 59(4): 225-249.

2. Carver JR, et al. American Society of Clinical Oncology clinical evidence review on the ongoing care of adult cancer survivors: Cardiac and pulmonary late effects. *J Clin Oncol.* 2007; 25(25): 3991-4008.

3. Browne BC, et al. HER-2 signaling and inhibition in breast cancer. *Curr Cancer Drug Targets.* 2009; 9(3): 419-438.

4. Hewitt ME, et al. *From cancer patient to cancer survivor: Lost in transition: An American Society of Clinical Oncology and Institute of Medicine Symposium.* Washington, DC: National Academies Press; 2006: vi, 189.

5. Mock V, et al. NCCN practice guidelines for cancer-related fatigue. *Oncology* (Williston Park). 2000; 14(11A): 151-161.

6. Curt G, et al. Impact of cancer-related fatigue on the lives of patients: New findings from the Fatigue Coalition. *Oncologist.* 2000; 5(5): 353-360.

7. Palesh OG, et al. Prevalence, demographics, and psychological associations of sleep disruption in patients with cancer: University of Rochester Cancer Center-Community Clinical Oncology Program. *J Clin Oncol.* 2010; 28(2): 292-298.

8. Davidson JR, et al. Sleep disturbance in cancer patients. *Soc Sci Med.* 2002; 54(9): 1309-1321.

9. Cohen L, et al. Psychological adjustment and sleep quality in a randomized trial of the effects of a Tibetan yoga intervention in patients with lymphoma. *Cancer.* 2004; 100(10): 2253-2260.

10. Ferrell BR, et al. Quality of life in long-term cancer survivors. *Oncol Nurs Forum.* 1995; 22(6): 915-922.

11. Deimling GT, et al. The health of older-adult, long-term cancer survivors. *Cancer Nurs.* 2005; 28(6): 415-424.

12. Keating NL, et al. Physical and mental health status of older long-term cancer survivors. *J Am Geriatr Soc.* 2005; 53(12): 2145-2152.

13. Hudson MM, et al. Health status of adult long-term survivors of childhood cancer: A report from the Childhood Cancer Survivor Study. *JAMA.* 2003; 290(12): 1583-1592.

14. Caraceni A, Weinstein SM. Classification of cancer pain syndromes. *Oncology* (Williston Park). 2001; 15(12): 1627-1640, 1642; discussion 1642-1643, 1646-1647.

15. Stjernsward J, Colleau SM, Ventafridda V. The World Health Organization Cancer Pain and Palliative Care Program. Past, present, and future. *J Pain Symptom Manage.* 1996; 12(2): 65-72.

16. Hequet O, et al. Subclinical late cardiomyopathy after doxorubicin therapy for lymphoma in adults. *J Clin Oncol.* 2004; 22(10): 1864-1871.

17. Shan K, Lincoff AM, Young JB. Anthracycline-induced cardiotoxicity. *Ann Intern Med.* 1996; 125(1): 47-58.

18. Steinherz LJ, et al. Cardiac toxicity 4 to 20 years after completing anthracycline therapy. *JAMA.* 1991; 266(12): 1672-1677.

19. Suter TM, Cook-Bruns N, Barton C. Cardiotoxicity associated with trastuzumab (Herceptin) therapy in the treatment of metastatic breast cancer. *Breast.* 2004; 13(3): 173-183.

20. Applefeld MM, et al. The late appearance of chronic pericardial disease in patients treated by radiotherapy for Hodgkin's disease. *Ann Intern Med.* 1981; 94(3): 338-341.

21. Gaya AM, Ashford RF. Cardiac complications of radiation therapy. *Clin Oncol (R Coll Radiol).* 2005; 17(3): 153-159.

22. Hirsch A, et al. Effect of ABVD chemotherapy with and without mantle or mediastinal irradiation on pulmonary function and symptoms in early-stage Hodgkin's disease. *J Clin Oncol.* 1996; 14(4): 1297-1305.

23. Theuws JC, et al. Effect of radiotherapy and chemotherapy on pulmonary function after treatment for breast cancer and lymphoma: A follow-up study. *J Clin Oncol.* 1999; 17(10): 3091-3100.

24. Lehne G, Johansen B, Fossa SD. Long-term follow-up of pulmonary function in patients cured from testicular cancer with combination chemotherapy including bleomycin. *Br J Cancer.* 1993; 68(3): 555-558.

25. Beinert T, et al. Late pulmonary impairment following allogeneic bone marrow transplantation. *Eur J Med Res.* 1996; 1(7): 343-348.

26. Cesario A, et al. Pre-operative pulmonary rehabilitation and surgery for lung cancer. *Lung Cancer.* 2007; 57(1): 118-119.

27. Spruit MA, et al. Exercise capacity before and after an 8-week multidisciplinary inpatient rehabilitation program in lung cancer patients: A pilot study. *Lung Cancer.* 2006; 52(2): 257-260.

28. Roach M, 3rd, et al. Radiation pneumonitis following combined modality therapy for lung cancer: Analysis of prognostic factors. *J Clin Oncol.* 1995; 13(10): 2606-2612.

29. Harris S. Radiotherapy for early and advanced breast cancer. *Int J Clin Pract.* 2001; 55(9): 609-612.

30. Tarbell NJ, Thompson L, Mauch P. Thoracic irradiation in Hodgkin's disease: Disease control and long-term complications. *Int J Radiat Oncol Biol Phys.* 1990; 18(2): 275-281.

31. Paice JA. Clinical challenges: Chemotherapy-induced peripheral neuropathy. *Semin Oncol Nurs.* 2009; 25(2 Suppl 1): S8-19.

32. Albers J, et al. Interventions for preventing neuropathy caused by cisplatin and related compounds. *Cochrane Database Syst Rev.* 2007(1): CD005228.

33. Dworkin RH, et al. Advances in neuropathic pain: Diagnosis, mechanisms, and treatment recommendations. *Arch Neurol.* 2003; 60(11): 1524-1534.

34. Rao RD, et al. Efficacy of gabapentin in the management of chemotherapy-induced peripheral neuropathy: A phase 3 randomized, double-blind, placebo-controlled, crossover trial (N00C3). *Cancer.* 2007; 110(9): 2110-2118.

35. Bezjak A, et al. Quality-of-life outcomes for adjuvant chemotherapy in early-stage non-small-cell lung cancer: Results from a randomized trial JBR.10. *J Clin Oncol.* 2008; 26(31): 5052-5059.

36. Kollmannsberger C, et al. Late toxicity following curative treatment of testicular cancer. *Semin Surg Oncol.* 1999; 17(4): 275-281.

37. Efstathiou E, Logothetis CJ. Review of late complications of treatment and late relapse in testicular cancer. *J Natl Compr Canc Netw.* 2006; 4(10): 1059-1070.

38. Castellon SA, et al. Neurocognitive performance in breast cancer survivors exposed to adjuvant chemotherapy and tamoxifen. *J Clin Exp Neuropsychol.* 2004; 26(7): 955-969.

39. Taillibert S, Voillery D, Bernard-Marty C. Chemobrain: Is systemic chemotherapy neurotoxic? *Curr Opin Oncol.* 2007; 19(6): 623-627.

40. Sinard RJ, et al. Hypothyroidism after treatment for nonthyroid head and neck cancer. *Arch Otolaryngol Head Neck Surg.* 2000; 126(5): 652-657.

41. Smith GL, et al. Hypothyroidism in older patients with head and neck cancer after treatment with radiation: A population-based study. *Head Neck.* 2009; 31(8): 1031-1038.

42. Crew KD, et al. Prevalence of joint symptoms in postmenopausal women taking aromatase inhibitors for early-stage breast cancer. *J Clin Oncol.* 2007; 25(25): 3877-3883.

43. Crew KD, et al. Randomized, blinded, sham-controlled trial of acupuncture for the management of aromatase inhibitor-associated joint symptoms in women with early-stage breast cancer. *J Clin Oncol.* 2010; 28(7): 1154-1160.

44. Galvao DA, et al. Changes in muscle, fat and bone mass after 36 weeks of maximal androgen blockade for prostate cancer. *BJU Int.* 2008; 102(1): 44-47.

45. Petrek JA, et al. Lymphedema in a cohort of breast carcinoma survivors 20 years after diagnosis. *Cancer.* 2001; 92(6): 1368-1377.

46. Hayes SC, Reul-Hirche H, Turner J. Exercise and secondary lymphedema: Safety, potential benefits, and research issues. *Med Sci Sports Exerc.* 2009; 41(3): 483-489.

47. McKenzie DC, Kalda AL. Effect of upper extremity exercise on secondary lymphedema in breast cancer patients: A pilot study. *J Clin Oncol.* 2003; 21(3): 463-466.

48. Schmitz KH, et al. Physical Activity and Lymphedema (the PAL trial): Assessing the safety of progressive strength training in breast cancer survivors. *Contemp Clin Trials.* 2009; 30(3): 233-245.

49. Schmitz KH, et al. Weight lifting in women with breast-cancer-related lymphedema. *N Engl J Med.* 200; 361(7): 664-673.

50. Schmitz KH, et al. Weight lifting for women at risk for breast-cancer-related lymphedema: A randomized trial. *JAMA.* 304(24): 2699-2705.

51. Engel J, et al. Quality of life in rectal cancer patients: A four-year prospective study. *Ann Surg.* 2003; 238(2): 203-213.

52. Grumann MM, et al. Comparison of quality of life in patients undergoing abdominoperineal extirpation or anterior resection for rectal cancer. *Ann Surg.* 2001; 233(2): 149-156.

53. Camilleri-Brennan J, Steele RJ. Quality of life after treatment for rectal cancer. *Br J Surg.* 1998; 85(8): 1036-1043.

54. Ramsey SD, et al. Quality of life in long-term survivors of colorectal cancer. *Am J Gastroenterol.* 2002; 97(5): 1228-1234.

55. Oberlin O, et al. Long-term evaluation of Ifosfamide-related nephrotoxicity in children. *J Clin Oncol.* 2009; 27(32): 5350-5355.

56. Skinner R, et al. Persistent nephrotoxicity during 10-year follow-up after cisplatin or carboplatin treatment in childhood: Relevance of age and dose as risk factors. *Eur J Cancer.* 2009; 45(18): 3213-3219.

57. Jones DP, et al. Renal late effects in patients treated for cancer in childhood: A report from the Children's Oncology Group. *Pediatr Blood Cancer.* 2008; 51(6): 724-731.

58. Castellino S, et al. Hepato-biliary late effects in survivors of childhood and adolescent cancer: A report from the Children's Oncology Group. *Pediatr Blood Cancer.* 2010; 54(5): 663-669.

59. Hijiya N, et al. Cumulative incidence of secondary neoplasms as a first event after childhood acute lymphoblastic leukemia. *JAMA.* 2007; 297(11): 1207-1215.

60. Perkins JL, et al. Nonmelanoma skin cancer in survivors of childhood and adolescent cancer: A report from the childhood cancer survivor study. *J Clin Oncol.* 2005; 23(16): 3733-3741.

61. Deyo RA, Mirza SK, Martin BI. Back pain prevalence and visit rates: Estimates from U.S. national surveys, 2002. *Spine* (Phila Pa 1976). 2006; 31(23): 2724-2727.

62. Hart LG, Deyo RA, Cherkin DC. Physician office visits for low back pain. Frequency, clinical evaluation, and treatment patterns from a U.S. national survey. *Spine* (Phila Pa 1976). 1995; 20(1): 11-19.

63. Pengel LH, et al. Acute low back pain: Systematic review of its prognosis. *BMJ.* 2003; 327(7410): 323.

CHAPTER 3

Lifestyle Factors Associated With Cancer Incidence, Recurrence, and Survival

Heather K. Neilson, MSc, and Christine M. Friedenreich, PhD

Content in this chapter covered in the CET exam outline includes the following:

- Knowledge of how lifestyle factors, including nutrition, physical activity, and heredity, influence hypothesized mechanisms of cancer etiology.

Age, sex, and genetics are well-known, unavoidable risk factors for cancer; however, modifiable risk factors also exist. Remarkably, roughly one third of cancer deaths worldwide may actually be preventable.[1] Generally speaking, for Americans, the most important behaviors for reducing cancer risk are limiting exposures to UV radiation, not using tobacco, avoiding infectious agents, exercising, eating well, and maintaining a healthy body weight.[2] This chapter provides an overview of the scientific literature on the effect of body weight, diet, and physical activity on the risk of developing cancer and, after a cancer diagnosis, the effect of these factors on cancer recurrence and survival.

Effect of Body Weight

In developed countries, smoking, alcohol use, and overweight (body mass index [BMI] of 25.0 to 29.9 kg/m²) and obesity (BMI ≥ 30.0) are likely the three most important, preventable risk factors for cancer,[1] whereas obesity is considered a major risk factor for cancer death.[3, 4] Hence, as the obesity epidemic grows, widespread increases in cancer incidence and mortality can be expected. Current evidence supports the fact that higher BMI is related to increased risks for cancers of the esophagus (adenocarcinoma), colon, breast

(in postmenopausal women), endometrium, and kidney.[5-8] In 30 European countries in 2002, overweight and obesity alone were responsible for an estimated 10 to 40% of these five cancers,[9] whereas in the United States for a similar time period, 21 to 57% of these cancers could be attributed to overweight and obesity[10] (see figure 3.1). It is also probable, but less certain, that higher BMI increases the risk of gallbladder, liver, pancreatic, and ovarian cancer; aggressive prostate cancer; and possibly other cancers as well.[5, 11-14]

Not only is body weight an important cause of cancer, but also emerging evidence implies that it may also be a key factor in cancer prognosis. For example, studies over the past decade suggest that obesity increases the risk of recurrence or death, or both, from breast cancer,[16, 17] colon cancer,[18, 19] possibly prostate cancer,[20, 21] and maybe other cancers as well. In one American study in which more than 900,000 adults were followed for 16 years, higher BMI was associated with increased mortality rates from cancers of the esophagus, colon and rectum, liver, gallbladder, pancreas, kidney, stomach (in men), prostate, breast (in women), uterus, cervix, and ovary, as well as non-Hodgkin's lymphoma, multiple myeloma, and leukemia (in men).[3] The following sections discuss five cancers that are convincingly associated with body weight in terms of cancer risk, as well as the related evidence on cancer recurrence and survival.

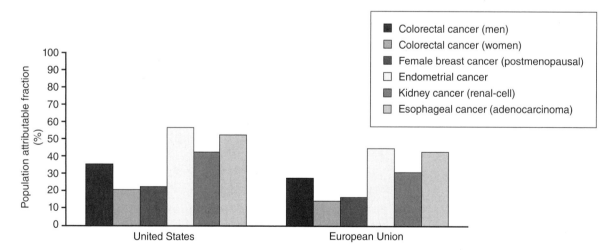

Figure 3.1 Percentage of adult cancers attributable to overweight and obesity in the United States and European Union. The population attributable fraction is the percentage of disease in a population that would be prevented if a given risk factor (e.g., overweight and obesity) were eliminated.[15]

Data from Calle and Kaaks 2004.[10]

Breast Cancer

It is now well established by extensive research that postmenopausal breast cancer risk is higher for overweight and obese women than for post-menopausal women of normal weight[5] and that the risk tends to increase with increasing BMI.[8] Weight gain also increases risk, whereas intentional weight loss seems to reduce risk,[22–24] but these effects may only occur in nonusers of menopausal hormones. Among premenopausal women, generally the opposite holds true because higher body weight has been associated with a decreased breast cancer risk.[25, 26]

Interestingly, energy balance (i.e., energy intake versus energy expenditure) could be even more important than body weight in determining a woman's risk of breast cancer. One large research study showed that postmenopausal breast cancer risk was doubled when women with the highest BMI, highest caloric intake, and least amount of physical activity were compared to physically active women with the lowest BMI and caloric intake.[27] Similar effects may occur in premenopausal breast cancer as well.[28]

Body mass index has also been examined considerably over the past 30 years as a hypothesized prognosticator for breast cancer survivors. In general, most epidemiologic evidence suggests poorer outcomes with higher BMI in both pre- and postmenopausal women. Most studies associate overweight and obesity, and also postdiagnosis weight gain, with an increased risk of breast cancer recurrence and shortened survival times.[16, 29, 30]

Colon Cancer

The overall evidence from research studies is now convincing that higher BMI increases the risk of colon and colorectal cancer, with the association being somewhat stronger in men than in women.[31–33] Most studies of colon or colorectal cancer suggest an increasing risk with higher BMI. In addition, when comparing groups with the highest BMI to those with the lowest BMI, the risk is approximately doubled. Moreover, the relation with BMI does not seem to depend on the subsite of the tumor (i.e., proximal or distal colon).[31, 32] Overall, study findings on BMI have been more consistent and suggest a greater increase in risk for colon cancer than for rectal cancer,[5, 32, 33] although an increased risk of rectal cancer with higher BMI might exist in men.[32]

Much less research has addressed colon cancer prognosis in relation to BMI, but the overall evidence generally supports poorer outcomes in those who are obese.[21] One study, for example, found colon cancer deaths and recurrences (combined with second primaries) to be more common in patients with BMI ≥ 35 compared to those of normal weight.[18] In another study, deaths from colorectal cancer were more likely to occur in patients with higher percent body fat, higher body weight, and larger waist circumference.[19] Another study showed that obese women diagnosed with colon cancer had a higher average mortality rate over time than women of normal weight diagnosed with colon cancer, but this same association was not found for men.[34] Despite these relatively recent findings, more research is needed before any firm conclusions can be drawn surrounding BMI and colon cancer prognosis.

Endometrial Cancer

The strongest and most consistent evidence supporting an association with elevated BMI exists for endometrial cancer. The proportion of endometrial cancer in the United States attributed to overweight and obesity was estimated at 57%,[10] and more recently in Europe at 40%.[9] In other words, more than half of all endometrial cancer cases in the United States have been attributed to body weight (see figure 3.1), making obesity a key modifiable risk factor for endometrial cancer.[35] Our own review of the scientific literature describing more than 40 studies of BMI and endometrial cancer risk in women revealed a two- to fourfold increase in risk when groups of women with the highest BMI were compared to those with the lowest BMI. The lowest BMI category was typically defined as BMI < 25 or another cut-point within the normal range for BMI (18.5 to 24.9).

In most studies, risk tended to increase with increasing BMI.[6] One group estimated that for every 5 kg/m² increase in BMI, the risk of endometrial cancer increases by 60%; however, in women with BMI > 27 kg/m² the increase could be much greater.[36] In addition, the association was stronger in women who never used hormone replacement therapy.[36] Some evidence suggests that substantial weight gain over the adult lifetime (from age 18 to age 75) also increases risk; however, this effect may only occur in women who never used menopausal hormonal therapy.[37, 38]

Although much less research has addressed BMI and long-term prognosis for endometrial cancer, some studies following endometrial cancer patients have related higher BMI to worsened prognosis. Those studies showed that obesity, and particularly morbid obesity (BMI > 40),[3] in women with endometrial cancer may be linked to higher risk of death.[39] However, because other studies have not found obesity to be a negative prognostic factor in endometrial cancer,[21] more research is needed to clarify the association.

Kidney Cancer

Convincing evidence implicates obesity as a key risk factor for kidney cancer, particularly renal cell carcinoma. Some studies suggest a stronger link with BMI in women than in men.[6] Our own review of the scientific literature revealed relatively consistent results across studies and, overall, a two- to threefold increase in risk for those with the highest BMI compared to those with the lowest BMI. Risk also tends to increase with increasing BMI, with an estimated 5 to 7% increase in risk for every unit increase in BMI (1 kg/m^2) in both men and women.[40–42]

Paradoxically, recent studies of recurrence and survival from renal cell carcinoma have generally revealed better or equivalent outcomes for overweight and obese patients compared to normal weight patients.[43–45] However, given the small number of studies that have investigated the relation between BMI and kidney cancer prognosis, more long-term studies are needed to confirm these findings.

Esophageal Cancer

Present evidence suggests that higher BMI increases the risk of esophageal adenocarcinoma,[46, 47] especially in those with abdominal obesity.[48] An estimated 52% of incidences of esophageal adenocarcinoma in the United States have been attributed to overweight and obesity[10] (see figure 3.1), and approximately 40% in Europe.[9] In a combined analysis of research studies, every 5 kg/m^2 increase in BMI was associated with a 52 to 54% higher risk of esophageal adenocarcinoma.[46] In contrast, higher BMI appears to *decrease* the risk of squamous cell carcinoma and possibly also prolong survival of this disease.[46] Studies that examined the effect of BMI on survival and recurrence from esophageal adenocarcinoma are very sparse, but one study that followed patients following esophagectomy found no association with BMI.[49] More research is needed to confirm those findings.

Biologic Mechanisms

The reasons overweight and obese people are at higher risk for various cancers are not yet fully understood; however, many hypotheses have been proposed (see table 3.1).[10, 50] In general, the most well-studied mechanisms involve sex steroids, insulin and insulin-like growth factors (IGFs), and adipokines,[51] which are biologically active substances derived from fat (e.g., leptin). Future studies in humans will be extremely important for testing these mechanisms and others, and also for understanding how mechanisms interact to alter cancer risk.

Recommendations for Body Weight and Cancer

In 2006 the American Cancer Society published guidelines on nutrition and physical activity for preventing cancer[13] and also for cancer survivors.[52] With respect to body weight, it recommended the following:

- **For cancer prevention:** Maintain a healthy body weight (BMI 18.5 to 24.9) throughout life by balancing caloric intake with physical activity, avoiding excessive weight gain throughout life, and achieving and maintaining a healthy weight if currently overweight or obese.[13]
- **For cancer survivors:** Throughout the cancer continuum, strive to achieve and maintain a healthy weight.[52]

Furthermore, the World Cancer Research Fund and the American Institute for Cancer Research recommend that for preventing cancer, people should avoid increases in waist circumference throughout adulthood.[5]

TABLE 3.1 Hypothesized Biologic Mechanisms Possibly Explaining the Increased Risk of Cancer in Overweight and Obese People

Type of cancer	Effects of overweight and obesity
Breast cancer	↑ estrogen, ↑ testosterone, ↓ SHBG ↑ leptin, ↓ adiponectin, ↑ insulin, ↑ IGF, ↑ cholesterol Immune system dysfunction ↑ inflammatory cytokines
Colon cancer	↑ leptin, ↑ insulin, ↑ IGF, ↑ cholesterol ↑ inflammatory cytokines ↑ oxidative stress
Endometrial cancer	↑ estrogen, ↑ testosterone, ↓ SHBG ↑ leptin, ↑ insulin, ↑ IGF, ↑ cholesterol
Kidney cancer	↑ estrogen, ↑ testosterone, ↓ SHBG ↑ renal atherosclerosis ↑ hypertension-induced injury to renal tubules ↑ oxidative stress
Esophageal cancer	↑ leptin, ↑ insulin, ↑ IGF, ↑ cholesterol ↑ intra-abdominal pressure, ↑ gastroesophageal reflux disease ↑ Barrett's esophagus ↑ esophageal transit time, ↑ exposure time
All cancers	↑ pool of cells to undergo malignant transformation ↑ energy intake, ↓ physical activity ↑ concentration of growth factors or carcinogens in adipose tissue

IGF = insulin-like growth factors; SHBG = sex hormone binding globulin

Adapted from Ballard-Barbash et al. 2006.[50]

Take-Home Message

There is now strong evidence that increased body weight and body mass index, and high waist circumference, are related to an increase in risk of several cancers as well as possibly being associated with poorer chances of survival after cancer. People should be advised to maintain body weight within a normal range throughout life to reduce cancer risk and improve their chances of survival after cancer.

Effect of Exercise

Considerable scientific evidence suggests that physical activity reduces the risk of several cancer types with the evidence classified as convincing or probable for colon, breast, and endometrial cancers; possible for prostate, ovarian, and lung cancers; and null or insufficient for other cancers.[53] There is also increasing evidence that physical activity improves some health indicators and quality of life after diagnosis,[52, 54–56] although there have not yet been any reported clinical trials on the effect of postdiagnosis physical activity on the risk of cancer recurrence or survival.[52, 56] Challenges of these trials include the possibility of group differences in prognostic factors and treatments; the stresses of diagnosis, treatment, and recovery on a patient's ability to exercise; and the need for a large trial to detect statistically significant differences between exercise and control groups.

The following sections review the scientific literature on cancer sites that have been studied most extensively in relation to physical activity. Epidemiologic research relating physical activity to ovarian[57, 58] and lung cancers[59] are described elsewhere (see citations noted here). It is noteworthy that much of the epidemiologic evidence is based on studies that used questionnaires to estimate physical activity levels. Many factors must be considered when selecting a questionnaire,[60] including its validity for the research question being asked.

Colon Cancer

The most consistent and strong evidence for a role of physical activity in cancer etiology exists for colon cancer. An average risk reduction of about 25 to 30% is observed in both men and women who undertake the highest level of assessed physical activity compared to the lowest level of activity in studies that have examined these associations[55, 61–63] (activity levels were not uniformly defined). These findings are likely to be independent of body weight changes. There is evidence for a dose–response effect with more benefit being observed for higher levels of activity, as defined in each study. These results have been observed in studies conducted in a variety of populations around the world, using varying methods for assessing physical activity and with various study designs.

Although 52 studies of physical activity and colon cancer have been identified,[64] some aspects of this etiologic association remain unclear including whether the benefits of physical activity depend on menopausal hormone therapy use, dietary intake, or BMI. In addition, the time in life when physical activity is most beneficial for colon cancer prevention is unknown; greater risk reductions may result from higher activity levels over the lifetime as opposed to more recent activity.[64] It is also unclear whether physical activity has a differential effect on various regions of the colon.[64]

Based on the overall evidence from studies of recreational activity, about 30 to 60 minutes per day of moderate- to vigorous-intensity physical activity may be needed to lower colon cancer risk significantly.[13] An even greater benefit for colon cancer risk reduction may exist for vigorous-intensity activity,[13] but the magnitude of this benefit is unclear.[64]

Relatively recent research has been conducted on the role of leisure-time activity in improving colon cancer survival.[19, 65–68] Four cohort studies conducted by Meyerhardt and colleagues[65–68] all showed better survival among colorectal cancer survivors who were more physically active postdiagnosis. In addition, in the Melbourne Collaborative Cohort Study, prediagnosis exercise was associated with better disease-specific survival.[19]

The largest prognostic study to date was conducted in 832 men and women with stage III colon cancer.[65] In that study 18 to 26.9 MET-hours per week of postdiagnosis leisure-time activity lowered the risk of cancer recurrence or death by 49% compared with those who did less than 3 MET-hours per week. Furthermore, significant trends were found relating increasing activity levels to improved disease-free, recurrence-free, and overall survival. A minimum of 18 MET-hours per week of leisure activity improved disease-free survival rates regardless of sex, BMI, number of positive lymph nodes, chemotherapy type, age, or baseline performance status.

Breast Cancer

Extensive research has been conducted on the etiologic role of physical activity in relation to breast cancer risk, with the majority of studies concluding that women who are more physically active have a lower risk compared to sedentary women.[55, 69, 70] Across 73 studies, the average risk reduction was about 25% for the highest versus the lowest activity categories compared,[70] and there is consistent evidence of a dose–response effect, with greater risk decreases observed with higher levels of activity. All types of activity are beneficial, with somewhat stronger effects observed overall for recreational and household activity.[70] As well, the effect appears to be significant more often in postmenopausal women and, on average, and is stronger in normal weight women, non-Caucasians, women without a family history of breast cancer, and women who are parous. Effects are also stronger for activity done over the lifetime or after menopause, activity of moderate or vigorous intensity, or activity of longer duration (hours per week).[70]

Based on previous research, at least four hours per week of moderate- to vigorous-intensity activity may be necessary to reduce risk significantly.[55] A few aspects of this association remain unclear, including whether the benefit of physical activity depends on the histologic type of the tumor, the hormone receptor status, and other molecular aspects.

The role of physical activity in breast cancer survival has been examined in 15 observational studies conducted thus far.[71–85] Eight of these studies suggested that higher physical activity levels were associated with a significantly decreased risk of breast cancer mortality[74–78, 83] or overall mortality,[84, 85] implying that physically active people with breast cancer may have improved prognosis with fewer recurrences and deaths compared with sedentary survivors. The largest prognostic studies to date were conducted in the Breast Cancer Family Registry[85] and the Collaborative Women's Longevity Study[76] with each study enrolling more than 4,000 breast cancer survivors. The latter study found a 51% decrease in breast cancer mortality among the most physically active as well as evidence for a dose–response effect of decreasing the risk of breast cancer death with increasing levels of total recreational activity postdiagnosis.[76] In the Breast Cancer Family Registry study, all-cause mortality was decreased by 23 to 29% in women who were recreationally active three years prediagnosis compared to inactive women, whereas no association was found with lifetime physical activity.[85]

Endometrial Cancer

Twenty of the 25 published epidemiologic studies[86–105] suggest a protective effect from physical activity in endometrial cancer risk; no association was reported in five studies.[106–110] Overall, evidence suggests about a 20 to 30% decreased risk for the most active versus the least active study participants; also, activity of light to moderate intensity may lower risk, whereas sitting time may increase risk.[58] Despite these findings, recent reviews of this literature[58, 111, 112] have emphasized the need for further research studies that have more detailed assessments of lifetime physical activity and that consider all types and parameters of activity. Furthermore, it remains somewhat unclear how independent this association is from BMI or whether this effect depends on menopausal hormone therapy use.

No observational studies have been published on the role of exercise in endometrial cancer survival, but one randomized controlled trial examined how a six-month intervention of lifestyle counseling could influence physical activity levels, dietary habits, weight loss, and quality of life in endometrial

cancer survivors.[113] This study was able to achieve more weight loss and increased exercise levels in the intervention group than in the control group and demonstrated that this type of lifestyle intervention is feasible and could result in sustained behavior change over a yearlong period.

Prostate Cancer

There is inconsistent evidence regarding the association between physical activity and prostate cancer, with about one third (16 out of 42) of the studies conducted thus far indicating a protective effect.[11, 55, 114] The magnitude of the risk reduction is modest, on average around 9%,[115] and there remains a lack of clarity on whether the benefit from physical activity varies according to other factors such as age, race, family history, and BMI. The effect of physical activity may also be more restricted to advanced prostate cancers. Some evidence is emerging that higher levels of lifetime physical activity may decrease prostate cancer risk.[116, 117] Both occupational and recreational activities have been associated with decreased prostate cancer risk.

The inconsistency across prostate cancer studies may be attributed to several factors. First, prostate cancer is a slow-growing tumor with a long latency period, and a large percentage of men die with evidence of undiagnosed prostate cancer. Therefore, some studies may have been unable to detect a difference in physical activity levels between the cancer patients and the "healthy" control populations because of latent, nonclinical prostate cancer among the controls. Second, healthier, physically active men may be more likely to be screened for prostate cancer, and hence more likely to be diagnosed, than less active men. As a result, some study populations might not have accurately reflected the general population of cancer patients, and true risk reductions were attenuated. Finally, it has been hypothesized[115] that studies including a greater proportion of screen-detected, early-stage prostate cancer cases might reveal weaker associations between physical activity and prostate cancer risk than studies of advanced prostate cancer. A study by Littman and colleagues[118] found a strong inverse association between physical activity and prostate cancer risk in men with no history of recent PSA testing, but no association was found in men with a history of recent PSA testing. Another study[114] showed no difference in risk based on PSA screening history, casting doubt on this hypothesis.

Only one observational study has reported on physical activity and prostate cancer survival.[119] In that study of 2,705 nonmetastatic prostate cancer survivors from the Health Professionals Follow-Up Study, men who engaged in leisure-time physical activity postdiagnosis had significantly lower risks of all-cause and prostate cancer mortality; significant trends were noted, with increasing MET-hours per week corresponding with greater reductions in risk. Men reporting at least three hours per week of vigorous activity (versus less than one hour per week) had a 61% lower risk of death from prostate cancer.

Biologic Mechanisms

Physical activity likely has an effect on cancer risk through multiple, interrelated biologic mechanisms that include, primarily, an effect on body composi-

tion, endogenous sex hormones and metabolic factors, inflammation, insulin resistance, and possibly immune function, though less is known about this mechanism.[120] Some mechanisms are hypothesized to be common across most cancer sites, whereas others are specific to a subset of cancer sites. For example, for colon cancer, physical activity promotes a more rapid gastrointestinal transit time thereby reducing the length of time that the colonic mucosa is exposed to carcinogens. Some commonly hypothesized biologic mechanisms linking physical activity to cancer risk are summarized in table 3.2.

Recommendations for Physical Activity

The most current recommendations for cancer prevention and cancer survival related to physical activity have been developed by the World Cancer Research Fund and the American Institute for Cancer Research in their 2007 report,[5] the Ameri-

TABLE 3.2 Hypothesized Biologic Mechanisms Possibly Explaining the Decreased Risk of Cancer in Physically Active People

Type of cancer	Effects of physical activity
Colon cancer	↓ body fat ↓ insulin, ↓ IGF-1 ↓ leptin, ↑ adiponectin ↓ transit time through bowel ↑ vitamin D
Postmenopausal breast cancer	↓ body fat ↓ sex hormones ↓ insulin ↓ leptin, ↑ adiponectin ↑ vitamin D
Endometrial cancer	↓ body fat ↓ sex hormones ↓ insulin, ↓ IGF-1 ↓ leptin, ↑ adiponectin
Prostate cancer	↓ testosterone ↓ insulin, ↓ IGF-1 ↓ leptin, ↑ adiponectin
Most cancers	↓ chronic low-grade inflammation Improved immune function ↓ oxidative stress, ↑ antioxidant defense, enhanced DNA repair

IGF-1 = insulin-like growth factor-1

can Cancer Society,[13, 52] and an American College of Sports Medicine roundtable discussion.[121] These recommendations are similar, based on the largely observational epidemiologic research that has examined the links between physical activity and cancer risk. Because very limited research has been done on cancer survival, in general, these national and international agencies are recommending that the guidelines for prevention also be followed for survival with some treatment- and disease-specific modifications.

- **For cancer prevention:** Be moderately physically active, equivalent to brisk walking, for at least 30 minutes every day. As fitness improves, aim for 60 minutes or more of moderate, or for 30 minutes or more of vigorous, physical activity every day. Limit sedentary habits such as watching television.[5]

- **For cancer survival:** No specific recommendations have yet been prescribed for cancer survivors because research done on these populations has been insufficient. Hence, following the recommendations for cancer prevention and avoiding inactivity is likely appropriate,[5, 52, 55, 121] with specific adaptations based on disease and treatment-related adverse effects.[121]

Take-Home Message

Strong evidence suggests that physical activity reduces the risk of colon, breast, and endometrial cancers; the evidence for other cancers is more limited. The role of physical activity in cancer survival is emerging, and there is increasing evidence that physical activity may increase the chances of survival of breast and colon cancers. Although the optimal type, dose, and timing of activity are not entirely clear, patients can be advised to aim for 60 minutes or more of moderate, or 30 minutes or more of vigorous, physical activity every day and to limit sedentary behavior. The risks associated with specific cancers and cancer treatments should be considered when prescribing exercise to survivors.

Effect of Diet

An unhealthy diet could account for up to 30% of all cancers in developing countries[2] and perhaps 35% of cancer deaths in the United States.[122] Hence, along with tobacco use, diet is one of the most important modifiable risk factors for cancer. Given the diverse and complex nature of the human diet, however, it is also one of the most difficult factors to study in large human populations. Numerous instruments for dietary assessment have been developed and validated.[123] As in physical activity assessment, the choice of instrument depends largely on the intended purpose. A vast body of epidemiologic research has addressed a wide array of research questions related to cancer and diet in an attempt to disentangle individual dietary effects. Here we highlight some of the strongest associations identified thus far,[5, 7] although more associations will undoubtedly emerge in the future.

Sugar, Fast Foods, and Other Energy-Dense Foods

High-calorie foods and drinks are suspected risk factors for cancer given their contributions to weight gain, overweight, and obesity. The risks deriving from specific aspects of an energy-dense diet, however, are not as clear. Foods containing high amounts of sugar, for example, may be associated with increased colorectal cancer risk, and biologic mechanisms have been proposed, but the overall evidence in humans is currently limited and merely suggestive.[5]

In terms of fat intake, evidence from a substantial number of human studies has provided only limited, but suggestive evidence for increased risk of cancers of the lung, breast, colorectum,[5] and possibly prostate.[124, 125] Despite plausible biologic mechanisms for these cancers, the overall findings surrounding fat intake and cancer incidence are inconsistent. Notably, dietary fat has been studied in relation to breast cancer recurrence and survival in two large randomized controlled trials. Findings from the Women's Intervention Nutrition Study[126] and the Women's Healthy Eating and Living study[127] have suggested limited prognostic gain from lowering dietary fat, although there may be some decrease in recurrence rates for certain subgroups of postmenopausal women. More limited evidence suggests that the aggressiveness of prostate tumors and deaths from prostate cancer may be related to higher total and saturated fat intakes.[128]

Fruits and Vegetables

A plant-based diet rich in fruits, vegetables, and whole grains is continually recommended for the prevention of various cancers.[5, 7, 13, 52] In a comprehensive review of published literature on this subject, a variety of fruits and vegetables appeared likely to prevent cancer, although the evidence was not fully convincing (see table 3.3).[5]

Compared to cancer incidence, far fewer studies have examined fruit and vegetable intake in relation to cancer prognosis. Very limited data support a decreased risk of recurrence or progression of prostate cancer, for example, with higher intake of tomatoes or lycopene.[129] Vegetable intake has been linked to longer survival from ovarian cancer[130] and advanced lung cancer,[131, 132] but again, these findings are very preliminary. The effects on breast cancer prognosis are also unclear.[17] In the Women's Healthy Eating and Living randomized controlled trial of breast cancer patients, long-term adoption of a low-fat diet high in fruits, vegetables, and fiber had no effect on breast cancer recurrence or survival.[127]

Fruits and vegetables could prevent cancer through multiple, interrelated mechanisms. Promotion of a healthy body weight, prevention of oxidative stress and DNA damage, and the ability to alter the activities of carcinogen-activating enzymes are just a few possible mediating pathways to prevention. Higher intake may also favorably alter immune function, inflammation, and cellular growth.[5, 133]

Fiber

According to one international report on cancer prevention,[5] a diet high in fiber may well reduce the risk of colorectal cancer. Yet, at least one pooled analysis of research on this subject found no effect from fiber beyond the effects of other dietary risk factors.[134] Part of the difficulty in studying fiber intake in humans may be that intake is too low to observe any benefit.[135, 136] The Polyp Prevention Trial, conducted in the United States, explored the effect of increasing dietary fiber intake over four years (and also lowering fat and increasing fruit and vegetable intakes) in people who had previously experienced one or more colorectal adenomas. Adenoma recurrence was significantly lowered among the most compliant study participants,[137] implying that a high-fiber diet may also lower the risk of colorectal cancer recurrences.

The reasons that fiber may be protective are unclear, but several mechanisms have been proposed.[5] High fiber intake favorably alters the quality of the feces by diluting its contents, increasing its weight, and shortening transit time through the colon. The outcome of these effects is decreased contact between potential fecal carcinogens and

TABLE 3.3   Fruits and Vegetables That Probably Prevent Cancer

Fruits and vegetables	Cancers probably affected
Nonstarchy vegetables	Stomach, esophagus, mouth, pharynx, and larynx
Allium vegetables	Stomach
Garlic	Colorectum
Fruits	Lung, stomach, esophagus, mouth, pharynx, and larynx
Foods containing folate	Pancreas
Foods containing carotenoids	Mouth, pharynx, larynx, and lung
Foods containing beta-carotene	Esophagus
Foods containing lycopene	Prostate
Foods containing vitamin C	Esophagus
Foods containing selenium	Prostate

Reprinted in part, by permission, from World Cancer Research Fund and the American Institute for Cancer Research, 2007, Foods and drinks. In *Food, nutrition, physical activity, and the prevention of cancer: A global perspective* (Washington, DC: American Institute for Cancer Research), 76. Available: www.dietandcancerreport.org/downloads/chapters/chapter_04.pdf

colonic cells. As well, fiber fermentation products (e.g., butyrate) produced in the gut can help promote healthy cellular growth. Furthermore, intakes of fiber and folate are correlated, and hence, the observed effects may actually be from folate.

Red Meat and Processed Meat

There is convincing evidence that consumption of red meat and processed meat (i.e., preserved by smoking, curing, salting, or with preservatives) increases the risk of colorectal cancer.[5, 63] Very few studies, however, have examined the effect of diet on colorectal cancer recurrence and survivorship. In one follow-up study of patients with stage III colon cancer, postdiagnosis intake of a "Western diet" (high intake of red and processed meats, sweets, French fries, and refined grains) was associated with higher risks of recurrence and death, whereas a "prudent diet" (fruits, vegetables, legumes, fish, poultry, and whole grains) was not associated with an increased risk.[138] Whether these findings are attributable to meat intake specifically, however, is unknown.

Red and processed meats might increase cancer risk because potentially carcinogenic N-nitroso compounds are formed in the stomach and gut following their ingestion. Cooking at high temperatures produces potentially carcinogenic by-products, and the heme iron content of meats may also promote DNA damage and cancer in the colon. Moreover, processed meats are high in salt, which also encourages the formation of N-nitroso compounds.[5, 13] In addition, higher meat consumption may coincide with low intakes of fruits, vegetables, and fiber, which may decrease cancer risk.

Alcohol

There is now a wealth of convincing evidence[5] that total alcohol intake, irrespective of the source, increases the risk of cancers of the mouth, pharynx, larynx, esophagus, colorectum (in men)[63] and breast in both pre- and postmenopausal women.[138–140] With respect to breast cancer, the increased risk from alcohol appears to be the most elevated in women with low folate intake.[141] It is less convincing, but still probable, that alcohol consumption increases the risk of liver cancer and of colorectal cancer in

women. Alcohol in small quantities does not appear to prevent cancer as it does cardiovascular disease.[5] The effect of alcohol intake on cancer prognosis has been studied in relation to breast cancer; however, the effect remains uncertain. Alcohol intake has not been associated with breast cancer recurrence or overall survival in most studies of women diagnosed with breast cancer.[17]

Alcohol may increase cancer risk via multiple pathways.[5, 13] Some of its metabolites and by-products, for example, may be carcinogenic. Alcohol also acts as a solvent, which facilitates the entry of other cancer-causing compounds (e.g., as found in tobacco) into cells. Hence, for certain cancers, the combined cancer-causing effects of alcohol and tobacco are worse than they would be for either substance alone. Furthermore, alcohol may indirectly alter normal cell cycles, affect the metabolism of other carcinogens, increase circulating hormone levels, and reduce folate levels.

Salt

Total salt intake and the intake of salted and salty foods are probably associated with stomach cancer, and intake of Cantonese-style salted fish appears to increase the risk of nasopharyngeal cancer.[5] Salt intake could plausibly cause stomach cancer by damaging the stomach lining, increasing the formation of N-nitroso compounds, which are potentially carcinogenic, or interacting with other carcinogens. It is also hypothesized that salt intake and *Heliobacter pylori* infection might act synergistically to increase risk.[142] Salted fish may increase the risk of cancer of the nasopharynx because of its N-nitrosamine content.[5]

Dietary Supplements

In their report on diet and cancer prevention, the World Cancer Research Fund and the American Institute for Cancer Research[5] do not recommend dietary supplements for the purpose of preventing cancer. Instead, they recommend that proper nutrition be attained through the intake of foods alone. Although evidence suggests that some supplement use may help prevent cancer, high doses can actually cause cancer in certain subgroups of the population. For example, convincing evidence supports a causal role for high-dose beta-carotene supplement use in lung cancer, depending on smoking status and genetics.[5] The American Cancer Society similarly advises cancer survivors to avoid very high doses of vitamins, minerals, and other dietary supplements; they state that although low doses may be useful, they should only be taken with advice from a health care provider.[52]

Recommendations for Diet and Cancer

The pool of scientific evidence on diet and cancer is already vast and continues to expand; however, much uncertainty remains. In the meantime, therefore, it is recommended that the general population consume whole foods, follow a healthy dietary pattern, and be mindful of total caloric intake and body weight.[13] More specific recommendations are outlined in the sidebar Dietary Recommendations for Preventing Cancer. If they can, and unless otherwise advised, cancer survivors should follow cancer prevention recommendations for diet, weight, and physical activity.[5]

Take-Home Message

Diet and cancer is a prolific area of research, but still, much uncertainty exists, particularly with regard to cancer recurrence and survival. A variety of plausible diet-related mechanisms have been proposed, and in the context of whole food consumption, these mechanisms are likely intertwined. People should consume a plant-based, whole foods diet that is rich in fruits, vegetables, and whole grains for the prevention of cancers and for improved cancer prognosis.

Summary

A wealth of literature describes evidence relating cancer risk to body weight, physical activity, and various aspects of diet. Convincing evidence

---

Dietary Recommendations for Preventing Cancer

- Consume energy-dense foods sparingly.
- Avoid sugary drinks.
- Consume fast foods sparingly, if at all.
- Eat at least five portions or servings (at least 14 oz or 400 g) of a variety of nonstarchy vegetables and of fruits every day.
- Eat relatively unprocessed cereals (grains), pulses (legumes), or both, with every meal.
- Limit refined starchy foods. If you consume starchy roots or tubers as staples, you should also make sure you consume sufficient nonstarchy vegetables, fruits, and pulses (legumes).
- If you eat red meat, consume less than 16 oz (500 g) a week; very little, if any, of that should be processed.
- If you consume alcoholic drinks, limit consumption to no more than two drinks a day if you are a man and one drink a day if you are a woman.
- Avoid salt-preserved, salted, or salty foods; preserve foods without using salt.
- Limit your consumption of processed foods with added salt to ensure an intake of less than 6 g (2.4 g sodium) a day.
- Do not eat moldy cereals (grains) or pulses (legumes).[†]
- Dietary supplements are not recommended for cancer prevention.

[†]Convincing evidence supports a causal relation between aflatoxin exposure and liver cancer in humans.[5] Aflatoxin is a potent liver toxin and carcinogen produced by certain molds or fungi that grow on grains, legumes, nuts, and seeds under warm, humid conditions. Despite existing regulations and control measures to prevent human aflatoxin exposure in developed countries, exposure is rampant in developing countries where control measures are not feasible or practical.[143]

Adapted from World Cancer Research Fund and the American Institute for Cancer Research 2007.

supports causal associations between overweight and obesity and five cancers; preventive roles for physical activity in cancers of the colon, breast, and endometrium; and both helpful and harmful effects from various aspects of diet on numerous cancer sites. The overall evidence describing these effects in cancer survivors, however, is weak if not lacking altogether. Consequently, international and U.S. recommendations for cancer survivors are to follow the advice given to the general population for cancer prevention, while accounting for the risks associated with specific cancers and their treatments. In brief, these recommendations include maintaining a healthy body weight; exercising *at minimum* 30 minutes per day, five days per week and at moderate intensity (but preferably more); and eating a whole foods diet that is rich in fruits, vegetables, and grains and low in fat and added sugars, red and processed meats, salt, and alcohol.

Although much is known about body weight, physical activity, and diet in relation to cancer risk, many aspects of these associations remain unclear. More research is needed to understand the biologic mechanisms explaining past findings and how certain population subgroups (e.g., based on gender, race, hormone use, histologic subtypes of tumor, and genotypes) might be uniquely affected by these behaviors.

Finally, although we have described associations currently supported by the strongest scientific evidence, it is recognized that other risk factors are also important in cancer causation. Additional research on these modifiable lifestyle risk factors will increase our understanding of how the risk of developing these cancers might be reduced even more. A large percentage of cancer is preventable through changes in lifestyle that are achievable for most of the population. Hence, clinicians should disseminate the most current public health recommendations on diet and physical activity to help achieve the benefits in cancer prevention that are now clearly recognized.

References

1. Danaei G, Vander HS, Lopez AD, Murray CJ, Ezzati M. Causes of cancer in the world: Comparative risk assessment of nine behavioural and environmental risk factors. *Lancet*. 2005; 366: 1784-1793.

2. Mackay J, Jemal A, Lee NC, Parkin DM. *Risk Factors: The Cancer Atlas*. Atlanta: The American Cancer Society; 2006: chap. 2.

3. Calle EE, Rodriguez C, Walker-Thurmond K, Thun MJ. Overweight, obesity, and mortality from cancer in a prospectively studied cohort of U.S. adults. *N Engl J Med*. 2003; 348: 1625-1638.

4. McGee DL. Body mass index and mortality: A meta-analysis based on person-level data from twenty-six observational studies. *Ann Epidemiol*. 2005; 15: 87-97.

5. World Cancer Research Fund and the American Institute for Cancer Research. *Food, Nutrition, Physical Activity, and the Prevention of Cancer: A Global Perspective*. Washington, DC: American Institute for Cancer Research; 2007.

6. IARC Working Group, World Health Organization. Weight control and physical activity— IACR handbook for cancer prevention. Vol. 6. Lyon, France: IARC Press; 2002.

7. Key TJ, Schatzkin A, Willett WC, Allen NE, Spencer EA, Travis RC. Diet, nutrition and the prevention of cancer. *Public Health Nutr*. 2004; 7: 187-200.

8. Renehan AG, Tyson M, Egger M, Heller RF, Zwahlen M. Body-mass index and incidence of cancer: A systematic review and meta-analysis of prospective observational studies. *Lancet*. 2008; 371: 569-578.

9. Renehan AG, Soerjomataram I, Tyson M, Egger M, Zwahlen M, Coebergh JW, Buchan I. Incident cancer burden attributable to excess body mass index in 30 European countries. *Int J Cancer*. 2010; 126: 692-702.

10. Calle EE, Kaaks R. Overweight, obesity and cancer: Epidemiological evidence and proposed mechanisms. *Nat Rev Cancer*. 2004; 4: 579-591.

11. Pan SY, DesMeules M. Energy intake, physical activity, energy balance, and cancer: Epidemiologic evidence. *Methods Mol Biol*. 2009; 472: 191-215.

12. Olsen CM, Green AC, Whiteman DC, Sadeghi S, Kolahdooz F, Webb PM. Obesity and the risk of epithelial ovarian cancer: A systematic review and meta-analysis. *Eur J Cancer*. 2007; 43: 690-709.

13. Kushi LH, Byers T, Doyle C, Bandera EV, McCullough M, McTiernan A, Gansler T, Andrews KS, Thun MJ. American Cancer Society Guidelines on Nutrition and Physical Activity for cancer prevention: Reducing the risk of cancer with healthy food choices and physical activity. *CA Cancer J Clin*. 2006; 56: 254-281.

14. Bergstrom A, Pisani P, Tenet V, Wolk A, Adami HO. Overweight as an avoidable cause of cancer in Europe. *Int J Cancer*. 2001; 91: 421-430.

15. Rockhill B, Newman B, Weinberg C. Use and misuse of population attributable fractions. *Am J Public Health*. 1998; 88: 15-19.

16. Chlebowski RT, Aiello E, McTiernan A. Weight loss in breast cancer patient management. *J Clin Oncol*. 2002; 20: 1128-1143.

17. Rock CL, Demark-Wahnefried W. Nutrition and survival after the diagnosis of breast cancer: A review of the evidence. *J Clin Oncol*. 2002; 20: 3302-3316.

18. Dignam JJ, Polite BN, Yothers G, Raich P, Colangelo L, O'Connell MJ, Wolmark N. Body mass index and outcomes in patients who receive adjuvant chemotherapy for colon cancer. *J Natl Cancer Inst*. 2006; 98: 1647-1654.

19. Haydon AM, Macinnis RJ, English DR, Giles GG. Effect of physical activity and body size on survival after diagnosis with colorectal cancer. *Gut*. 2006; 55: 62-67.

20. Denmark-Wahnefried W, Moyad MA. Dietary intervention in the management of prostate cancer. *Curr Opin Urol*. 2007; 17: 168-174.

21. Rock CL. Energy balance and cancer prognosis: Colon, prostate and other cancers. In: McTiernan A, ed. *Cancer Prevention and Management Through Exercise and Weight Control*. Boca Raton, FL; CRC Press; 2006: chap. 28.

22. Eliassen AH, Colditz GA, Rosner B, Willett WC, Hankinson SE. Adult weight change and risk of postmenopausal breast cancer. *JAMA*. 2006; 296: 193-201.

23. Harvie M, Howell A, Vierkant RA, Kumar N, Cerhan JR, Kelemen LE, Folsom AR, Sellers TA. Association of gain and loss of weight before and after menopause with risk of postmenopausal breast cancer in the Iowa women's health study. *Cancer Epidemiol Biomarkers Prev*. 2005; 14: 656-661.

24. Ahn J, Schatzkin A, Lacey JV, Jr., Albanes D, Ballard-Barbash R, Adams KF, Kipnis V, Mouw T, Hollenbeck AR, Leitzmann MF. Adiposity, adult weight change, and postmenopausal breast cancer risk. *Arch Intern Med*. 2007; 167: 2091-2102.

25. Friedenreich CM. Review of anthropometric factors and breast cancer risk. *Eur J Cancer Prev*. 2001; 10: 15-32.

26. van den Brandt PA, Spiegelman D, Yaun SS, Adami HO, Beeson L, Folsom AR, Fraser G, Goldbohm RA, Graham S, Kushi L, Marshall JR, Miller AB, et al. Pooled analysis of prospective cohort studies on height, weight, and breast cancer risk. *Am J Epidemiol*. 2000; 152: 514-527.

27. Chang SC, Ziegler RG, Dunn B, Stolzenberg-Solomon R, Lacey JV, Jr., Huang WY, Schatzkin A, Reding D, Hoover RN, Hartge P, Leitzmann MF. Association of energy intake and energy balance with postmenopausal breast cancer in the prostate, lung, colorectal, and ovarian cancer screening trial. *Cancer Epidemiol Biomarkers Prev*. 2006; 15: 334-341.

28. Silvera SA, Jain M, Howe GR, Miller AB, Rohan TE. Energy balance and breast cancer risk: A prospective cohort study. *Breast Cancer Res Treat*. 2006; 97: 97-106.

29. Ryu SY, Kim CB, Nam CM, Park JK, Kim KS, Park J, Yoo SY, Cho KS. Is body mass index the prognostic factor in breast cancer?: A meta-analysis. *J Korean Med Sci*. 2001; 16: 610-614.

30. Carmichael AR. Obesity and prognosis of breast cancer. *Obes Rev*. 2006; 7: 333-340.

31. Harriss DJ, Atkinson G, George K, Cable NT, Reilly T, Haboubi N, Zwahlen M, Egger M, Renehan AG. Lifestyle factors and colorectal cancer risk (1): Systematic review and meta-analysis of associations with body mass index. *Colorectal Dis*. 2009; 11: 547-563.

32. Larsson SC, Wolk A. Obesity and colon and rectal cancer risk: A meta-analysis of prospective studies. *Am J Clin Nutr*. 2007; 86: 556-565.

33. Moghaddam AA, Woodward M, Huxley R. Obesity and risk of colorectal cancer: A meta-analysis of 31 studies with 70,000 events. *Cancer Epidemiol Biomarkers Prev*. 2007; 16: 2533-2547.

34. Meyerhardt JA, Catalano PJ, Haller DG, Mayer RJ, Benson AB, III, Macdonald JS, Fuchs CS. Influence of body mass index on outcomes and treatment-related toxicity in patients with colon carcinoma. *Cancer*. 2003; 98: 484-495.

35. Linkov F, Edwards R, Balk J, Yurkovetsky Z, Stadterman B, Lokshin A, Taioli E. Endometrial hyperplasia, endometrial cancer and prevention: Gaps in existing research of modifiable risk factors. *Eur J Cancer*. 2008; 44: 1632-1644.

36. Crosbie EJ, Zwahlen M, Kitchener HC, Egger M, Renehan AG. Body mass index, hormone replacement therapy, and endometrial cancer risk: A meta-analysis. *Cancer Epidemiol Biomarkers Prev*. 2010; 19: 3119-3130.

37. Chang SC, Lacey JV, Jr., Brinton LA, Hartge P, Adams K, Mouw T, Carroll L, Hollenbeck A, Schatzkin A, Leitzmann MF. Lifetime weight history and endometrial cancer risk by type of menopausal hormone use in the NIH-AARP diet and health study. *Cancer Epidemiol Biomarkers Prev*. 2007; 16: 723-730.

38. Park SL, Goodman MT, Zhang ZF, Kolonel LN, Henderson BE, Setiawan VW. Body size, adult BMI gain and endometrial cancer risk: The multiethnic cohort. *Int J Cancer*. 2009; 126: 490-499.

39. Fader AN, Arriba LN, Frasure HE, von G, V. Endometrial cancer and obesity: Epidemiology, biomarkers, prevention and survivorship. *Gynecol Oncol*. 2009; 114: 121-127.

40. Bergstrom A, Hsieh CC, Lindblad P, Lu CM, Cook NR, Wolk A. Obesity and renal cell cancer—A quantitative review. *Br J Cancer*. 2001; 85: 984-990.

41. Ildaphonse G, George PS, Mathew A. Obesity and kidney cancer risk in men: A meta-analysis (1992-2008). *Asian Pac J Cancer Prev*. 2009; 10: 279-286.

42. Mathew A, George PS, Ildaphonse G. Obesity and kidney cancer risk in women: A meta-analysis (1992-2008). *Asian Pac J Cancer Prev*. 2009; 10: 471-478.

43. Donat SM, Salzhauer EW, Mitra N, Yanke BV, Snyder ME, Russo P. Impact of body mass index on survival

of patients with surgically treated renal cell carcinoma. *J Urol.* 2006; 175: 46-52.

44. Haferkamp A, Pritsch M, Bedke J, Wagener N, Pfitzenmaier J, Buse S, Hohenfellner M. The influence of body mass index on the long-term survival of patients with renal cell carcinoma after tumour nephrectomy. *BJU Int.* 2008; 101: 1243-1246.

45. Parker AS, Lohse CM, Cheville JC, Thiel DD, Leibovich BC, Blute ML. Greater body mass index is associated with better pathologic features and improved outcome among patients treated surgically for clear cell renal cell carcinoma. *Urology.* 2006; 68: 741-746.

46. Smith M, Zhou M, Whitlock G, Yang G, Offer A, Hui G, Peto R, Huang Z, Chen Z. Esophageal cancer and body mass index: Results from a prospective study of 220,000 men in China and a meta-analysis of published studies. *Int J Cancer.* 2008; 122: 1604-1610.

47. Kubo A, Corley DA. Body mass index and adenocarcinomas of the esophagus or gastric cardia: A systematic review and meta-analysis. *Cancer Epidemiol Biomarkers Prev.* 2006; 15: 872-878.

48. Corley DA, Kubo A, Zhao W. Abdominal obesity and the risk of esophageal and gastric cardia carcinomas. *Cancer Epidemiol Biomarkers Prev.* 2008; 17: 352-358.

49. Morgan MA, Lewis WG, Hopper AN, Escofet X, Harvard TJ, Brewster AE, Crosby TD, Roberts SA, Clark GW. Prognostic significance of body mass indices for patients undergoing esophagectomy for cancer. *Dis Esophagus.* 2007; 20: 29-35.

50. Ballard-Barbash R, Friedenreich C, Slattery M, Thune I. Obesity and body composition. In: Schottenfeld D, Fraumeni JF, eds. *Cancer Epidemiology and Prevention.* 3rd ed. New York: Oxford University Press; 2006: chap. 22.

51. Renehan AG, Roberts DL, Dive C. Obesity and cancer: Pathophysiological and biological mechanisms. *Arch Physiol Biochem.* 2008; 114: 71-83.

52. Doyle C, Kushi LH, Byers T, Courneya KS, Mark-Wahnefried W, Grant B, McTiernan A, Rock CL, Thompson C, Gansler T, Andrews KS. Nutrition and physical activity during and after cancer treatment: An American Cancer Society guide for informed choices. *CA Cancer J Clin.* 2006; 56: 323-353.

53. Friedenreich CM, Neilson HK, Lynch BM. State of the epidemiological evidence on physical activity and cancer prevention. *Eur J Cancer.* 2010; 46: 2593-2604.

54. Schmitz KH, Holtzman J, Courneya KS, Masse LC, Duval S, Kane R. Controlled physical activity trials in cancer survivors: A systematic review and meta-analysis. *Cancer Epidemiol Biomarkers Prev.* 2005; 14: 1588-1595.

55. Physical Activity Guidelines Advisory Committee. *Physical Activity Guidelines Advisory Committee Report, 2008.* 2008.

56. Courneya KS, Friedenreich CM. Physical activity and cancer: An introduction. In: Courneya KS, Friedenreich CM, eds. *Physical Activity and Cancer.* Berlin: Springer-Verlag; 2011: v. 186, chap. 1.

57. Moorman PG, Jones LW, Akushevich L, Schildkraut JM. Recreational physical activity and ovarian cancer risk and survival. *Ann Epidemiol.* 2011; 21: 178-187.

58. Cust AE. Physical activity and gynecologic cancer prevention. *Recent Results Cancer Res.* 2011; 186: 159-185.

59. Emaus A, Thune I. Physical activity and lung cancer prevention. *Recent Results Cancer Res.* 2011; 186: 101-133.

60. Terwee CB, Mokkink LB, van Poppel MN, Chinapaw MJ, van MW, de Vet HC. Qualitative attributes and measurement properties of physical activity questionnaires: A checklist. *Sports Med.* 2010; 40: 525-537.

61. Lee IM, Oguma Y. Physical activity. In: Schottenfeld D, Fraumeni JF, eds. *Cancer Epidemiology and Prevention.* 3rd ed. New York: Oxford University Press; 2006: chap. 23.

62. Wolin KY, Yan Y, Colditz GA, Lee IM. Physical activity and colon cancer prevention: A meta-analysis. *Br J Cancer.* 2009; 100: 611-616.

63. Huxley RR, Ansary-Moghaddam A, Clifton P, Czernichow S, Parr CL, Woodward M. The impact of dietary and lifestyle risk factors on risk of colorectal cancer: A quantitative overview of the epidemiological evidence. *Int J Cancer.* 2009; 125: 171-180.

64. Wolin KY, Tuchman H. Physical activity and gastrointestinal cancer prevention. *Recent Results Cancer Res.* 2011; 186: 73-100.

65. Meyerhardt JA, Heseltine D, Niedzwiecki D, Hollis D, Saltz LB, Mayer RJ, Thomas J, Nelson H, Whittom R, Hantel A, Schilsky RL, Fuchs CS. Impact of physical activity on cancer recurrence and survival in patients with stage III colon cancer: Findings from CALGB 89803. *J Clin Oncol.* 2006; 24: 3535-3541.

66. Meyerhardt JA, Giovannucci EL, Holmes MD, Chan AT, Chan JA, Colditz GA, Fuchs CS. Physical activity and survival after colorectal cancer diagnosis. *J Clin Oncol.* 2006; 24: 3527-3534.

67. Meyerhardt JA, Ogino S, Kirkner GJ, Chan AT, Wolpin B, Ng K, Nosho K, Shima K, Giovannucci EL, Loda M, Fuchs CS. Interaction of molecular markers and physical activity on mortality in patients with colon cancer. *Clin Cancer Res.* 2009; 15: 5931-5936.

68. Meyerhardt JA, Giovannucci EL, Ogino S, Kirkner GJ, Chan AT, Willett W, Fuchs CS. Physical activity and male colorectal cancer survival. *Arch Intern Med.* 2009; 169: 2102-2108.

69. Monninkhof EM, Elias SG, Vlems FA, van der Tweel I, Schuit AJ, Voskuil DW, van Leeuwen FE. Physical activity and breast cancer: A systematic review. *Epidemiology*. 2007; 18: 137-157.

70. Lynch BM, Neilson HK, Friedenreich CM. Physical activity and breast cancer prevention. *Recent Results Cancer Res*. 2011; 186: 13-42.

71. Abrahamson PE, Gammon MD, Lund MJ, Britton JA, Marshall SW, Flagg EW, Porter PL, Brinton LA, Eley JW, Coates RJ. Recreational physical activity and survival among young women with breast cancer. *Cancer*. 2006; 107: 1777-1785.

72. Borugian MJ, Sheps SB, Kim-Sing C, Van PC, Potter JD, Dunn B, Gallagher RP, Hislop TG. Insulin, macronutrient intake, and physical activity: Are potential indicators of insulin resistance associated with mortality from breast cancer? *Cancer Epidemiol Biomarkers Prev*. 2004; 13: 1163-1172.

73. Dal ML, Zucchetto A, Talamini R, Serraino D, Stocco CF, Vercelli M, Falcini F, Franceschi S. Effect of obesity and other lifestyle factors on mortality in women with breast cancer. *Int J Cancer*. 2008; 123: 2188-2194.

74. Enger SM, Bernstein L. Exercise activity, body size and premenopausal breast cancer survival. *Br J Cancer*. 2004; 90: 2138-2141.

75. Friedenreich CM, Gregory J, Kopciuk KA, Mackey JR, Courneya KS. Prospective cohort study of lifetime physical activity and breast cancer survival. *Int J Cancer*. 2009; 124: 1954-1962.

76. Holick CN, Newcomb PA, Trentham-Dietz A, Titus-Ernstoff L, Bersch AJ, Stampfer MJ, Baron JA, Egan KM, Willett WC. Physical activity and survival after diagnosis of invasive breast cancer. *Cancer Epidemiol Biomarkers Prev*. 2008; 17: 379-386.

77. Holmes MD, Chen WY, Feskanich D, Kroenke CH, Colditz GA. Physical activity and survival after breast cancer diagnosis. *JAMA*. 2005; 293: 2479-2486.

78. Irwin ML, Smith AW, McTiernan A, Ballard-Barbash R, Cronin K, Gilliland FD, Baumgartner RN, Baumgartner KB, Bernstein L. Influence of pre- and postdiagnosis physical activity on mortality in breast cancer survivors: The health, eating, activity, and lifestyle study. *J Clin Oncol*. 2008; 26: 3958-3964.

79. Rohan TE, Fu W, Hiller JE. Physical activity and survival from breast cancer. *Eur J Cancer Prev*. 1995; 4: 419-424.

80. Sternfeld B, Weltzien E, Quesenberry CP, Jr., Castillo AL, Kwan M, Slattery ML, Caan BJ. Physical activity and risk of recurrence and mortality in breast cancer survivors: Findings from the LACE study. *Cancer Epidemiol Biomarkers Prev*. 2009; 18: 87-95.

81. Emaus A, Veierod MB, Tretli S, Finstad SE, Selmer R, Furberg AS, Bernstein L, Schlichting E, Thune I. Metabolic profile, physical activity, and mortality in breast cancer patients. *Breast Cancer Res Treat*. 2010; 121: 651-660.

82. Hellmann SS, Thygesen LC, Tolstrup JS, Gronbaek M. Modifiable risk factors and survival in women diagnosed with primary breast cancer: Results from a prospective cohort study. *Eur J Cancer Prev*. 2010; 19(5): 366-373.

83. West-Wright CN, Henderson KD, Sullivan-Halley J, Ursin G, Deapen D, Neuhausen S, Reynolds P, Chang E, Ma H, Bernstein L. Long-term and recent recreational physical activity and survival after breast cancer: The California Teachers Study. *Cancer Epidemiol Biomarkers Prev*. 2009; 18: 2851-2859.

84. Bertram LA, Stefanick ML, Saquib N, Natarajan L, Patterson RE, Bardwell W, Flatt SW, Newman VA, Rock CL, Thomson CA, Pierce JP. Physical activity, additional breast cancer events, and mortality among early-stage breast cancer survivors: Findings from the WHEL Study. *Cancer Causes Control*. 2011; 22: 427-435.

85. Keegan TH, Milne RL, Andrulis IL, Chang ET, Sangaramoorthy M, Phillips KA, Giles GG, Goodwin PJ, Apicella C, Hopper JL, Whittemore AS, John EM. Past recreational physical activity, body size, and all-cause mortality following breast cancer diagnosis: Results from the breast cancer family registry. *Breast Cancer Res Treat*. 2010; 123: 531-542.

86. Zheng W, Shu XO, McLaughlin JK, Chow WH, Gao YT, Blot WJ. Occupational physical activity and the incidence of cancer of the breast, corpus uteri, and ovary in Shanghai. *Cancer*. 1993; 71: 3620-3624.

87. Moradi T, Nyren O, Bergstrom R, Gridley G, Linet M, Wolk A, Dosemeci M, Adami HO. Risk for endometrial cancer in relation to occupational physical activity: A nationwide cohort study in Sweden. *Int J Cancer*. 1998; 76: 665-670.

88. Terry P, Baron JA, Weiderpass E, Yuen J, Lichtenstein P, Nyren O. Lifestyle and endometrial cancer risk: A cohort study from the Swedish Twin Registry. *Int J Cancer*. 1999; 82: 38-42.

89. Colbert LH, Lacey JV, Jr., Schairer C, Albert P, Schatzkin A, Albanes D. Physical activity and risk of endometrial cancer in a prospective cohort study (United States). *Cancer Causes Control*. 2003; 14: 559-567.

90. Furberg AS, Thune I. Metabolic abnormalities (hypertension, hyperglycemia and overweight), lifestyle (high energy intake and physical inactivity) and endometrial cancer risk in a Norwegian cohort. *Int J Cancer*. 2003; 104: 669-676.

91. Schouten LJ, Goldbohm RA, van den Brandt PA. Anthropometry, physical activity, and endometrial cancer risk: Results from the Netherlands Cohort Study. *J Natl Cancer Inst*. 2004; 96: 1635-1638.

92. Friberg E, Mantzoros CS, Wolk A. Physical activity and risk of endometrial cancer: A population-based prospective cohort study. *Cancer Epidemiol Biomarkers Prev.* 2006; 15: 2136-2140.

93. Friedenreich C, Cust A, Lahmann PH, Steindorf K, Boutron-Ruault MC, Clavel-Chapelon F, Mesrine S, Linseisen J, Rohrmann S, Pischon T, Schulz M, Tjonneland A, et al. Physical activity and risk of endometrial cancer: The European prospective investigation into cancer and nutrition. *Int J Cancer.* 2007; 121: 347-355.

94. Patel AV, Feigelson HS, Talbot JT, McCullough ML, Rodriguez C, Patel RC, Thun MJ, Calle EE. The role of body weight in the relationship between physical activity and endometrial cancer: Results from a large cohort of US women. *Int J Cancer.* 2008; 123: 1877-1882.

95. Gierach GL, Chang SC, Brinton LA, Lacey JV, Jr., Hollenbeck AR, Schatzkin A, Leitzmann MF. Physical activity, sedentary behavior, and endometrial cancer risk in the NIH-AARP Diet and Health Study. *Int J Cancer.* 2009; 124: 2139-2147.

96. Conroy MB, Sattelmair JR, Cook NR, Manson JE, Buring JE, Lee IM. Physical activity, adiposity, and risk of endometrial cancer. *Cancer Causes Control.* 2009; 20: 1107-1115.

97. Sturgeon SR, Brinton LA, Berman ML, Mortel R, Twiggs LB, Barrett RJ, Wilbanks GD. Past and present physical activity and endometrial cancer risk. *Br J Cancer.* 1993; 68: 584-589.

98. Levi F, La Vecchia C, Negri E, Franceschi S. Selected physical activities and the risk of endometrial cancer. *Br J Cancer.* 1993; 67: 846-851.

99. Hirose K, Tajima K, Hamajima N, Takezaki T, Inoue M, Kuroishi T, Kuzuya K, Nakamura S, Tokudome S. Subsite (cervix/endometrium)-specific risk and protective factors in uterus cancer. *Jpn J Cancer Res.* 1996; 87: 1001-1009.

100. Goodman MT, Hankin JH, Wilkens LR, Lyu LC, McDuffie K, Liu LQ, Kolonel LN. Diet, body size, physical activity, and the risk of endometrial cancer. *Cancer Res.* 1997; 57: 5077-5085.

101. Moradi T, Weiderpass E, Signorello LB, Persson I, Nyren O, Adami HO. Physical activity and post-menopausal endometrial cancer risk (Sweden). *Cancer Causes Control.* 2000; 11: 829-837.

102. Salazar-Martinez E, Lazcano-Ponce EC, Lira-Lira GG, Escudero-De los RP, Salmeron-Castro J, Larrea F, Hernandez-Avila M. Case-control study of diabetes, obesity, physical activity and risk of endometrial cancer among Mexican women. *Cancer Causes Control.* 2000; 11: 707-711.

103. Littman AJ, Voigt LF, Beresford SA, Weiss NS. Recreational physical activity and endometrial cancer risk. *Am J Epidemiol.* 2001; 154: 924-933.

104. Matthews CE, Xu WH, Zheng W, Gao YT, Ruan ZX, Cheng JR, Xiang YB, Shu XO. Physical activity and risk of endometrial cancer: A report from the Shanghai endometrial cancer study. *Cancer Epidemiol Biomarkers Prev.* 2005; 14: 779-785.

105. Friedenreich CM, Cook LS, Magliocco AM, Duggan MA, Courneya KS. Case-control study of lifetime total physical activity and endometrial cancer risk. *Cancer Causes Control.* 2010; 21: 1105-1116.

106. Pukkala E, Poskiparta M, Apter D, Vihko V. Life-long physical activity and cancer risk among Finnish female teachers. *Eur J Cancer Prev.* 1993; 2: 369-376.

107. Dosemeci M, Hayes RB, Vetter R, Hoover RN, Tucker M, Engin K, Unsal M, Blair A. Occupational physical activity, socioeconomic status, and risks of 15 cancer sites in Turkey. *Cancer Causes Control.* 1993; 4: 313-321.

108. Shu XO, Hatch MC, Zheng W, Gao YT, Brinton LA. Physical activity and risk of endometrial cancer. *Epidemiology.* 1993; 4: 342-349.

109. Olson SH, Vena JE, Dorn JP, Marshall JR, Zielezny M, Laughlin R, Graham S. Exercise, occupational activity, and risk of endometrial cancer. *Ann Epidemiol.* 1997; 7: 46-53.

110. Tavani A, Bravi F, Dal ML, Zucchetto A, Bosetti C, Pelucchi C, Montella M, Franceschi S, La VC. Physical activity and risk of endometrial cancer: An Italian case-control study. *Eur J Cancer Prev.* 2009; 18: 303-306.

111. Voskuil DW, Monninkhof EM, Elias SG, Vlems FA, van Leeuwen FE. Physical activity and endometrial cancer risk: A systematic review of current evidence. *Cancer Epidemiol Biomarkers Prev.* 2007; 16: 639-648.

112. Cust AE, Armstrong BK, Friedenreich CM, Slimani N, Bauman A. Physical activity and endometrial cancer risk: A review of the current evidence, biologic mechanisms and the quality of physical activity assessment methods. *Cancer Causes Control.* 2007; 18: 243-258.

113. von Gruenigen V, Courneya KS, Gibbons HE, Kavanagh MB, Waggoner SE, Lerner E. Feasibility and effectiveness of a lifestyle intervention program in obese endometrial cancer patients: A randomized trial. *Gynecol Oncol.* 2008; 109: 19-26.

114. Moore SC, Peters TM, Ahn J, Park Y, Schatzkin A, Albanes D, Ballard-Barbash R, Hollenbeck A, Leitzmann MF. Physical activity in relation to total, advanced, and fatal prostate cancer. *Cancer Epidemiol Biomarkers Prev.* 2008; 17: 2458-2466.

115. Leitzmann MF. Physical activity and genitourinary cancer prevention. *Recent Results Cancer Res.* 2011; 186: 43-71.

116. Friedenreich CM, McGregor SE, Courneya KS, Angyalfi SJ, Elliott FG. Case-control study of lifetime total physical activity and prostate cancer risk. *Am J Epidemiol.* 2004; 159: 740-749.

117. Orsini N, Bellocco R, Bottai M, Pagano M, Andersson SO, Johansson JE, Giovannucci E, Wolk A. A prospective study of lifetime physical activity and prostate cancer incidence and mortality. *Br J Cancer*. 2009; 101: 1932-1938.

118. Littman AJ, Kristal AR, White E. Recreational physical activity and prostate cancer risk (United States). *Cancer Causes Control*. 2006; 17: 831-841.

119. Kenfield SA, Stampfer MJ, Giovannucci E, Chan JM. Physical activity and survival after prostate cancer diagnosis in the health professionals follow-up study. *J Clin Oncol*. 2011; 29: 726-732.

120. McTiernan A. Mechanisms linking physical activity with cancer. *Nat Rev Cancer*. 2008; 8: 205-211.

121. Schmitz KH, Courneya KS, Matthews C, mark-Wahnefried W, Galvao DA, Pinto BM, Irwin ML, Wolin KY, Segal RJ, Lucia A, Schneider CM, von G, V, et al. American College of Sports Medicine roundtable on exercise guidelines for cancer survivors. *Med Sci Sports Exerc*. 2010; 42: 1409-1426.

122. Doll R, Peto R. The causes of cancer: Quantitative estimates of avoidable risks of cancer in the United States today. *J Natl Cancer Inst*. 1981; 66: 1191-1308.

123. Willett W. Foreword. The validity of dietary assessment methods for use in epidemiologic studies. *Br J Nutr*. 2009; 102 Suppl 1: S1-S2.

124. Kushi L, Giovannucci E. Dietary fat and cancer. *Am J Med*. 2002; 113 Suppl 9B: 63S-70S.

125. Kolonel LN, Nomura AM, Cooney RV. Dietary fat and prostate cancer: Current status. *J Natl Cancer Inst*. 1999; 91: 414-428.

126. Chlebowski RT, Blackburn GL, Thomson CA, Nixon DW, Shapiro A, Hoy MK, Goodman MT, Giuliano AE, Karanja N, McAndrew P, Hudis C, Butler J, et al. Dietary fat reduction and breast cancer outcome: Interim efficacy results from the Women's Intervention Nutrition Study. *J Natl Cancer Inst*. 2006; 98: 1767-1776.

127. Pierce JP, Natarajan L, Caan BJ, Parker BA, Greenberg ER, Flatt SW, Rock CL, Kealey S, Al-Delaimy WK, Bardwell WA, Carlson RW, Emond JA, et al. Influence of a diet very high in vegetables, fruit, and fiber and low in fat on prognosis following treatment for breast cancer: The Women's Healthy Eating and Living (WHEL) randomized trial. *JAMA*. 2007; 298: 289-298.

128. Berkow SE, Barnard ND, Saxe GA, Ankerberg-Nobis T. Diet and survival after prostate cancer diagnosis. *Nutr Rev*. 2007; 65: 391-403.

129. Chan JM, Gann PH, Giovannucci EL. Role of diet in prostate cancer development and progression. *J Clin Oncol*. 2005; 23: 8152-8160.

130. Nagle CM, Purdie DM, Webb PM, Green A, Harvey PW, Bain CJ. Dietary influences on survival after ovarian cancer. *Int J Cancer*. 2003; 106: 264-269.

131. Sun AS, Ostadal O, Ryznar V, Dulik I, Dusek J, Vaclavik A, Yeh HC, Hsu C, Bruckner HW, Fasy TM. Phase I/II study of stage III and IV non-small cell lung cancer patients taking a specific dietary supplement. *Nutr Cancer*. 1999; 34: 62-69.

132. Sun AS, Yeh HC, Wang LH, Huang YP, Maeda H, Pivazyan A, Hsu C, Lewis ER, Bruckner HW, Fasy TM. Pilot study of a specific dietary supplement in tumor-bearing mice and in stage IIIB and IV non-small cell lung cancer patients. *Nutr Cancer*. 2001; 39: 85-95.

133. IARC Working Group. *IARC Handbook of Cancer Prevention, Volume 8: Fruit and Vegetables*. Lyon, France: IARC Press; 2003.

134. Park Y, Hunter DJ, Spiegelman D, Bergkvist L, Berrino F, van den Brandt PA, Buring JE, Colditz GA, Freudenheim JL, Fuchs CS, Giovannucci E, Goldbohm RA, et al. Dietary fiber intake and risk of colorectal cancer: A pooled analysis of prospective cohort studies. *JAMA*. 2005; 294: 2849-2857.

135. Ryan-Harshman M, Aldoori W. Diet and colorectal cancer: Review of the evidence. *Can Fam Physician*, 2007; 53: 1913-1920.

136. Rock CL. Primary dietary prevention: Is the fiber story over? *Recent Results Cancer Res*. 2007; 174: 171-177.

137. Sansbury LB, Wanke K, Albert PS, Kahle L, Schatzkin A, Lanza E. The effect of strict adherence to a high-fiber, high-fruit and -vegetable, and low-fat eating pattern on adenoma recurrence. *Am J Epidemiol*. 2009; 170: 576-584.

138. Meyerhardt JA, Niedzwiecki D, Hollis D, Saltz LB, Hu FB, Mayer RJ, Nelson H, Whittom R, Hantel A, Thomas J, Fuchs CS. Association of dietary patterns with cancer recurrence and survival in patients with stage III colon cancer. *JAMA*. 2007; 298: 754-764.

139. Hamajima N, Hirose K, Tajima K, Rohan T, Calle EE, Heath CW, Jr., Coates RJ, Liff JM, Talamini R, Chantarakul N, Koetsawang S, Rachawat D, et al. Alcohol, tobacco and breast cancer—Collaborative reanalysis of individual data from 53 epidemiological studies, including 58,515 women with breast cancer and 95,067 women without the disease. *Br J Cancer*. 2002; 87: 1234-1245.

140. Smith-Warner SA, Spiegelman D, Yaun SS, van den Brandt PA, Folsom AR, Goldbohm RA, Graham S, Holmberg L, Howe GR, Marshall JR, Miller AB, Potter JD, et al. Alcohol and breast cancer in women: A pooled analysis of cohort studies. *JAMA*. 1998; 279: 535-540.

141. Larsson SC, Giovannucci E, Wolk A. Folate and risk of breast cancer: A meta-analysis. *J Natl Cancer Inst*. 2007; 99: 64-76.

142. Wang XQ, Terry PD, Yan H. Review of salt consumption and stomach cancer risk: Epidemiological and biological evidence. *World J Gastroenterol.* 2009; 15: 2204-2213.

143. Williams JH, Phillips TD, Jolly PE, Stiles JK, Jolly CM, Aggarwal D. Human aflatoxicosis in developing countries: A review of toxicology, exposure, potential health consequences, and interventions. *Am J Clin Nutr.* 2004; 80: 1106-1122.

CHAPTER 4

Benefits of Physical Activity After a Cancer Diagnosis

Kristin L. Campbell, BSc PT, PhD

Content in this chapter covered in the CET exam outline includes the following:

- Knowledge of physiologic outcomes that may be improved by exercise training among cancer survivors.

- Knowledge of symptoms and psychological attributes that may be improved by exercise training among cancer survivors.

- Knowledge of lymph, immunologic, cardiac, neurologic, and hematologic systems as they pertain to cancer-specific exercise issues.

- Knowledge of acute and chronic effects of exercise on temperature regulation and the adverse thermoregulatory/vasomotor symptoms (e.g., hot flashes) experienced by many cancer survivors.

The understanding of the role of physical activity after a cancer diagnosis has expanded greatly in the past 20 years. Traditionally, during and following cancer treatment, people were told by health care providers and well-intentioned family members to rest and conserve energy. However, it is now understood that physical activity can help to alleviate many of the effects of cancer treatment; therefore, survivors should be encouraged to engage in physical activity, as able, both during and following treatment.[1]

Initially, much of the research on the benefits of physical activity for survivors came from the exercise psychology literature, with documented improvements in quality of life and feelings of well-being. The research has since expanded to include awareness that survivors can achieve the same physiological benefits of physical activity as those in the general population. However, cancer treatments, including surgery, chemotherapy, radiation, and hormonal therapies, do affect survivors' physiological responses to physical activity, and also cause side effects that are unique to this population. Fitness professionals need to understand these unique factors when prescribing physical activity and monitoring the response to physical activity of cancer survivors.

The evidence supporting the benefits of physical activity following a cancer diagnosis comes predominantly from studies in female breast cancer survivors, both during and following treatment (chemotherapy, radiation, or both), and prostate cancer survivors, with limited research regarding colon and gynecological cancer survivors. The response to physical activity of other survivor groups may differ depending on the cancer site and the associated treatment approach. The summary of the evidence used to develop the consensus guidelines in the 2010 "American College of Sports Medicine Roundtable on Exercise Guidelines for Cancer Survivors" is divided by cancer type (see table 4.1).[1]

Fitness professionals should seek specific information on the type of treatments and associated side effects when working with particular cancer groups. Furthermore, the timing related to treatment(s) may change the types of exercise that clients can engage in and their response to exercise. The goals of a physical activity intervention for people receiving treatment (i.e., surgery, chemotherapy, radiation, or a combination of these) differ from those of people who have completed treatment (but may still be receiving hormonal treatment). In addition, the median age of cancer diagnosis is 65 to 69 years of age, requiring that fitness professionals have familiarity working with older populations.

Many cancer survivors will be deconditioned following surgery and cancer treatments. Fitness professionals should be familiar with working with people with lower baseline exercise capacities. Finally, the research on the beneficial effect of physical activity on cancer survivors has focused on those undergoing treatment and following treatment for earlier-stage cancers. The role of physical activity in survivors with metastatic cancer or in the palliative setting is beyond the scope of this chapter. The exercise center intake form in figure 4.1 is included as an example of pertinent client information.

Take-Home Message
Although cancer survivors will not expect fitness professionals to be experts on cancer treatment, such professionals will need to understand the basic aspects of cancer treatment, which are commonly surgery, chemotherapy, and radiation. Those working with a particular cancer group should get to know some of the specific issues and common treatments their clients face.

Physiological Effects of Exercise Training

The health-related physical fitness components are cardiorespiratory fitness, muscular endurance, muscular strength, flexibility, and body composition.[3] Improving these components is a goal of exercise interventions. When developing an exercise prescription, fitness professionals should take into account whether the person is still receiving treatment or has completed treatment. Exercise has been shown to result in improvements or maintenance of physiological and psychological factors during treatments such as chemotherapy and radiation. Greater improvements, however, are generally seen when exercise is undertaken following comple-

TABLE 4.1 Summary of the Evidence of the Safety and Efficacy of Exercise Training by Cancer Site

	Cancer site						
	Breast (during treatment)	Breast (following treatment)	Prostate	Colon	Gynecological	Hematologic cancer (no HSCT)	Hematologic cancer (HSCT)
Safety	A	A	A	--	--	--	A
Aerobic fitness	A	A	A	--	--	A	C
Muscular strength	A	A	A	--	--	--	C
Flexibility	--	A	--	--	--	--	--
Body composition	B	B	B	--	--	--	--
Quality of life	B	B	B	--	--	--	C
Fatigue	B	B	A	--	--	B	C
Other psychosocial factors	B (anxiety)	B (depression) B (anxiety) B (body image)	--	--	--	--	--
Other	--	A (physical function) C (pain) A (safety for lymphedema onset or worsening)	B (physical function)	--	--	--	--

Evaluation of evidence based on the categories outlined by the National Heart, Lung and Blood Institute:[2] A (overwhelming data from randomized controlled trials); B (few randomized controlled trials exist, or they are small and the results are inconsistent); C (results stem from uncontrolled, nonrandomized, and/or observational studies); – (not sufficient evidence).

Abbreviation: HSCT = hematopoietic stem cell transplantation

Adapted, by permission, from K.H. Schmitz et al., 2010, "American College of Sports Medicine roundtable on exercise guidelines for cancer survivors," *Medicine and Science in Sports and Exercise* 42 (7): 1409-1426.

tion of active treatment.[4] This should not dissuade people from starting or maintaining an exercise program during treatment, but clear expectations about the anticipated responses will help to align the goals of both the survivor and the fitness professional.

Cardiorespiratory Fitness

There is consistent evidence that aerobic exercise training improves cardiorespiratory fitness in cancer survivors, with the strongest evidence from studies in breast (during and following cancer treatment) and prostate cancer survivors.[1] However, in general, this effect may be stronger after treatment.[4-6] Cardiorespiratory fitness has been measured as peak oxygen consumption ($\dot{V}O_2$peak) or by using functional tests, such as the 6- or 12-minute walk test, in breast cancer,[4,7] prostate cancer,[8] hematologic cancers,[9] and mixed cancer survivors.[6]

The exercise prescriptions in these studies have followed basic exercise physiology principles and

Figure 4.1 Exercise Center Intake Form

Name: _____ Date (DD/MM/YR): _____

Date of birth (DD/MM/YR): _____ Age: _____

Emergency Contact

Name: _____ Relationship: _____

Home phone number: _____ Cell phone number: _____

Medical History—Cancer

1. What was the date of your cancer diagnosis (MM/YR)? _____

2. What type of cancer were you diagnosed with (e.g., breast, lung)? _____

3. What stage was your cancer? ☐ 0 ☐ I ☐ II ☐ III ☐ IV ☐ Undetermined ☐ Don't know

4. If applicable, which side of the body was your cancer on? ☐ Left ☐ Right ☐ Both ☐ N/A

5. What types of cancer treatments have you received or will you receive in the future?

   Surgery ☐ No ☐ Current ☐ Completed: date (MM/YR):___/___
   ☐ Future/planned: date (MM/YR):___/___

   Chemotherapy ☐ No ☐ Current ☐ Completed: date (MM/YR):___/___
   ☐ Future/planned: date (MM/YR):___/___

   Radiation ☐ No ☐ Current ☐ Completed: date (MM/YR):___/___
   ☐ Future/planned: date (MM/YR):___/___

   Type of surgery (if known): _____

6. Please provide any other comments you have about your cancer or cancer treatment (if applicable):

   _____

   _____

Medical History—General

7. Do you have any other current medical conditions? (Please check all that apply.)

   ☐ Hypertension (high blood pressure)

   ☐ Diabetes

   ☐ High cholesterol

   ☐ Arthritis or joint pain

   ☐ Other (specify): _____

8. Please list your current medications and supplements, including any medications that are part of your cancer treatment, such as hormone therapy. (Please provide the names as best as you can remember them and what they are for.) _____

   _____

   _____

9. Please list any injuries you have had (past or present) and how they may limit your physical activity (if applicable). _____

_____

_____

_____

For Staff Use: Medical Notes

_____

_____

_____

_____

_____

_____

General Information

10. What is your main goal related to starting an exercise program?

    □ Physical fitness

    □ Achieve a particular goal (i.e., start a new activity, participate in an event) (specify): _____

_____

    □ Lose weight

    □ Other (specify): _____

11. Do you anticipate any barriers to starting an exercise program?

    □ Lack of time

    □ Lack of enjoyment from exercise

    □ Lack of self-discipline

    □ Lack of equipment

    □ Fatigue or feeling unwell

    □ Weather

    □ Financial

    □ Other responsibilities (e.g., family, job, volunteer position)

    □ Other (specify): _____

12. Do you have any specific cancer-related concerns about exercise?

    □ Type of exercise that is safe during or following cancer treatment

    □ Risk of infection at the fitness center or public facilities

    □ Risk of developing lymphedema

    □ Knowledge of fitness center staff related to working with cancer survivors

    □ Other (specify): _____

(continued)

Exercise Center Intake Form *(continued)*

13. What types of physical activities do you currently do or have done in the past?

_____

_____

_____

For Staff Use: General Notes

_____

_____

_____

_____

_____

_____

_____

_____

_____

_____

_____

_____

_____

_____

_____

_____

_____

_____

From ACSM, 2012, *ACSM's guide to exercise and cancer survivorship* (Champaign, IL: Human Kinetics). Developed by S. Neil, A. Kirkham and K. Campbell.

have used a variety of aerobic exercise prescriptions, as follows:

- Frequency: Two to five days per week
- Intensity: 50 to 75% of measured or predicted maximum heart rate
- Type: Walking primarily, along with other aerobic activities
- Time: 10 to 60 minutes per session
- Duration of program: 6 to 26 weeks

Frequency and Intensity

Although the wide range of reported exercise prescriptions used in the research to date, as well as the diversity of cancer types and related treatments, has made it difficult to develop specific exercise guidelines for each cancer type or treatment, the 2010 "American College of Sports Medicine Roundtable on Exercise Guidelines for Cancer Survivors" provides consensus guidelines.[1] These guidelines for cancer survivors are consistent with the 2008

U.S. Department of Health and Human Services (U.S. DHHS) "Physical Activity Guidelines for Americans."[10] Cancer survivors are encouraged to meet the U.S. DHHS guidelines for aerobic activity of 150 minutes per week of moderate-intensity exercise or 75 minutes of vigorous-intensity exercise (or an equivalent combination). However, if cancer survivors are unable to meet these recommendations as a result of their health status, the U.S. DHHS and the ACSM roundtable guidelines recommend that they "should be as active as their abilities and conditions allow" and, overall, "avoid inactivity."[1, 10]

Timing

The timing of the intervention either during or following cancer treatment may affect the degree of cardiorespiratory fitness improvement. The current research suggests that during treatment, aerobic exercise helps to maintain cardiorespiratory fitness or results in small improvements compared to a decline in fitness seen in people in control groups who are not exercising.

In a recent randomized controlled trial of aerobic exercise in breast cancer survivors during chemotherapy treatment (three days per week, 45 minutes per sessions at 60 to 80% of $\dot{V}O_2$max; median duration of the intervention was 17 weeks), those in the aerobic exercise groups had no change in cardiorespiratory fitness compared to a decline in $\dot{V}O_2$max of approximately 1.5 ml/kg/min, or 6%, seen in the control group.[11] In a randomized controlled trial of aerobic exercise in breast cancer survivors undergoing radiation treatment (three to five days per week, 20 to 45 minutes per session, 50 to 70% of maximum heart rate for seven weeks), the aerobic exercise group reported a 6% increase (3.2 ml/kg/min) in $\dot{V}O_2$max versus a 5% decrease (–0.6 ml/kg/min) in the stretching control group.[12]

Similar results have occurred in prostate cancer survivors receiving radiotherapy with or without androgen deprivation therapy (ADT), with a decline in $\dot{V}O_2$max of –1.4 ml/kg/min (–5%) in the usual care group compared to maintenance in the exercise groups (+0.14 ml/kg/min, or 0.5%, in the resistance group and +0.04 ml/kg/min, or 0.1%, in the aerobic group).[13] The aerobic exercise intervention was three day per week, 15 to 45 minutes per session, at 50 to 75% of $\dot{V}O_2$max for 24 weeks.

Take-Home Message
During treatment, cancer survivors are encouraged to continue with their usual physical activity, but may need to reduce the duration or intensity, or both, depending on how they are feeling. A good rule of thumb may be that if a client is used to running marathons, a good goal for exercise during treatment may be to aim for running 3 to 6 miles (5 to 10 km).

This "blunting" of the negative effects of adjuvant cancer treatment (i.e., chemotherapy, radiation, or both) as a result of aerobic exercise (i.e., no or small improvement in the intervention group and a decline in the control group) has also been observed in other studies that measured cardiorespiratory fitness using the 12-minute walking test, with improvements ranging from +38 to +328 meters in the aerobic exercise groups, compared to a decline or smaller increase in the usual care groups (–91 to +42 m).[14–18] However, this response may differ according to the type of treatment, particularly treatment that includes chemotherapy.

In one randomized controlled trial that enrolled breast cancer survivors in an aerobic exercise intervention at the start of treatment (with or without chemotherapy), predicted $\dot{V}O_2$max was relatively unchanged in women receiving chemotherapy, whereas there was an improvement in those not receiving chemotherapy (1 and 3 ml/kg/min in the self-directed and supervised interventions groups, respectively).[19] Furthermore, emerging evidence in mixed cancer survivors[20] and those with lymphoma[21] shows that highly structured aerobic interventions that include higher-intensity intervals can be safe for people undergoing chemotherapy and may result in greater increases in cardiorespiratory fitness—namely 10% in 9 weeks in the mixed cancer survivors, and an increase of 4 to 5 ml/kg/min in 12 weeks in the lymphoma survivors.

The observed decline in cardiorespiratory fitness with cancer treatment has been attributed to factors such as reduced levels of usual physical activity, anemia, tachycardia, dehydration, and cardiac dysfunction. Fitness professionals may find the Exercise and Energy Weekly Log (figure 4.2) helpful, especially when working with clients who are receiving cancer treatment. This tool allows clients to track their level of fatigue over time, as well as during exercise sessions. The fitness professional can use this information to alter the exercise prescription.

Take-Home Message

A client still on active treatment may have reduced tolerance for exercise on specific days (e.g., the day of treatment or the days immediately following a treatment session). Exercise prescription may need to be temporarily modified on these days. It is also worth remembering that as treatments progress, exercise tolerance may decrease as a result of the cumulative effects of the treatment.

In contrast, more consistent improvements in aerobic fitness have been noted in interventions that take place following cancer treatment. Randomized controlled trials in cancer survivors following treatment have revealed aerobic fitness improvements (measured as $\dot{V}O_2max$) ranging from 2.2 to 7.3 ml/kg/min in the exercise group (7 to 19%), whereas controls showed little change or declines of up to 1.7 ml/kg/min, or 6%.[22-27] Similarly, improvements have also been noted during the 6-minute walk test, the 1-mile or 2-kilometer walk test, and cycle ergometer tests.

Specificity of Training

The method of prescription used in research studies of aerobic exercise interventions in cancer populations has varied substantially. Training principles such as specificity, overload, progression, and initial fitness level to guide the prescription have not been applied universally. Some interventions have employed home-based walking programs with targeted frequency (i.e., days per week) and duration (i.e., minutes per week) goals,[17] whereas others have been individualized based on maximal aerobic fitness testing to determine specific workloads.[2]

The earliest aerobic research for cancer survivors focused on safety. This may explain the wide variety

in approaches to exercise prescription that have been used and the varied results of the interventions. The overall safety of exercise for cancer survivors has now been established, as noted in the 2010 ACSM roundtable guidelines.[1] The research focus should now move toward exercise prescriptions that are specifically designed to elicit a training response and that report adherence to the intervention that includes information on the prescribed intensity or duration of exercise rather than documenting attendance alone (i.e., frequency). The exercise program intensity should be great enough to safely stimulate improvements in cardiorespiratory fitness and functional status. Baseline assessments of cardiorespiratory fitness can facilitate development of the most appropriate and effective exercise prescription for survivors. The 2010 ACSM roundtable guidelines provide information on specific preexercise medical assessments and exercise testing for cancer survivors and overall support the safety of aerobic exercise for cancer survivors.[1]

In summary, physical activity levels, along with cardiorespiratory fitness and functional capacity levels, tend to decrease with cancer treatment, especially chemotherapy. The overall goal of exercise during treatment may be to maintain cardiorespiratory fitness or functional capacity, rather than improve it. The period following completion of cancer treatment may be a better time to focus on improving cardiorespiratory fitness. Specific recommendations for developing an appropriate

Take-Home Message

Following cancer treatment, some survivors may want to get back to their prediagnosis physical activities quickly. After treatment, which usually lasts 6 to 12 months, regaining fitness takes time. To avoid feelings of frustration on the part of client or excessive fatigue for several days following an exercise session, the fitness professional should start the client's exercise program slowly (starting with 10 to 15 minutes per session) and aim for consistency (three to five days per week) while monitoring the client's response and altering the prescription as needed.

Figure 4.2 Exercise and Energy Weekly Log

Name: _____   Date (DD/MM-DD/MM/YR): _____

For each section, please check the appropriate box daily.

Number of hours of sleep last night.	Monday	Tuesday	Wednesday	Thursday	Friday	Saturday	Sunday
12+							
10-11							
8-9							
6-7							
4-5							
<4							

How would you describe the quality of sleep you experienced last night?

Very deep							
Normal							
Restless							
Bad with breaks							
I did not sleep							

Did you take any sort of sleeping aid?

Yes/No							
Name							

How would you describe the severity of the fatigue you are experiencing today? (0 = None; 10 = Severe)

0-10							

How would you describe your interest level in physical activity today?

Very high							
Good							
Low							
No interest							

Comments: _____
_____
_____
_____
_____

(continued)

Home Exercise Log

	Monday	Tuesday	Wednesday	Thursday	Friday	Saturday	Sunday
Activity	• Walking • Bicycling • Other: _____	• Walking • Bicycling • Other: _____	• Walking • Bicycling • Other: _____	• Walking • Bicycling • Other: _____	• Walking • Bicycling • Other: _____	• Walking • Bicycling • Other: _____	• Walking • Bicycling • Other: _____
Time (minutes)							
Average heart rate							
RPE (6-20)							
Comments							

	Monday	Tuesday	Wednesday	Thursday	Friday	Saturday	Sunday
Activity	• Walking • Bicycling • Other: _____	• Walking • Bicycling • Other: _____	• Walking • Bicycling • Other: _____	• Walking • Bicycling • Other: _____	• Walking • Bicycling • Other: _____	• Walking • Bicycling • Other: _____	• Walking • Bicycling • Other: _____
Time (minutes)							
Average heart rate							
RPE (6-20)							
Comments							

From ACSM, 2012, *ACSM's guide to exercise and cancer survivorship* (Champaign, IL: Human Kinetics). Adapted from T. Bompa, 2009, *Periodization training: Theory and methodology;* and Piper Fatigue Scale.

exercise prescription are found in chapter 6. However, further research is needed to establish the most effective exercise methods for cancer survivors.

Muscular Strength and Endurance

Resistance exercise training has been effective in improving muscular strength and endurance in cancer survivors,[28] with the majority of research being in those with breast cancer,[11, 29] prostate cancer,[30] and head and neck cancer.[31, 32] Muscular strength has been measured as 1-repetition maximum (1RM) or 6- to 7-repetition maximum to estimate 1RM. Muscular endurance has been measured as the number of repetitions of a certain weight in a set time. Assessing baseline muscular strength and endurance is important for developing the most appropriate and effective prescription for cancer survivors.

Research studies with cancer survivors have used a variety of resistance prescriptions, [28] as follows:

- Frequency: One to five sessions per week (primarily two or three)
- Number of exercises: Varied numbers involving large muscle groups (primarily five to nine)
- Sets: One to three sets
- Repetitions: 8 to 12 reps
- Intensity: 25 to 85% of 1RM
- Duration of program: 3 to 52 weeks

The 2010 ACSM roundtable guidelines for resistance training exercise for cancer survivors are also consistent with the 2008 U.S. DHHS "Physical Activity Guidelines for Americans."[1] Cancer survivors are encouraged to meet the U.S. DHHS guidelines of two or three weekly sessions that include exercises for the major muscle groups,[10] as able.

Strong evidence of the benefit of resistance training has been reported in breast cancer and prostate survivors during and following cancer treatment.[1] The role of resistance training following surgery for breast cancer has been controversial; traditionally, practitioners have advised people not to lift more than 10 pounds (4.5 kg) and to limit repetitive upper-extremity activities.[33, 34] These limitations were aimed at reducing the risk of developing upper-extremity lymphedema, swelling that can affect the arm and trunk following breast cancer

surgery and treatment. Results from recent research have suggested that progressive resistance training improves muscular strength, muscular endurance, and functional ability, without increasing the risk of developing upper-extremity lymphedema[11, 29] or exacerbating preexisting lymphedema.[35]

Schmitz and colleagues[35] studied breast cancer survivors with preexisting lymphedema. The exercise group had an increase in strength, measured as 1RM, of 29.4% for the bench press (versus 4.1% in controls) and 32.5% for the leg press (versus 7.6% in controls). The exercise group reported a significant improvement in lymphedema symptoms. Also, exacerbations of lymphedema were nominal in the exercise group, which also had fewer exacerbations compared to the control group. The key message stressed in this study was adhering to proper form and progressing the exercises slowly. To achieve this, the study included supervision by trained instructors for the first 13 weeks. Also, the intensity started low and progressed slowly by the smallest increment to reduce the risks of worsening lymphedema. In addition, participants wore compression sleeves during their resistance exercise sessions, and symptoms of worsening lymphedema (i.e., swelling, feelings of heaviness) were closely monitored.

Resistance training has also been encouraged for prostate cancer survivors undergoing androgen deprivation therapy, which lowers testosterone levels. The treatment-associated reduction in muscle mass and muscle strength can compromise physical function, particularly in older men.[30, 36-38] In a study that compared a 12-week resistance training program and a usual care group during ADT treatment, the exercise group had a significant increase in upper- and lower-body muscular strength (1RM) and endurance (number of repetitions of 70% 1RM) compared to the control group, [36] with an 11% improvement in 1RM chest press (versus 1% in controls) and 37% improvement in the 1RM leg press (versus 7% in controls).

Resistance training has also been studied in head and neck cancer survivors. Resistance training in this population may be particularly important because of the associated shoulder dysfunction, which is a well-recognized complication of the neck dissection surgeries commonly used. The shoulder dysfunction is due to damage to or resection of the spinal accessory nerves and surrounding muscles, such as the trapezius muscle. A small randomized controlled trial compared a 12-week standard care program that included range-of-motion, stretching, and shoulder-strengthening exercises with elastic resistance bands with a 12-week progressive resistance program based on individual baseline strength testing. Both groups improved muscular strength and endurance, but the individualized, progressive program resulted in greater improvements in 1RM for the seated row (37% versus 15% in the standard care group) and the chest press (45% versus 24% in the standard care group).[32]

Timing

The majority of resistance training programs for people with cancer have been undertaken following cancer treatment and have reported benefits.[28] However, research on the benefits of resistance training during chemotherapy treatment is limited. During chemotherapy, an improvement in strength was reported in breast cancer survivors who were randomized to a resistance exercise program compared to those randomized to an aerobic exercise program or control group (the only group to maintain their usual lifestyle).[11] In addition, the resistance group in this study also had a better chemotherapy completion rate than the aerobic exercise or control group did. A better chemotherapy completion rate means that people were more likely to receive their prescribed chemotherapy dose on schedule, instead of experiencing the delays commonly seen with chemotherapy. A better chemotherapy completion rate is an outcome that may be of particular interest to the clinical oncology community (i.e., oncologists) because delivery of the prescribed chemotherapy dose is linked to improved clinical outcomes. Improvements in upper- and lower-body strength were also noted in prostate cancer survivors who took part in a resistance program during radiation therapy[13] and during androgen deprivation therapy.[36]

Specificity of Training

As with aerobic interventions, issues with specificity also exist for resistance interventions. Baseline testing has not been used universally. A generic approach to prescribing resistance exercise that does not take baseline strength into account may result in an exercise prescription that is too easy (and therefore results in less improvement) or too hard (limiting improvement and possibility increasing the risk of injury).

The 1-repetition maximum (1RM) test has been employed during recent exercise studies with breast, prostate, and head and neck cancer survivors to determine the appropriate exercise prescription for program.[32, 35, 36] This information has then been used to develop an exercise prescription in a variety of ways. The initial intensity for head and neck cancer survivors was set at 25 to 30% of 1RM and progressed to 60 to 70% of 1RM. The protocol included both double- and single-limb (arm) exercises, because strength was disproportionally reduced on the treatment side as a result of surgery or radiation.[32] This study included both men and women, making an individualized approach even more important than in studies of a single sex. For breast cancer survivors with or without lymphedema, the goal of the program by Schmitz and colleagues[35] was to progress slowly to avoid acute injury to the arm. Damage to the arm has been suggested as a risk factor for lymphedema (see chapter 6). The authors did not set an upper limit for resistance.

Supervision is another key feature in achieving specificity of resistance training. Supervision initially or for the entire study can ensure that clients use proper form and an appropriate progression. Home-based programs are more difficult to monitor for proper form or appropriate progression of resistance, which may limit clients' gains in strength and endurance.

Finally, adherence and compliance to the prescribed intensity and progression have not been well documented in the literature, which limits the ability to determine the overall expected effect of resistance programs for cancer survivors. Further research is needed to continue the development of feasible and effective resistance programs for cancer survivors.

Flexibility

A reduction in range of motion following surgery for cancer is common, and treatment to improve range of motion is usually done by physical therapists. However, the role flexibility plays in recovery from cancer treatments is an important issue. Currently, there is little research on the effect of exercise interventions on flexibility in cancer survivors, but the evidence that is available reports an improvement in upper- and lower-body flexibility with exercise interventions in cancer survivors following treatment.[6]

In addition, recent research has examined the role of yoga as part of the physical activity prescription for survivors, especially breast cancer survivors.[39] The majority of yoga studies have focused on quality of life, fatigue, and psychological benefits. Improvements, however, in sit-and-reach distances have been reported in a pilot study of yoga in breast cancer survivors following active treatment.[40] Overall, this component of fitness has not been a focus of exercise intervention research in cancer survivors to date.

Body Composition

The issues around body composition differ by cancer type and type of cancer treatment. Weight gain is commonly seen after a diagnosis of breast cancer, particularly with chemotherapy and radiation treatment.[41] The cause of this weight gain appears to be a combination of a reduction in usual physical activity level, acceleration into menopause of previously premenopausal women, and a possible side effect of hormonal therapies such as aromatase inhibitors.[42, 43] Weight loss intervention studies in breast cancer survivors following treatment have revealed some short-term success using combinations of individual or group dietitian-led counseling, and commercially available programs, with or without the inclusion of exercise. Exercise interventions in breast cancer survivors, without a dietary component or designed goal of weight loss, have resulted in weight maintenance but not weight loss or reduction in BMI.[4] More information is needed to determine the most effective method for weight loss for this population because of the unique factors that contribute to weight gain. Furthermore, the goal of achieving a healthy body weight is commonly delayed until the completion of adjuvant treatment.

Significant increases in fat mass and decreases in lean muscle mass have been consistently noted in prospective studies of men receiving androgen deprivation therapy, with greater changes seen with longer durations of androgen deprivation therapy.[44] Observed decreases in strength and associated function, such as 4-meter walk velocity, have implications for overall physical function and a concomitant increase in fat mass that may put these people at higher risk for developing metabolic syndrome and cardiovascular disease.[44]

Six intervention studies of prostate cancer survivors have shown an improvement in weight control and the prevention of increased fat mass, along with a maintenance or increase of lean mass,[13, 30, 36, 45-47] whereas five other intervention studies showed no benefit.[38, 48-51] A three-arm randomized controlled trial compared the effects of a 24-week intervention (with a usual care group, resistance exercise group, and aerobic exercise group) in men with prostate cancer, the majority of whom were receiving androgen deprivation therapy. In addition to improving strength, the resistance exercise intervention also prevented an increase in body fat (measured by dual-energy X-ray absorptiometry) seen in the other two intervention groups. Lean mass was not measured.[13] This suggests that resistance training may be of great benefit to men receiving androgen deprivation therapy for prostate cancer treatment to prevent or minimize the commonly observed body composition changes associated with such treatment.

Finally, weight loss and cachexia (muscle wasting) may be an issue for survivors of other cancers, such as lung cancer. Beneficial effects of resistance training alone or in combination with nutritional support to reduce muscle wasting have been suggested, but currently little research has been done on cancer survivors with cachexia.[52, 53]

Psychological Benefits of Exercise Training

The most commonly reported psychological domains in research of physical activity in cancer survivors are quality of life and fatigue. Let's take a closer look at those two areas.

Quality of Life

Improvements in quality of life have been reported with exercise interventions in breast cancer survivors both during and following treatment,[4] measured by the general version of the function assessment of cancer therapy scale (FACT-G) and the breast cancer–specific scale (FACT-B). However, in other reviews of the literature, improvements in quality of life are noted to be stronger or present only with interventions undertaken following active cancer treatment.[1] During treatment, especially chemotherapy, quality of life scores appear to vary considerably among individuals, which may account for the lack in observed improvement in quality of life with exercise interventions compared to interventions undertaken following treatment.[11]

However, improvements in quality of life have been noted in prostate cancer survivors participating in exercise interventions during treatment.[8] Resistance training mitigated the decline in quality of life, compared to the usual lifestyle control group, in two recent randomized controlled trials in men receiving radiation with or without ADT[13] or ADT alone[38] for prostate cancer. In prostate cancer, quality of life has been strongly linked to physical function. Resistance training may help to maintain muscle mass and preserve physical function.[37]

In observational studies, positive associations between physical activity and quality of life have also been noted in other cancer survivor groups— namely, multiple myeloma; brain, ovarian, endometrial, bladder, colorectal, and lung cancer; and non-Hodgkin's lymphoma.[54] However, randomized controlled trials are needed in these diverse populations to better understand the link between physical activity and improved quality of life.

Fatigue

Fatigue is a common side effect of cancer treatment that can linger following the completion of treatment. Decreased fatigue has been noted with exercise in cancer survivors,[5] and breast cancer survivors, specifically.[4] However, these effects appear to be stronger with interventions undertaken following treatment.[4,5] Of seven randomized controlled trials of exercise interventions aimed at decreasing fatigue during chemotherapy, four reported a significant effect, and three, including the largest of these studies, showed no effect.[1] In exercise interventions that have assessed fatigue in breast cancer survivors following treatment, of the nine randomized controlled trials, four reported decreased fatigue, four reported no effect on fatigue, and one reported worsening fatigue.[1]

In contrast, both resistance training and aerobic exercise have been shown to mitigate the increase in fatigue observed in prostate cancer survivors. A reduction in fatigue has been reported in exercise trials in prostate cancer survivors undergoing androgen deprivation therapy (two randomized controlled trials), radiation therapy (one randomized controlled trial), or both (one randomized

controlled trial), but no effect was seen in a low-intensity home-based randomized controlled trial.[1] The etiology of cancer-related fatigue is not fully understood. Anemia and other factors should be medically managed. However, beyond these factors, low levels of energy can lead to lower levels of physical activity, resulting in deconditioning. This then becomes a vicious cycle. The goal of physical activity interventions in relation to fatigue is to maintain or improve physical function, when possible, and to limit the associated deconditioning.

Physical activity prescriptions for those with significant fatigue may require a number of modifications, including the following:

- Slower progression, breaking physical activity into several short bouts throughout the day
- Engaging in physical activity at times of the day when the person has more energy
- Careful monitoring of fatigue levels over time with adjustment to the prescription if fatigue is worsening rather than improving

Other Psychosocial Factors

Less evidence is available regarding the effect of physical activity on other psychological factors, such as anxiety, depression, self-esteem, happiness, and body image. Some improvements have been noted; however, the evidence from randomized controlled trials and controlled clinical trials is weak (for interventions both during and following active treatment).[55]

In a randomized controlled trial (which was the first to focus on adults with lymphoma), a 12-week aerobic exercise intervention resulted in improved quality of life, decreased fatigue, increased feelings of happiness, and decreased feelings of depression, compared to the usual care control group. These improvements were maintained at six months postintervention.[21] Furthermore, these improvements were similar in patients receiving chemotherapy and those who had completed active treatment. In a three-arm randomized controlled trial in breast cancer survivors during chemotherapy, improvements in self-esteem were noted in both the aerobic exercise intervention group versus control and in the resistance exercise intervention group versus control.[11] This study also found that improvements in psychosocial factors may be associated with exercise preference. Only the people who reported that they preferred resistance training before randomization and then were randomized to the resistance group had an improvement in quality of life. More research into the effect of exercise preferences is needed.

In general, physical activity may be valuable in attenuating the decline in quality of life seen with cancer treatment, and greater improvements may result from exercise interventions undertaken following treatment. Some improvements in other psychosocial factors have been noted but not universally. Improvements may differ among patient populations, treatment timing, the measurement tool(s) used, and other factors.

Take-Home Message

Cancer survivors may experience depression or be under significant stress. When prescribing an exercise program, fitness professionals may need to encourage clients or make themselves more accessible to clients as they begin the program. A follow-up phone call, for example, to a client who misses an exercise session may be warranted.

Cancer-Specific Exercise Issues by Body System

The effect of cancer treatments on various body systems is well documented (see chapter 2). These effects may influence how survivors respond to exercise and what types of exercise may be appropriate.

Lymphatic System

The lymphatic system can be disrupted by lymph node dissection surgery or radiation therapy. The result of disrupting the lymph nodes is improper clearance of lymph fluid, which can cause swelling of the affected area. Upper-extremity and upper-trunk lymphedema following breast cancer surgery is the most well-known site of lymphedema, but surgery to the abdomen (e.g., for ovarian cancer),

groin, or leg can cause lower-extremity lymphedema, and lymphedema can be found in the face and neck following head and neck cancer surgery.

Lymph is propelled by the rhythmic contraction of smooth muscle in the walls of the larger lymph vessels. The system also depends on the "auxiliary pumps," such as skeletal muscle contraction and breathing, to enhance flow, both of which increase with physical activity. Therefore, exercise is thought to assist lymphatic flow. The skeletal muscle acts as a pump, and may improve lymphatic function in women with upper-extremity lymphedema. Upper-extremity activity has been shown to increase lymph flow in healthy controls, women with breast cancer, and women with breast cancer–related lymphedema.[56-58] Regular physical activity (resistance, aerobic, or both) may help the lymph system to better handle the stresses of activities of daily living and bouts of activity, although the mechanism is unclear.[35, 58] Lane and colleagues[58] suggest that regular physical activity may result in the development of new lymphatic vessels that help to drain lymph fluid in the arm, but more research in this area is needed.

In breast cancer survivors, seven randomized controlled trials of upper-body aerobic exercise or resistance exercise have reported that the intervention did not contribute to the onset or worsening of lymphedema.[1] The largest of these randomized controlled trials tested the safety of weightlifting in breast cancer survivors with lymphedema. The exercise group experienced fewer lymphedema flares or exacerbations (i.e., 14% compared to 29% in the control group). Those in the control group also required more medical treatment for these exacerbations (195 treatments versus 77 in the exercise group).[35]

The use of compression sleeves during exercise to prevent the development of upper-extremity lymphedema has been suggested. Although no research supports a benefit to this, using a compression sleeve may encourage breast cancer survivors who are concerned about the possible development of lymphedema to participate in exercise. In women with preexisting lymphedema, the use of a compression sleeve during physical activity has been advocated.[35] In a small pilot study that examined upper-extremity limb volume after a short bout of upper-extremity activity, those with lymphedema who wore a compression sleeve on the affected arm had a smaller increase in limb volume in their affected limb than in their unaffected limb. This suggested that the sleeve attenuated the normal increase in limb volume that occurs with exercise. This might help to alleviate stress on the lymph system in the affected limb.[59] More research on the role of compressions sleeves during physical activity is needed.

Much less is known about the effects of exercise on lower-extremity or facial lymphedema, and to date, there is no evidence that aerobic or resistance exercise reduces the risk of lymphedema or exacerbates existing lymphedema in these areas. A better understanding of the role of exercise and lower-extremity lymphedema may be especially relevant for gynecological cancer survivors and others who have had lymph nodes removed or radiation to the lymph nodes in the groin.[1]

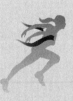

Take-Home Message

Many breast cancer survivors worry about developing lymphedema. Fitness professionals should check in with their clients about any new symptoms of heaviness, pain, or swelling in the arm on the side of surgery. If new symptoms develop, clients should check in with a lymphedema specialist or physician prior to continuing resistance training.

Immune System

Immune suppression is common with cancer treatment, especially chemotherapy. Some are concerned that exercise, especially higher-intensity exercise, could exacerbate this immunosuppression, and in turn delay treatment delivery schedules and increase susceptibility to infection. The inverted J-shape relationship between intensity of exercise training and immune function suggests a reduction in immune function with overtraining, exhaustive exercise, or both, in athletes.[60] However, research on the effect of exercise on the immune system in cancer survivors is limited.

Two randomized controlled trials examined the effect of exercise on immune function in breast cancer survivors following treatment. One showed no difference in the concentration of circulating lymphocytes or natural killer (NK) cell cytotoxic activity following an eight-week mixed aerobic and resistance exercise intervention,[61] whereas the other reported a significant improvement in NK cell activity following a 15-week aerobic intervention.[62]

Immune function is an especially important issue for people receiving high-dose chemotherapy and hematopoietic stem cell transplantation (HSCT) as part of cancer treatment. Early evidence from a nonrandomized controlled trial suggests that a mixed aerobic and resistance exercise program for three months following transplantation did not facilitate faster recovery of measured immune parameters, but neither did it hinder it compared to a nonrandomized control group.[63] When randomized controlled trials and other study designs are included, the overall results have been mixed with either no change in immune function or improvements in some measures of immune function (e.g., natural kill cell cytolytic activity, monocyte function, proportion of circulating granulocytes, and duration of neutropenia) with aerobic or resistance training either during or following treatment.[6, 7, 28, 64] However, the majority of interventions have focused on moderate-intensity exercise. Therefore, little research exists on the effect of higher volume and intensity of activity in cancer survivors, both of which have been linked to immunosuppression in athletes.

Take-Home Message

Cancer survivors, especially during treatment, are strongly advised to avoid situations in which they may be at risk of infection. Fitness professionals should ensure that the exercise space is clean and that appropriate infection control measures are strictly followed, such as cleaning equipment between clients and avoiding situations in which survivors are in close contact with others who may have colds or coughs. If the program takes place in a public gym setting, dedicated class times for cancer survivors only will avoid interactions with the general public.

Cardiovascular System

Cancer survivors may be at higher risk for developing or worsening preexisting chronic diseases such as cardiovascular disease (CVD), as a result of a sedentary lifestyle prior to diagnosis or a decrease in physical activity following treatment. Furthermore, there is emerging concern that current hormonal treatments, such as aromatase inhibitors in breast cancer survivors and androgen deprivation therapy in prostate cancer survivors, may promote the development of insulin resistance, metabolic syndrome, and unfavorable cholesterol patterns. An increased risk of metabolic syndrome is also now being documented in survivors of childhood cancer.

Investigators conducting aerobic physical activity interventions with breast cancer survivors have reported improvements in CVD risk factors, such as cardiorespiratory fitness[4, 5, 7, 55] and blood levels of the systemic inflammatory marker C-reactive protein,[65] with trends toward reductions in resting heart rate and systolic blood pressure.[65] Although these findings may have implications for the risk of cardiovascular disease in cancer survivors, more research on the role of exercise to counteract these side effects is needed.

Cancer treatment can also have deleterious effects on the heart itself. Commonly used chemotherapy agents, particularly anthracyclines, are noted to be cardiotoxic (i.e., have a deleterious effect on the heart and its function), causing myocardial damage and thus affecting the contractility of the heart. In addition, newer biological therapies, such as trastuzumab (or Herceptin), are also associated with an increase in cardiotoxicity. An echocardiogram is commonly used before, during, and after chemotherapy treatment to monitor the effects of these drugs on cardiac function, particularly left ventricular ejection fraction (LVEF) (i.e., the percentage of blood expelled from the left ventricle during a systolic contraction).[66] The incidence of cardiotoxicity with anthracyclines is reported to be less than 10%, with higher risk in older people (over 65 years) and those taking higher doses of the agents.[67]

Fitness professionals should note whether their clients have received cancer treatments that can affect cardiac function. In addition, some clients may be aware that their cardiac function has been affected by treatment (i.e., a reduction in left ventricular ejection fraction noted on an echocardiogram); however, cardiotoxicity is commonly asymptomatic. Although this does not prohibit engaging in exercise, fitness professionals should recognize the signs of cardiac insufficiency and individualize exercise interventions for people with known reduced cardiac function.

There has been little research regarding the ability of physical activity to counteract treatment-induced cardiotoxicity. Although aerobic physical activity has been effective in reversing left ventricular remodeling in patients with heart failure, a recent study of aerobic activity for women with breast cancer receiving adjuvant trastuzumab failed to demonstrate a prevention of left ventricular dimensional and functional reductions (i.e., ejection fraction).[68] Overall, more research is needed to better understand the role of physical activity in improving CVD risk factors and counteracting treatment-induced cardiotoxicity in breast cancer survivors.

Nervous System

The most common neurological effect of cancer treatment is chemotherapy-induced peripheral neuropathy. Although the mechanism is not fully understood, some chemotherapy drugs can cause damage to peripheral nerves. Damage generally occurs first in sensory nerves and starts in the longest nerves (i.e., those to the feet and toes).[69] Following are common symptoms:

- Numbness or reduced sensation
- Painful sensation, such as burning or tingling
- Increased pain sensitivity to nonpainful stimuli

There is no evidence that physical activity can improve these symptoms. Peripheral neuropathies in the feet can impair balance secondary to decreased sensation or proprioception and can increase the risk of exercise-related falls. Neuropathy also affects fingers and hands and may make holding weights difficult and painful. Depending on the severity of neuropathy, exercises may need to be individualized. Cancer survivors with foot neuropathies should be cautious when performing weight-bearing activities (e.g., walking on a treadmill). Stationary bicycles and recumbent steppers and ergometers are good exercise modalities for people experiencing loss of balance, loss of sensory input, or lower-extremity pain.

Cancer survivors with severe finger and hand neuropathy may need spotters when they lift weights.

In addition, people with primary brain cancers, metastases to the brain, or tumors affecting the spinal cord (e.g., spinal cord compression) may be impaired in their ability to safely engage in physical activity. People with these conditions may have impairments in balance, cognitive processing, and ambulation, with a subsequent risk of falling. This content is beyond the scope of this chapter.

Hematological System

Exercise is thought to stimulate improvement in hematological response, such as an increased hemoglobin level; however, the observed response is quite heterogeneous in the general population. Anemia (i.e., a deficiency in the amount of oxygen-carrying hemoglobin in the red blood cells) is a common side effect of cancer treatment and can result in fatigue and reduce physical function. Neutropenia (i.e., a reduction in neutrophils, which are white blood cells important for combating infection) is another common side effect of cancer treatments, along with a reduction in platelets levels (thrombopenia). Exercise may play a role in improving these hematological issues in cancer survivors; however, the research is limited to date.

Dimeo and colleagues[70] compared people receiving high-dose chemotherapy and stem cell transplantation; one group used cycle ergometers attached to their beds (30 minutes per day), and the other group did not exercise. The exercise group had a reduction in the duration of neutropenia and thrombopenia, as well as fewer days of hospitalization. In a small randomized controlled trial during radiation treatment, breast cancer survivors in the aerobic exercise intervention had a 6.3% increase in $\dot{V}O_2$max compared to a 4.6% decline in those in the placebo stretching control group. The exercise group also had increases in red blood cell count, hematocrit, and hemoglobin, whereas those in the control group experienced declines in these blood measures.[71]

A small randomized controlled trial of breast cancer survivors posttreatment showed no change in hemoglobin concentration or hematocrit over an eight-week combined aerobic and resistance intervention compared to control.[25] More research regarding the role of exercise on hematological factors and the relationship these responses might have on treatment decisions (as well as physiological and psychological outcomes) seems warranted.

Effects of Cancer Medications or Treatments on Designing an Exercise Program

Cancer survivors may face additional challenges to participating in exercise programming related specifically to cancer treatment or ongoing medications that are commonly prescribed to cancer survivors following chemotherapy or radiation. Three issues that exercise specialists should be aware of are (1) thermoregulatory, or vasomotor, symptoms related to abrupt changes in hormone levels; (2) musculoskeletal effects that can cause joint pain; and (3) issues around bone health and the fact that some cancer survivors may have an increased risk for osteopenia and osteoporosis.

Thermoregulatory, or Vasomotor, Symptoms

Hot flashes are common side effects of abrupt changes in hormonal levels (i.e., premature menopause in premenopausal women undergoing treatment for breast cancer or medical or surgical androgen ablation in men undergoing treatment for prostate cancer). Hot flashes are sudden feelings of heat, sudden sweating, and change in skin color (to pink or red). Hormonal replacement therapy is highly effective in alleviating vasomotor symptoms associated with menopause, but is contraindicated in breast cancer survivors.[72]

Research on the role of physical activity in helping to alleviate these symptoms has been limited. Observational studies of people without cancer suggest that women who are more physically active report lower rates of hot flashes.[73] However, exercise intervention studies in postmenopausal women have reported mixed results,[74] with some reporting an increase in the severity of hot flashes in the exercise group compared to the control group.[75] This increase in symptoms has been attributed to an increase in core body temperature during exercise and a further reduction in systemic levels of the female hormone estrogen secondary to the associated weight loss during the study. Postmenopausal women convert other steroid hormones to estrogen in fat tissue. A loss of body fat can reduce estrogen levels further, exacerbating the hot flashes. Research on hot flashes in men, due to either reduced testosterone with normal aging or secondary to ADT, is very limited, and no physical activity intervention studies have been reported.

Fitness professionals should explain to clients the negative effects that high ambient temperature, relative humidity, and heavy clothing can have on exercise responses, tolerance, and symptoms of hot flashes.[76] Ambient temperature is thought to contribute to the frequency and severity of hot flashes, so access to fans or air-conditioning may be helpful in counteracting the rise in body temperature associated with physical activity. In addition, loose-fitting clothing and materials that allow air circulation around the skin may also be helpful.

Musculoskeletal Effects

Arthralgia, or joint pain, is a commonly reported side effect of many types of cancer treatments, including chemotherapy drugs (such as taxanes, cyclophospamide, and cisplatin), colony-stimulating factors (used to treat neutropenia), and hormonal therapies (particularly aromatase inhibitors such as anastrozole, letrozole and exemestane, which are widely used for breast cancer treatments). The cause of joint pain with these agents is not well understood; however, in the case of aromatase inhibitors, the resulting estrogen deficiency is thought to be a cause, and this is under investigation. Pharmaceutical treatments, such as nonsteroidal anti-inflammatory drugs (i.e., ibuprofen) to manage joint pain have been commonly used but have additional side effects.[77] In noncancer populations (i.e., people with osteoarthritis or fibromyalgia), exercise has been shown to improve joint pain, although the mechanism is not clear.[78] As a result, exercise is suggested as a possible treatment for cancer-related joint pain; however, no randomized trial data exist yet. In prescribing exercise for people experiencing cancer-related joint pain, fitness professionals should use the general aerobic and resistance training prescription for cancer survivors. They should also monitor their client's exercise responses and adjust the exercise dose (i.e., volume and intensity) and type

of activity accordingly if certain activities or doses worsen joint pain. Also, because joint pain can occur as a result of bone metastasis, a new onset of joint pain should be investigated before continuing exercise.

Bone Health

Bone loss is a potential health concern for cancer survivors (particularly breast and prostate cancer survivors receiving hormonal treatments). Bone mineral density is lower in men undergoing androgen deprivation therapy for prostate cancer than it is in age-matched controls. The severity of bone loss increases with the duration of androgen deprivation therapy.[44] Early menopause and hormonal therapy result in increased rates of osteoporosis and osteopenia in breast cancer survivors.[79, 80] Pharmaceutical treatments to reduce bone loss, such as bisphosphonates, although highly effective, are associated with side effects such as indigestion. Weight-bearing activities play an important role in bone health across the life span, by promoting an increase in bone mineral density. Mechanical stresses applied to bones stimulate the preservation of existing bone and the apposition of new bone minerals. Furthermore, by improving muscular strength and physical function, exercise may help prevent falls in people with osteopenia or osteoporosis.[81]

Two randomized controlled trials in breast cancer survivors have shown that moderate-intensity aerobic activity attenuated the bone loss in the spine or the whole body seen in the usual care control groups.[14, 82] Two recent randomized controlled trials examined the effects of exercise in comparison to or in addition to bisphosphonate treatment.[83, 84] In one 24-month randomized controlled trial, postmenopausal breast cancer survivors ($n = 249$) were randomized to medication only (a combination of a bisphosphonate drug called risedronate, plus calcium and vitamin D) or medication plus a resistance intervention designed to load the spine, hip, and forearms. Improvements in bone mineral density were noted in both groups. There was a greater increase in bone mineral density in the medication plus resistance intervention group compared to the medication only group, but this was not statistically significant.[84] The second study was a 12-month randomized controlled trial of women undergoing chemotherapy for breast cancer ($n = 62$); one group received zoledronic acid (an intravenous bisphosphonate drug), and the other maintained a home-based aerobic physical activity program (mainly walking). In addition, each participant received calcium and vitamin D.[83] The group receiving the bisphosphonate drug maintained bone density, whereas the aerobic group had significant declines. However, the compliance to the prescribed intervention, choice of interventions type, and intensity of physical activity in these trials may have been insufficient to initiate a skeletal response. The majority of other studies that have reported on bone health–related outcomes have not chosen an intervention that is aimed specifically at bone health, but rather, examined this as a secondary outcome.

The role of physical activity in improving bone health, alone or in conjunction with medications, is an important future area for research. Preliminary results suggest that weight-bearing exercise may improve bone health in breast and prostate cancer survivors. In the absence of conclusive findings in cancer survivors, fitness professionals should follow the recommendations outlined in the ACSM position stand on bone health.[85]

Summary

Research suggests that physical activity is generally safe and effective for cancer survivors. The goal(s) of the prescribed physical activity and the associated prescription(s) may differ depending on treatment timing, the type of cancer, and the acute or long-term side effects of treatment. However, overall, cancer survivors can obtain physiological, psychosocial, and health benefits by being physically active. Promoting physical activity in the cancer survivor population is of particular importance because physical activity levels tend to decrease at the time of diagnosis. However, more research is needed to (1) determine optimal testing and prescription methods for survivors; (2) understand the role of physical activity in other cancer types, beyond breast and prostate; and (3) address the role of physical activity on acute and long-term side effects as cancer treatment continues to evolve.

References

1. Schmitz KH, Courneya KS, Matthews C, Demark-Wahnefried W, Galvao DA, Pinto BM, et al. American College of Sports Medicine roundtable on exercise guidelines for cancer survivors. *Med Sci Sports Exerc.* 2010; 42(7): 1409-1426.

2. Clinical guidelines on the identification, evaluation, and treatment of overweight and obesity in adults: The evidence report. National Institutes of Health. *Obes Res.* 1998; 6 Suppl 2: 51S-209S.

3. Thompson WR, Gordon NF, Pescatello LS, eds. *ACSM's Guidelines for Exercise Testing and Prescription.* 8th ed. Baltimore: Wolters Kluwer Lippincott Williams & Wilkins; 2009.

4. McNeely ML, Campbell KL, Rowe BH, Klassen TP, Mackey JR, Courneya KS. Effects of exercise on breast cancer patients and survivors: A systematic review and meta-analysis. *CMAJ,* 2006; 175(1): 34-41.

5. Conn VS, Hafdahl AR, Porock DC, McDaniel R, Nielsen PJ. A meta-analysis of exercise interventions among people treated for cancer. *Support Care Cancer.* 2006; 14(7): 699-712.

6. Speck RM, Courneya KS, Masse LC, Duval S, Schmitz KH. An update of controlled physical activity trials in cancer survivors: A systematic review and meta-analysis. *J Cancer Surviv.* 2010; e-pub.

7. Markes M, Brockow T, Resch KL. Exercise for women receiving adjuvant therapy for breast cancer. *Cochrane Database Syst Rev.* 2006; (4): CD005001.

8. Thorsen L, Courneya KS, Stevinson C, Fossa SD. A systematic review of physical activity in prostate cancer survivors: Outcomes, prevalence, and determinants. *Support Care Cancer.* 2008; 16(9): 987-997.

9. Liu RD, Chinapaw MJ, Huijgens PC, van Mechelen W. Physical exercise interventions in haematological cancer patients, feasible to conduct but effectiveness to be established: A systematic literature review. *Cancer Treat Rev.* 2009; 35(2): 185-192.

10. Committee. PAGA. Physical Activity Guidelines Advisory Committee Report. In: *Services* UDHHS, ed. Washington, DC; 2008.

11. Courneya KS, Segal RJ, Mackey JR, Gelmon K, Reid RD, Friedenreich CM, et al. Effects of aerobic and resistance exercise in breast cancer patients receiving adjuvant chemotherapy: A multicenter randomized controlled trial. *J Clin Oncol.* 2007; 25(28): 4396-4404.

12. Drouin JS, Armstrong H, Krause S, Orr J, Birk TJ, Hryniuk WM. Effects of aerobic exercise training on peak aerobic capacity, fatigue and psychological factors during radiation for breast cancer. *Rehab Oncol.* 2005; 23(1): 11-17.

13. Segal RJ, Reid RD, Courneya KS, Sigal RJ, Kenny GP, Prud'Homme DG, et al. Randomized controlled trial of resistance or aerobic exercise in men receiving radiation therapy for prostate cancer. *J Clin Oncol.* 2009; 27(3): 344-351.

14. Schwartz AL, Winters-Stone K, Gallucci B. Exercise effects on bone mineral density in women with breast

cancer receiving adjuvant chemotherapy. *Oncol Nurs Forum.* 2007; 34(3): 627-633.

15. Campbell A, Mutrie N, White F, McGuire F, Kearney N. A pilot study of a supervised group exercise programme as a rehabilitation treatment for women with breast cancer receiving adjuvant treatment. *Eur J Oncol Nurs.* 2005; 9(1): 56-63.

16. Mock V, Burke MB, Sheehan P, Creaton EM, Winningham ML, McKenney-Tedder S, et al. A nursing rehabilitation program for women with breast cancer receiving adjuvant chemotherapy. *Oncology Nursing Forum.* 1994; 21(5): 899-907; discussion 908.

17. Mock V, Frangakis C, Davidson NE, Ropka ME, Pickett M, Poniatowski B, et al. Exercise manages fatigue during breast cancer treatment: A randomized controlled trial. *Psycho-Oncology.* 2005; 14(6): 464-477.

18. Mutrie N, Campbell AM, Whyte F, McConnachie A, Emslie C, Lee L, et al. Benefits of supervised group exercise programme for women being treated for early stage breast cancer: Pragmatic randomised controlled trial. *BMJ.* 2007; 334(7592): 517.

19. Segal R, Evans W, Johnson D, Smith J, Colletta S, Grayton J, et al. Structured exercise improved physical functioning in women with stage I and II breast cancer: Results of a randomized controlled trial. *J Clin Oncol.* 2001; 19(3): 657-665.

20. Adamsen L, Quist M, Andersen C, Moller T, Herrstedt J, Kronborg D, et al. Effect of a multimodal high intensity exercise intervention in cancer patients undergoing chemotherapy: A randomised controlled trial. *BMJ.* 2009; 339: b3410.

21. Courneya KS, Sellar CM, Stevinson C, McNeely ML, Peddle CJ, Friedenreich CM, et al. Randomized controlled trial of the effects of aerobic exercise on physical functioning and quality of life in lymphoma patients. *J Clin Oncol.* 2009; 27(27): 4605-4612.

22. Burnham TR, Wilcox A. Effects of exercise on physiological and psychological variables in cancer survivors. *Med Sci Sports Exerc.* 2002; 34(12): 1863-1867.

23. Courneya KS, Mackay JR, Bell GJ, Jones LW, Field CJ, Fairey AS. Randomized controlled trial of exercise training in postmenopausal breast cancer survivors: Cardiopulmonary and quality of life outcomes. *J Clin Oncol.* 2003; 21(9): 1660-1668.

24. Daley AJ, Crank H, Saxton JM, Mutrie N, Coleman R, Roalfe A. Randomized trial of exercise therapy in women treated for breast cancer. *J Clin Oncol.* 2007; 25(13): 1713-1721.

25. Herrero F, San Juan AF, Fleck SJ, Balmer J, Perez M, Canete S, et al. Combined aerobic and resistance training in breast cancer survivors: A randomized, controlled pilot trial. *Int J Sports Med,* 2006; 27(7): 573-580.

26. Rogers LQ, Hopkins-Price P, Vicari S, Pamenter R, Courneya KS, Markwell S, et al. A randomized trial to increase physical activity in breast cancer survivors. *Med Sci Sports Exerc.* 2009; 41(4): 935-946.

27. Thorsen L, Skovlund E, Stromme SB, Hornslien K, Dahl AA, Fossa SD. Effectiveness of physical activity on cardiorespiratory fitness and health-related quality of life in young and middle-aged cancer patients shortly after chemotherapy. *J Clin Oncol.* 2005; 23(10): 2378-2388.

28. De Backer IC, Schep G, Backx FJ, Vreugdenhil G, Kuipers H. Resistance training in cancer survivors: A systematic review. *Int J Sports Med.* 2009; 30(10): 703-712.

29. Cheema B, Gaul CA, Lane K, Fiatarone Singh MA. Progressive resistance training in breast cancer: A systematic review of clinical trials. *Breast Cancer Res Treat.* 2008; 109(1): 9-26.

30. Galvao DA, Nosaka K, Taaffe DR, Spry N, Kristjanson LJ, McGuigan MR, et al. Resistance training and reduction of treatment side effects in prostate cancer patients. *Med Sci Sports Exerc.* 2006; 38(12): 2045-2052.

31. McNeely ML, Parliament M, Courneya KS, Seikaly H, Jha N, Scrimger R, et al. A pilot study of a randomized controlled trial to evaluate the effects of progressive resistance exercise training on shoulder dysfunction caused by spinal accessory neurapraxia/neurectomy in head and neck cancer survivors. *Head Neck.* 2004; 26(6): 518-530.

32. McNeely ML, Parliament MB, Seikaly H, Jha N, Magee DJ, Haykowsky MJ, et al. Effect of exercise on upper extremity pain and dysfunction in head and neck cancer survivors: A randomized controlled trial. *Cancer.* 2008; 113(1): 214-222.

33. Harris SR, Niesen-Vertommen SL. Challenging the myth of exercise-induced lymphedema following breast cancer: A series of case reports. *Journal of Surgl Oncol.* 2000; 74: 95-99.

34. Lane K, Jespersen D, McKenzie DC. The effect of a whole body exercise programme and dragon boat training on arm volume and arm circumference in women treated for breast cancer. *Eur J Cancer Care (Engl).* 2005; 14(4): 353-358.

35. Schmitz KH, Ahmed RL, Troxel A, Cheville A, Smith R, Lewis-Grant L, et al. Weight lifting in women with breast-cancer-related lymphedema. *N Engl J Med.* 2009; 361(7): 664-673.

36. Galvao DA, Taaffe DR, Spry N, Joseph D, Newton RU. Combined resistance and aerobic exercise program reverses muscle loss in men undergoing androgen suppression therapy for prostate cancer without bone metastases: A randomized controlled trial. *J Clin Oncol.* 2010; 28(2): 340-347.

37. Galvao DA, Taaffe DR, Spry N, Newton RU. Exercise can prevent and even reverse adverse effects of androgen suppression treatment in men with prostate cancer. *Prostate Cancer Prostatic Dis.* 2007; 10(4): 340-346.

38. Segal RJ, Reid RD, Courneya KS, Malone SC, Parliament MB, Scott CG, et al. Resistance exercise in men receiving androgen deprivation therapy for prostate cancer. *J Clin Oncol.* 2003; 21(9): 1653-1659.

39. Smith KB, Pukall CF. An evidence-based review of yoga as a complementary intervention for patients with cancer. *Psycho-Oncology.* 2009; 18(5): 465-475.

40. Culos-Reed SN, Carlson LE, Daroux LM, Hately-Aldous S. A pilot study of yoga for breast cancer survivors: Physical and psychological benefits. *Psycho-Oncology.* 2006; 15(10): 891-897.

41. Ingram C, Brown JK. Patterns of weight and body composition change in premenopausal women with early stage breast cancer: Has weight gain been overestimated? *Cancer Nurs.* 2004; 27(6): 483-490.

42. Garreau JR, Delamelena T, Walts D, Karamlou K, Johnson N. Side effects of aromatase inhibitors versus tamoxifen: The patients' perspective. *Am J Surg.* 2006; 192(4): 496-498.

43. Ingram C, Courneya KS, Kingston D. The effects of exercise on body weight and composition in breast cancer survivors: An integrative systematic review. *Oncol Nurs Forum.* 2006; 33(5): 937-947; quiz 948-950.

44. Harle LK, Maggio M, Shahani S, Braga-Basaria M, Basaria S. Endocrine complications of androgen-deprivation therapy in men with prostate cancer. *Clin Adv Hematol Oncol.* 2006; 4(9): 687-696.

45. Culos-Reed SN, Robinson JW, Lau H, Stephenson L, Keats M, Norris S, et al. Physical activity for men receiving androgen deprivation therapy for prostate cancer: Benefits from a 16-week intervention. *Support Care Cancer.* 2010; 18(5): 591-599.

46. Demark-Wahnefried W, Clipp EC, Lipkus IM, Lobach D, Snyder DC, Sloane R, et al. Main outcomes of the FRESH START trial: A sequentially tailored, diet and exercise mailed print intervention among breast and prostate cancer survivors. *J Clin Oncol.* 2007; 25(19): 2709-2718.

47. Morey MC, Snyder DC, Sloane R, Cohen HJ, Peterson B, Hartman TJ, et al. Effects of home-based diet and exercise on functional outcomes among older, overweight long-term cancer survivors: RENEW: A randomized controlled trial. *JAMA.* 2009; 301(18): 1883-1891.

48. Carmack Taylor CL, Demoor C, Smith MA, Dunn AL, Basen-Engquist K, Nielsen I, et al. Active for Life After Cancer: A randomized trial examining a lifestyle physical activity program for prostate cancer patients. *Psycho-Oncology* 2006; 15(10): 847-862.

49. Culos-Reed SN, Robinson JL, Lau H, O'Connor K, Keats MR. Benefits of a physical activity intervention for men with prostate cancer. *J Sport Exerc Psychol.* 2007; 29(1): 118-127.

50. Demark-Wahnefried W, Clipp EC, Morey MC, Pieper CF, Sloane R, Snyder DC, et al. Lifestyle intervention development study to improve physical function in older adults with cancer: Outcomes from Project LEAD. *J Clin Oncol.* 2006; 24(21): 3465-3473.

51. Windsor PM, Nicol KF, Potter J. A randomized, controlled trial of aerobic exercise for treatment-related fatigue in men receiving radical external beam radiotherapy for localized prostate carcinoma. *Cancer.* 2004; 101(3): 550-557.

52. Mourtzakis M, Bedbrook M. Muscle atrophy in cancer: A role for nutrition and exercise. *Appl Physiol Nutr Metab.* 2009; 34(5): 950-956.

53. Little JP, Phillips SM. Resistance exercise and nutrition to counteract muscle wasting. *Appl Physiol Nutr Metab.* 2009; 34(5): 817-828.

54. Speed-Andrews AE, Courneya KS. Effects of exercise on quality of life and prognosis in cancer survivors. *Curr Sports Med Rep.* 2009; 8(4): 176-181.

55. Schmitz KH, Holtzman J, Courneya KS, Masse LC, Duval S, Kane R. Controlled physical activity trials in cancer survivors: A systematic review and meta-analysis. *Cancer Epidemiol Biomarkers Prev.* 2005; 14(7): 1588-1595.

56. Lane K, Worsley D, McKenzie D. Exercise and the lymphatic system: Implications for breast-cancer survivors. *Sports Med.* 2005; 35(6): 461-471.

57. Lane K, Worsley D, McKenzie DC. Lymphoscintigraphy to evaluate the effects of dynamic and isometric exercise on radioisotope clearance from the hands of healthy females. *Canadian J Appl Physiol.* 2003; 28(Suppl): S74.

58. Lane KN, Dolan LB, Worsley D, McKenzie DC. Upper extremity lymphatic function at rest and during exercise in breast cancer survivors with and without lymphedema compared with healthy controls. *J Appl Physiol.* 2007; 103(3): 917-925.

59. McNeely ML, Campbell KL, Courneya KS, Mackay JR. Effect of acute exercise on upper-limb volume in breast cancer survivors: A pilot study. *Physiotherapy Canada.* 2009; 61(4): 244-251.

60. Woods JA, Davis JM, Smith JA, Nieman DC. Exercise and cellular innate immune function. *Med Sci Sports Exerc.* 1999; 31(1): 57-66.

61. Nieman DC, Cook VD, Henson DA, Suttles J, Rejeski WJ, Ribisl PM, et al. Moderate exercise training and natural killer cell cytotoxic activity in breast cancer patients. *Int J Sports Med.* 1995; 16(5): 334-337.

62. Fairey AS, Courneya KS, Field CJ, Bell GJ, Jones LW, Mackey JR. Randomized controlled trial of exercise and blood immune function in postmenopausal breast cancer survivors. *J Appl Physiol.* 2005; 98(4): 1534-1540.

63. Hayes SC, Rowbottom D, Davies PS, Parker TW, Bashford J. Immunological changes after cancer treatment and participation in an exercise program. *Med Sci Sports Exerc.* 2003; 35(1): 2-9.

64. Fairey AS, Courneya KS, Field CJ, Mackey JR. Physical exercise and immune system function in cancer survivors: A comprehensive review and future directions. *Cancer.* 2002; 94(2): 539-551.

65. Fairey AS, Courneya KS, Field CJ, Bell GJ, Jones LW, Martin BS, et al. Effect of exercise training on C-reactive protein in postmenopausal breast cancer survivors: A randomized controlled trial. *Brain Behav Immun.* 2005; 19(5): 381-388.

66. Pai VB, Nahata MC. Cardiotoxicity of chemotherapeutic agents: Incidence, treatment and prevention. *Drug Saf.* 2000; 22(4): 263-302.

67. Bird BR, Swain SM. Cardiac toxicity in breast cancer survivors: Review of potential cardiac problems. *Clin Cancer Res.* 2008; 14(1): 14-24.

68. Haykowsky MJ, Mackey JR, Thompson RB, Jones LW, Paterson DI. Adjuvant trastuzumab induces ventricular remodeling despite aerobic exercise training. *Clin Cancer Res.* 2009; 15(15): 4963-4967.

69. Wickham R. Chemotherapy-induced peripheral neuropathy: A review and implications for oncology nursing practice. *Clin J Oncol Nurs.* 2007; 11(3): 361-376.

70. Dimeo F, Fetscher S, Lange W, Mertelsmann R, Keul J. Effects of aerobic exercise on the physical performance and incidence of treatment-related complications after high-dose chemotherapy. *Blood.* 1997; 90(9): 3390-3394.

71. Drouin JS, Young TJ, Beeler J, Byrne K, Birk TJ, Hryniuk WM, et al. Random control clinical trial on the effects of aerobic exercise training on erythrocyte levels during radiation treatment for breast cancer. *Cancer.* 2006; 107(10): 2490-2495.

72. Kontos M, Agbaje OF, Rymer J, Fentiman IS. What can be done about hot flushes after treatment for breast cancer? *Climacteric.* 2010; 13(1): 4-21.

73. Daley A, MacArthur C, Mutrie N, Stokes-Lampard H. Exercise for vasomotor menopausal symptoms. *Cochrane Database Syst Rev.* 2007; (4): CD006108.

74. Lindh-Astrand L, Nedstrand E, Wyon Y, Hammar M. Vasomotor symptoms and quality of life in previously sedentary postmenopausal women randomised to physical activity or estrogen therapy. *Maturitas.* 2004; 48(2): 97-105.

75. Aiello EJ, Yasui Y, Tworoger SS, Ulrich CM, Irwin ML, Bowen D, et al. Effect of a yearlong, moderate-intensity exercise intervention on the occurrence and severity of menopause symptoms in postmenopausal women. *Menopause.* 2004; 11(4): 382-388.

76. Loprinzi CL, Wolf SL, Barton DL, Laack NN. Symptom management in premenopausal patients with breast cancer. *Lancet Oncol.* 2008; 9(10): 993-1001.

77. Burstein HJ. Aromatase inhibitor-associated arthralgia syndrome. *Breast.* 2007; 16(3): 223-234.

78. Fransen M, McConnell S. Exercise for osteoarthritis of the knee. *Cochrane Database Syst Rev.* 2008; (4): CD004376.

79. Winters-Stone KM, Nail L, Bennett JA, Schwartz A. Bone health and falls: Fracture risk in breast cancer survivors with chemotherapy-induced amenorrhea. *Oncol Nurs Forum.* 2009; 36(3): 315-325.

80. Chen Z, Maricic M, Pettinger M, Ritenbaugh C, Lopez AM, Barad DH, et al. Osteoporosis and rate of bone loss among postmenopausal survivors of breast cancer. *Cancer.* 2005; 104(7): 1520-1530.

81. Winters-Stone KM, Schwartz A, Nail LM. A review of exercise interventions to improve bone health in adult cancer survivors. *J Cancer Surviv.* 2010; 4(3): 187-201.

82. Irwin ML, Alvarez-Reeves M, Cadmus L, Mierzejewski E, Mayne ST, Yu H, et al. Exercise improves body fat, lean mass, and bone mass in breast cancer survivors. *Obesity.* 2009; 17(8): 1534-1541.

83. Swenson KK, Nissen MJ, Anderson E, Shapiro A, Schousboe J, Leach J. Effects of exercise vs bisphosphonates on bone mineral density in breast cancer patients receiving chemotherapy. *J Support Oncol.* 2009; 7(3): 101-107.

84. Waltman NL, Twiss JJ, Ott CD, Gross GJ, Lindsey AM, Moore TE, et al. The effect of weight training on bone mineral density and bone turnover in postmenopausal breast cancer survivors with bone loss: A 24-month randomized controlled trial. *Osteoporos Int.* 2010; 21(8): 1361-1369.

85. Kohrt WM, Bloomfield SA, Little KD, Nelson ME, Yingling VR. American College of Sports Medicine Position Stand: Physical activity and bone health. *Med Sci Sports Exerc.* 2004; 36(11): 1985-1996.

CHAPTER 5

Cardiorespiratory Fitness Testing in Clients Diagnosed With Cancer

Lee W. Jones, PhD, and Claudio Battaglini, PhD

Content in this chapter covered in the CET exam outline includes the following:

- Ability to obtain a basic history regarding cancer diagnosis (e.g., type, stage) and treatment (e.g., surgeries, systemic and targeted therapies).

- Knowledge of and the ability to recognize the adverse acute, chronic, and late effects of cancer treatments.

- Ability to obtain medical history for other health conditions (e.g., neurological, cardiovascular, musculoskeletal, pulmonary) that may cooccur and interact with adverse effects of cancer treatments.

- Knowledge of and ability to discuss physiologic systems affected by cancer and treatment and how this would affect the major components of fitness, including balance, agility, speed, flexibility, endurance, and strength.

- Knowledge of how cancer and its treatments may alter balance, agility, speed, flexibility, endurance, and strength in cancer survivors and ability to select/modify and interpret tests of these fitness elements.

- Knowledge of how cancer and its treatments may affect body composition in cancer survivors and ability to select/modify and interpret tests of body composition in cancer survivors.

- Knowledge of categories of patients that require medical clearance prior to testing or exercise prescription.

- Knowledge of cancer-specific relative and absolute contraindications to exercise testing.

- Knowledge of the combined effects of aging and cancer treatment on exercise capacity and selection of appropriate testing modalities and interpretation of results.

Research and clinical interest in the role of physical activity and structured exercise training interventions for cancer survivors has increased dramatically over the past decade (as described in chapter 4). Furthermore, exercise is becoming recognized as an integral component to manage the unique issues and concerns faced by the rapidly growing number of cancer survivors in the United States. With this growing interest comes an increased need for the assessment of cardiorespiratory fitness in this population. The objective measurement of cardiorespiratory fitness is gaining recognition as an outcome of significant importance in clients diagnosed with cancer.[1] Cardiorespiratory fitness testing in clients who have been diagnosed with cancer may be used to do the following:

- Evaluate the cardiorespiratory effects of medical treatments associated with a cancer diagnosis
- Prescribe and develop accurate exercise regimens for clients diagnosed with cancer
- Evaluate the efficacy of exercise training regimens on cardiorespiratory fitness

Several terms are used to describe cardiorespiratory fitness, including *exercise capacity, aerobic power, cardiorespiratory fitness,* and *exercise tolerance*; these terms are often used interchangeably.

Cardiorespiratory fitness reflects the integrative ability of the components of the cardiopulmonary system (i.e., heart, lungs, and blood system) to deliver oxygen to the metabolically active skeletal muscles.[2] In research and clinical settings, cardiorespiratory fitness is most commonly assessed using maximal exercise testing protocols (e.g., cardiopulmonary exercise test [CPET] and stress tests), whereas in nonclinical settings cardiorespiratory fitness is assessed using submaximal tests (e.g., walk tests, age-predicted heart rate tests).[3] Cardiorespiratory fitness is a primary health indicator in humans and has consistently been associated with morbidity and longevity in healthy people, as well

as in those with chronic diseases such as cardiovascular disease, type 2 diabetes, and respiratory disease.[4-8]

Administration of Cardiorespiratory Fitness Testing

Several critical steps must be followed when administering cardiorespiratory fitness testing. This section looks at those steps—specifically, the sequence of testing procedures and the selection and utility of testing.

Sequence of Testing Procedures

There are many factors to consider when assessing a cancer survivor's cardiorespiratory fitness. Major considerations include the client's demographic and medical characteristics, the client's needs and desires, the setting, and available equipment.[1] Fitness professionals must make sure to assess the presence and degree of currently experienced side effects that may affect test results, such as fatigue, anemia, neuropathy, pain, shortness of breath, radiation-induced heart disease, general cardiovascular issues, and cardiomyopathy from certain chemotherapies (primarily anthracyclines) and targeted therapies (e.g., Herceptin). Fitness professionals must also use care in comparing cancer survivors to age-matched norms to avoid discouraging clients. It is always advisable to refer clients to their primary oncologists or general practitioners for initial cardiovascular and general comorbidity screening. Further, clients with remarkable medical histories (e.g., hypertension, heart disease) should have a physician supervise a classic stress test to ensure optimal safety of exercise testing and training. Despite all of these

Take-Home Message
Given that this may be the first cardiorespiratory fitness test clients have performed, significant learning effects can be expected. In other words, clients will invariably record a higher fitness score on a repeat assessment because they are more comfortable with the testing procedures. Conducting two tests at baseline may ensure the most accurate preexercise training fitness measurement (and subsequent exercise prescription).

caveats, it is possible to provide a general outline of exercise testing.

The testing appointment should begin with an assessment of resting physiological parameters such as heart rate and blood pressure. Next, body weight and height as well as body composition (if appropriate) should be recorded according to standard guidelines. Finally, after an initial warm-up period (approximately five minutes), the cardiorespiratory fitness assessment (whichever test is most appropriate) can be initiated. The fitness professional should perform physiological assessments *only* after the patient has completed a physical activity questionnaire such as the Physical Activity Readiness Questionnaire (PAR-Q; figure 5.1) or PARmed-X.

Take-Home Message
Cancer therapy can drastically change heart rate response to exercise. Thus, fitness professionals should include additional parameters that provide supplemental assessments of exercise effort or stress such as blood pressure, rating of perceived exertion, and oxygen saturation.

Thoroughly evaluating a client's medical history prior to selecting a test to evaluate cardiorespiratory fitness will maximize safety. As with other chronic conditions, clients with cancer undergo a comprehensive medical and physical examination at diagnosis and prior to the initiation of cancer therapy (if appropriate). As such, the oncologist will likely have thorough knowledge of any major health complications or other comorbidities that can be potential contraindications for cardiorespiratory fitness testing. Thus, obtaining oncologist approval for cardiorespiratory testing should, in most circumstances, circumvent the need for additional evaluation. Cancer survivors are typically older and commonly present with a diverse range of cardiovascular or musculoskeletal complications (or both); thus, preexercise screening and the use of appropriate testing modalities are critical to maximize the safety of exercise testing, as well as the accurate interpretation of results for older cancer survivors.[9-11]

Following is one recommended sequence of cardiorespiratory fitness testing procedures:

1. Preactivity screening questionnaire (e.g., PAR-Q or PARmed-X) and other questionnaires to evaluate medical history

2. Resting heart rate

3. Resting blood pressure

4. Anthropometrics (e.g., body weight, circumferences)

5. Cardiorespiratory fitness testing (e.g., stress test, 6-minute walk test)

In addition to maximizing exercise testing safety, fitness professionals should also ensure that clients not engage in behaviors that influence the results of the cardiorespiratory fitness test itself. For example, clients should be asked to abstain from behaviors (e.g., drinking caffeinated beverages, smoking, exercising) that may alter heart rate and blood pressure responses to exercise.[3] Abstinence from medications that may alter these parameters is not required because exercise testing is not used for diagnostic purposes in clients with cancer. To this end, fitness professionals should be well versed in cancer-specific medications as well as general medications that may affect the exercise response. A questionnaire to the client's primary care physician to inquire about any exercise response–modifying medications that the client may be taking can facilitate this process. See figure 5.2 for an example of such a form.

Figure 5.1

Physical Activity Readiness
Questionnaire - PAR-Q
(revised 2002)

PAR-Q & YOU

(A Questionnaire for People Aged 15 to 69)

Regular physical activity is fun and healthy, and increasingly more people are starting to become more active every day. Being more active is very safe for most people. However, some people should check with their doctor before they start becoming much more physically active.

If you are planning to become much more physically active than you are now, start by answering the seven questions in the box below. If you are between the ages of 15 and 69, the PAR-Q will tell you if you should check with your doctor before you start. If you are over 69 years of age, and you are not used to being very active, check with your doctor.

Common sense is your best guide when you answer these questions. Please read the questions carefully and answer each one honestly: check YES or NO.

YES	NO	
☐	☐	1. Has your doctor ever said that you have a heart condition <u>and</u> that you should only do physical activity recommended by a doctor?
☐	☐	2. Do you feel pain in your chest when you do physical activity?
☐	☐	3. In the past month, have you had chest pain when you were not doing physical activity?
☐	☐	4. Do you lose your balance because of dizziness or do you ever lose consciousness?
☐	☐	5. Do you have a bone or joint problem (for example, back, knee or hip) that could be made worse by a change in your physical activity?
☐	☐	6. Is your doctor currently prescribing drugs (for example, water pills) for your blood pressure or heart condition?
☐	☐	7. Do you know of <u>any other reason</u> why you should not do physical activity?

If you answered

YES to one or more questions

Talk with your doctor by phone or in person BEFORE you start becoming much more physically active or BEFORE you have a fitness appraisal. Tell your doctor about the PAR-Q and which questions you answered YES.

- You may be able to do any activity you want — as long as you start slowly and build up gradually. Or, you may need to restrict your activities to those which are safe for you. Talk with your doctor about the kinds of activities you wish to participate in and follow his/her advice.
- Find out which community programs are safe and helpful for you.

NO to all questions

If you answered NO honestly to all PAR-Q questions, you can be reasonably sure that you can:

- start becoming much more physically active — begin slowly and build up gradually. This is the safest and easiest way to go.
- take part in a fitness appraisal — this is an excellent way to determine your basic fitness so that you can plan the best way for you to live actively. It is also highly recommended that you have your blood pressure evaluated. If your reading is over 144/94, talk with your doctor before you start becoming much more physically active.

DELAY BECOMING MUCH MORE ACTIVE:
- if you are not feeling well because of a temporary illness such as a cold or a fever — wait until you feel better; or
- if you are or may be pregnant — talk to your doctor before you start becoming more active.

PLEASE NOTE: If your health changes so that you then answer YES to any of the above questions, tell your fitness or health professional. Ask whether you should change your physical activity plan.

Informed Use of the PAR-Q: The Canadian Society for Exercise Physiology, Health Canada, and their agents assume no liability for persons who undertake physical activity, and if in doubt after completing this questionnaire, consult your doctor prior to physical activity.

No changes permitted. You are encouraged to photocopy the PAR-Q but only if you use the entire form.

NOTE: If the PAR-Q is being given to a person before he or she participates in a physical activity program or a fitness appraisal, this section may be used for legal or administrative purposes.

"I have read, understood and completed this questionnaire. Any questions I had were answered to my full satisfaction."

NAME _____

SIGNATURE _____ DATE _____

SIGNATURE OF PARENT _____ WITNESS _____
or GUARDIAN (for participants under the age of majority)

Note: This physical activity clearance is valid for a maximum of 12 months from the date it is completed and becomes invalid if your condition changes so that you would answer YES to any of the seven questions.

CSEP | SCPE
THE GOLD STANDARD IN EXERCISE SCIENCE AND PERSONAL TRAINING

© Canadian Society for Exercise Physiology www.csep.ca/forms

From ACSM, 2012, *ACSM's guide to exercise and cancer survivorship* (Champaign, IL: Human Kinetics). From Physical Activity Readiness Questionnaire (PAR-Q) © 2002. Reprinted with permission for the Canadian Society for Exercise Physiology. www.csep.ca/forms.asp

Figure 5.2   Medication List

Name: _____

Please check any medication you presently take on a regular basis and provide the following information.

Cancer-Specific Medications

If you are currently undergoing radiation therapy, please check the box in the following table and provide dose and schedule.

	Medication	Name of medication(s)	Dose and schedule	Date started	Date of discontinued use
☐	Chemotherapy				
☐	Immunotherapy				
☐	Hormonal therapy				
☐	Other cancer therapy				
☐	Radiation therapy				

Other Medications and Supplements

Please make sure to include over-the-counter drugs such as Tylenol, aspirin, and vitamins under *Other medicines.*

Baseline testing: _____   Date/time: _____

	Medication	Name of medication(s)	Dose and schedule	Date started	Date of discontinued use
☐	Medicine for heart				
☐	Medicine for blood pressure				
☐	Medicine for breathing or lungs				
☐	Medicine for diabetes				
☐	Medicine for ulcers				
☐	Medicine for arthritis				
☐	Other medicines				
☐	Supplements				

(continued)

Medication List *(continued)*

Follow-up testing:_____   Date/time:_____

	Medication	Name of medication(s)	Dose and schedule	Date started	Date of discontinued use
☐	Medicine for heart				
☐	Medicine for blood pressure				
☐	Medicine for breathing or lungs				
☐	Medicine for diabetes				
☐	Medicine for ulcers				
☐	Medicine for arthritis				
☐	Other medicines				
☐	Vitamins and supplements				

Fitness professional's comments: _____

_____

_____

_____

_____

_____

_____

_____

_____

_____

_____

_____

_____

Fitness professional's name (Please print):_____

Fitness professional's signature: _____

Date: _____

From ACSM, 2012, *ACSM's guide to exercise and cancer survivorship* (Champaign, IL: Human Kinetics).

Take-Home Message

Because cancer survivors are often older, have received some form of aggressive therapy, and may present with a diverse range of comorbid conditions, they may find a cardiorespiratory fitness test intimidating. Thus, fitness professionals may need to take extra time to fully describe the test procedures and provide appropriate encouragement and reassurance before, during, and after testing procedures.

Selection and Utility of Testing

Several methods are available for evaluating cardiorespiratory fitness in clients with cancer (table 5.1). This section discusses the use of laboratory-based tests such as cardiopulmonary exercise testing as well as field-based tests including the 6-minute walk test. This section also discusses various parameters to consider when choosing a test modality for the evaluation of cardiorespiratory fitness in a client diagnosed with cancer.

Take-Home Message

Because clients with cancer are typically older and have received treatments that may have affected their balance, fitness professionals should choose the most appropriate cardiorespiratory fitness test exercise modality and have at least two qualified exercise physiologists at every test.

The first major consideration is whether to perform a maximal (with direct or estimated measurement of gas exchange) or submaximal cardiorespiratory exercise test. Maximal cardiorespiratory tests can be divided into two categories: (1) direct measurement of oxygen consumption via incremental cardiopulmonary exercise test with gas exchange measurement (figure 5.3), or

(2) estimated measurement of oxygen consumption using standard formulas from the highest treadmill or cycle workload achieved (figure 5.4). Both types of maximal tests require that the client achieve volitional exhaustion or symptom limitation, and both provide an accurate determination of cardiorespiratory fitness. It is important to clarify that maximal cardiorespiratory tests are not used for cardiac or pulmonary diagnostic purposes in the oncology setting.[1] Once a maximal test is chosen, it is imperative that it be conducted in a clinical setting with the appropriate equipment and qualified personnel.

Submaximal tests predict cardiorespiratory fitness based on the workload achieved at a given predetermined submaximal heart rate. The decision to conduct maximal or submaximal exercise tests should be determined following the careful consideration of several factors including the purpose

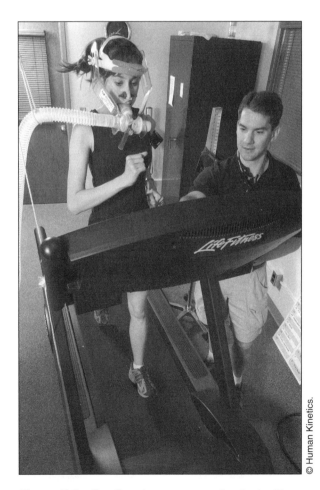

© Human Kinetics.

Figure 5.3 Cardiopulmonary exercise test with gas exchange collection.

TABLE 5.1 Exercise Test Modalities

	Maximal	
	CPET	**Stress Test**
Direct measurement of $\dot{V}O_2$	Yes	No
Estimated measurement of $\dot{V}O_2$	No	Yes, estimated from highest workload achieved during the test
Equipment	• Expired gas measurement system • Electronically braked cycle ergometer or motorized treadmill • 12-lead ECG • Pulse oximeter • BP monitoring	• Electronically braked cycle ergometer or motorized treadmill • 12-lead ECG • Pulse oximeter • BP monitoring
Cost	Relatively expensive	Reasonable
Test duration	8-12 minutes	8-20 minutes
Description of test	Incremental exercise with expired gas analysis until volitional exhaustion or symptom limitation.	Incremental exercise until volitional exhaustion or symptom limitation.

	Submaximal		
	Age-predicted HR	**6- or 12-minute walk test**	**Constant load test***
Direct measurement of $\dot{V}O_2$	No	No	No
Estimated measurement of $\dot{V}O_2$	Yes, estimated from the workload achieved at a predefined HR (70-85% HR_{max})	Yes, estimated from blood pressure and heart rate response during test	No
Equipment	• Electronically braked cycle ergometer or motorized treadmill • Heart rate monitor • Pulse oximeter • Stopwatch	• 30-meter hallway or corridor • Heart rate monitor • Pulse oximeter • Stopwatch	• Electronically braked cycle ergometer or motorized treadmill • Heart rate monitor • Pulse oximeter • Stopwatch
Cost	Reasonable	Inexpensive	Inexpensive
Test duration	8-20 minutes	6 or 12 minutes	5-30 minutes
Description of test	Incremental exercise until predefined HR (70-85% HR_{max}) achieved	Subject walks as far as possible in 6 or 12 minutes	Subject pedals for as long as possible at predetermined workload (50-70% $workload_{peak}$) measured during incremental CPET

*Can be performed only following a CPET (cardiopulmonary exercise test).

Adapted from L.W. Jones et al., 2008, "Cardiorespiratory exercise testing in clinical oncology research: systematic review and practice recommendations," *Lancet Oncology* 9(8): 757-765.

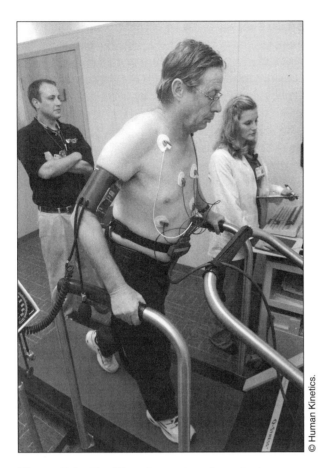

Figure 5.4 Traditional exercise stress test.

© Human Kinetics.

of testing (research investigation or exercise rehabilitation), the setting, and the patient population. These factors are reviewed in detail in the following sections.

Purpose of Testing

Cardiorespiratory fitness testing is predominantly used for research applications in the oncology setting. However, cancer exercise rehabilitation is becoming a more recognized component of clinical cancer management.[12] Thus, the need for cardiorespiratory fitness testing outside of predominantly research applications is likely to increase over the next decade.

In clients with cancer, cardiorespiratory fitness testing is used primarily to provide (1) an objective determination of peak oxygen consumption ($\dot{V}O_2$peak) or submaximal prediction of cardiorespiratory fitness, and (2) an exercise training prescription and cardiorespiratory fitness evaluation following exercise rehabilitation. In both settings, use of cardiopulmonary exercise testing, to assess

$\dot{V}O_2$peak, is recommended because it provides the most accurate assessment of cardiorespiratory fitness (figure 5.3). If cardiopulmonary exercise testing is not available, estimating $\dot{V}O_2$peak through stress testing is an excellent alternative (figure 5.4). Both cardiopulmonary exercise testing and traditional stress testing are reliable for identifying and detecting undiagnosed cardiovascular conditions, which submaximal cardiorespiratory fitness tests cannot do. It is noteworthy to mention that cardiopulmonary exercise testing procedures require regular equipment calibration to ensure that the test data are reliable and valid.

Despite the advantages of maximal cardiorespiratory fitness testing, submaximal testing (without gas exchange measurement) is also a valuable method to assess cardiorespiratory fitness in clients with cancer. These tests can be performed in a controlled laboratory, clinical setting, or field test (outside of a laboratory or clinic setting). Field tests include age-predicted heart rate tests and 6- or 12-minute walk tests; these tests are relatively easy and inexpensive to administer. Such testing may be appropriate in frail or elderly patients, or where appropriate medical supervision to conduct numerous tests in a nonclinic-based setting is not available.[1] However, the investigator or clinician must be cautious when interpreting the results of such tests. Submaximal testing relies on an extrapolation of cardiorespiratory fitness from the work rate achieved at a given submaximal heart rate. Thus, a significant potential for error exists because of the 10- to 12-beats-per-minute standard deviation in maximal heart rate in normal subjects as well as age-mediated errors in determining maximal heart rate.[3] There may be even greater variation in patients diagnosed with cancer who have been treated with cancer therapies or other medications that may affect heart rate control.[13-15]

Submaximal tests can also be used to assess functional capacity, in terms of distance walked or time to fatigue. For example, 6- or 12-minute walk tests provide a simple, safe, and inexpensive objective assessment that can be performed in numerous research and clinic settings. However, walking tests were originally designed to assess functional capacity in clients with severely compromised functional status, such as those with chronic heart failure or chronic obstructive pulmonary disease. As such, these types of tests may not be sensitive enough to evaluate the effects on clients who have been diagnosed with early-stage cancer and who do not have any additional comorbidity. A ceiling effect among these clients may occur because such tests are unable to sufficiently stress them to detect whether changes in cardiorespiratory fitness have transpired.[1] For information and practical guidelines on accurately administering a 6-minute walk test, please visit www.thoracic.org/statements/resources/pfet/sixminute.pdf.

Most important in choosing the appropriate fitness test is to make sure the test matches the client's goals. For example, if the client is new to exercise and has a goal of beginning a walking program, then a 6-minute walk test is much more appropriate than a maximal treadmill test.

Setting

The setting for the cardiorespiratory fitness test requires careful consideration. The two broad settings are clinically based (laboratory) facilities and nonclinically based (field) facilities. Because maximal cardiopulmonary exercise tests are relatively expensive and require specialized personnel and equipment and medical supervision, submaximal tests may be desirable in nonclinical settings. However, without appropriate medical supervision, even submaximal tests should only be conducted with clients classified as low risk of exercise-related adverse events. Ideally, cardiorespiratory fitness testing performed in a clinical setting should use cardiopulmonary exercise testing because these tests provide comprehensive and the most accurate information regarding cardiorespiratory fitness condition.

Patient Population

Clients with cancer vary widely in terms of prognosis, demographics, medical treatments, and extent of comorbid disease. Thus, fitness professionals should thoroughly consider each client's situation to select the most appropriate cardiorespiratory fitness test. In general, cardiopulmonary exercise testing is likely the best method to assess cardiorespiratory fitness in the majority of clients with cancer.

Literally hundreds of therapies are used in the oncology setting. Unfortunately, researchers do not currently have a good understanding of how these therapies affect the components that govern cardiorespiratory fitness.[2] Given that cardiopul-

monary exercise testing provides the safest and most robust assessment of cardiorespiratory fitness, selection of this test appears prudent. Special consideration should be given to clients currently undergoing some form of cancer therapy, especially those receiving chemotherapy or radiotherapy, or both, as these therapies can negatively affect several organ components that determine cardiorespiratory responses to exercise.

Exercise Testing Safety

Safety is a vital consideration when selecting tests to assess cardiorespiratory fitness in clients with cancer. Unfortunately, large-scale evaluations determining the safety of the various types of available cardiorespiratory tests for people with cancer have not been conducted.[9] Yet, previous research has indicated that maximal and submaximal exercise testing is, for the most part, a safe procedure for this population.[1] Nevertheless, many clients with cancer receive intensive medical therapies that may elevate the risk of an exercise test–related complication. Thus, fitness professionals must employ strict screening (eligibility) and testing procedures to optimize client safety. Specifically, the safety of cardiorespiratory fitness testing ultimately depends on two factors: (1) eligibility criteria and client selection, and (2) test administration and methodology.

Eligibility Criteria and Client Selection

Available absolute and relative contraindications to cardiorespiratory fitness testing published by the ASCM as well as other organizations (e.g., American Thoracic Society) are appropriate to apply to clients with cancer. However, added to these contraindications should be the presence of extensive skeletal and visceral metastases and untreated anemia (table 5.2).

As mentioned previously, for safety reasons, clients must be cleared for cardiorespiratory fitness testing by their oncologist or primary care physician. The information fitness professionals should have includes, but is not limited to, clinical diagnosis, stage of disease, prior or current treatments, physical activity profile, appropriate laboratory tests (e.g., hemoglobin [80-110 mg/dL]), complete blood counts), determination of exercise

TABLE 5.2   Absolute and Relative Contraindications for Exercise Testing

Absolute	Relative
Acute myocardial infarction (3-5 days)	Left main coronary stenosis or its equivalent
Unstable angina	Moderate stenotic valvular heart disease
Uncontrolled arrhythmias causing symptoms or hemodynamic compromise	Severe untreated arterial hypertension at rest (>200 mg Hg systolic, >120 mm Hg diastolic)
Syncope	Tachyarrhythmias or bradyarrhythmias
Active endocarditis	High-degree atrioventricular block
Acute myocarditis or pericarditis	Hypertrophic cardiomyopathy
Symptomatic severe aortic stenosis	Significant pulmonary hypertension
Uncontrolled heart failure	Advanced or complicated pregnancy
Acute pulmonary embolus or pulmonary infarction	Electrolyte abnormalities
Thrombosis of lower extremities	Orthopedic impairment that compromises exercise performance
Suspected dissecting aneurysm	Untreated anemia (hemoglobin level between 8 and 11 gm/dL)
Uncontrolled asthma	
Pulmonary edema	
Room air desaturation at rest ≤ 85%	
Respiratory failure	
Acute noncardiopulmonary disorder that may affect exercise performance or be aggravated by exercise (i.e., infection, renal failure, thyrotoxicosis)	
Mental impairment leading to inability to cooperate	
Evidence of extensive visceral or skeletal metastases, or both	

Adapted from American Thoracic Society/American College of Chest Physicians, 2003, "ATS/ACCP Statement on cardiopulmonary exercise testing." *American Journal of Respiratory and Critical Care Medicine* 167(2): 211-77.

contraindications, and oncologist or physician approval. Most of this information can come from routine oncology visits or from the client's medical history report.

A physical activity profile will help the fitness professional choose an appropriate cardiorespiratory exercise test protocol (maximal or submaximal) and modality (cycle ergometer or treadmill). In nonclinical settings, clients must receive physician clearance or complete a preexercise screening questionnaire (e.g., PAR-Q, PARmed-X) prior to testing.

Test Administration and Methodology

Once the fitness professional has determined whether cardiorespiratory testing is appropriate for the client, the next most important consideration is to ensure that the test chosen is administered correctly and safely. Choosing appropriate exercise equipment and testing protocols and monitoring patient exercise response play fundamental roles in ensuring a successful test.

Two types of exercise equipment can be used to evaluate cardiorespiratory fitness in clients with cancer: treadmill (see figure 5.2) and cycle ergometer (figure 5.5). For most laboratory settings, a treadmill is used when conducting maximal testing. If a treadmill is not available for use, then cycle ergometry is recommended.

Motor-driven treadmills provide progressively increasing exercise intensity through a combination of speed and grade (elevation) according to the selected protocol. Treadmill-based exercise tests are attractive because walking is a more natural and familiar activity than cycling for most people.

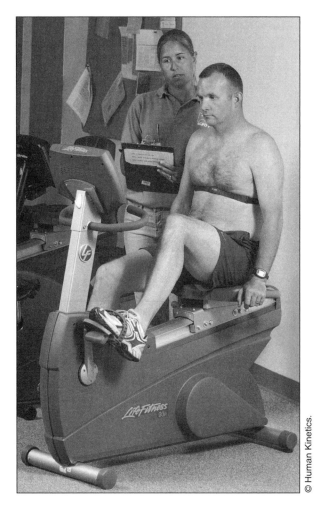

Figure 5.5 Cycle ergometer.

Exercise testing on a treadmill may elicit a higher physiological response, thus providing a more accurate assessment of cardiorespiratory fitness and increasing the possibility of uncovering potential underlying cardiac symptoms. Of course, safety is the highest priority. The main disadvantages of treadmill exercise testing are the difficulty of quantifying external work rate and the coordination and balance requirements. The latter point is an important consideration in older clients and those suffering cancer treatment–related toxicities that may affect balance and coordination. These toxicities may also alter heart rate and blood pressure responses to exercise.

In contrast, cardiorespiratory fitness testing administered on a cycle ergometer offers the following advantages:

• It is less likely to introduce movement and noise artifact into exercise response measures.

• It requires less coordination and balance than treadmill walking.

• Work rate is quantifiable.

Several protocol options are available to ensure the precise evaluation of oxygen consumption. Most protocols can be used with either a cycle ergometer or treadmill. Generally, protocols can be classified into two broad categories according to the application of workload:

• Constant increments (all clients use the same workload increments)

• Individualized increments (variable workload increments based on client characteristics)

Individualized protocols are recommended for clients with cancer given the expected large variation due to differences in cancer type, treatment, demographics, and the presence of other comorbidities. Multiple tests for the same client over a prolonged period of time should occur on the same exercise equipment and at the same time of the day, and preferably, should be administered by the same fitness professional.

Take-Home Message
Because a cardiorespiratory test will likely be a novel experience for the vast majority of clients with cancer, a follow-up phone call the day after testing is recommended to ensure that they are feeling well and not experiencing any unexpected signs or symptoms.

To maximize client safety during maximal or submaximal testing, it is critical that several physiological parameters be assessed before, during, and following the cardiorespiratory fitness assessment (table 5.1). In addition, the physiological responses to exercise will be very informative when designing a client-specific exercise training prescription (if appropriate).

Clearly, the level (extent) of physiological monitoring will be determined by the type of exercise test selected: maximal versus submaximal. For example, heart rate, blood pressure, pulse oximetry, and EKG monitoring are recommended for all clients prior to, during, and following maximal exercise testing.[3] Client monitoring with these devices will allow early detection of exercise-associated abnormalities or complications that may mandate test termination, while also providing detailed information on patient response to various exercise intensities.

Submaximal exercise responses during a maximal cardiopulmonary exercise test can also provide valuable data that can identify causes of poor cardiorespiratory fitness and assist with the individualization of exercise prescriptions. In addition, heart rate and pulse oximetry (capacity of the heart to deliver O_2 per beat) supply information regarding the cardiovascular response to exercise. However, EKG and physician monitoring are not required when conducting submaximal exercise tests in asymptomatic patients exercising within their normal levels of exercise. Nevertheless, even during field-based assessments such as 6- or 12-minute walk tests, heart rate and pulse oximetry are still advisable during exercise, as is blood pressure monitoring before and after testing.

Summary

Several tests are available to measure cardiorespiratory fitness in clients with cancer. The selection of a cardiorespiratory fitness test should be governed by several factors including the client's medical and demographic characteristics as well as the test setting and available equipment. Such considerations are critical for the safe, feasible, and precise assessment of cardiorespiratory fitness in clients with cancer. When correctly administered, cardiorespiratory fitness testing can be a valuable tool to aid in the comprehensive cardiovascular and functional assessment of clients with cancer as well as the design and monitoring of exercise prescriptions.

References

1. Jones LW, Eves ND, Haykowsky M, Joy AA, Douglas PS. Cardiorespiratory exercise testing in clinical oncology research: Systematic review and practice recommendations. *Lancet Oncol.* 2008; 9(8): 757-765.

2. Jones LW, Eves ND, Haykowsky M, Freedland SJ, Mackey JR. Exercise intolerance in cancer and the role of exercise therapy to reverse dysfunction. *Lancet Oncol.* 2009; 10(6): 598-605.

3. ATS/ACCP statement on cardiopulmonary exercise testing. *Am J Respir Crit Care Med.* 2003; 167(2): 211-277.

4. Kavanagh T, Mertens DJ, Hamm LF, et al. Prediction of long-term prognosis in 12,169 men referred for cardiac rehabilitation. *Circulation.* 2002; 106(6): 666-671.

5. Myers J, Prakash M, Froelicher V, Do D, Partington S, Atwood JE. Exercise capacity and mortality among men referred for exercise testing. *N Engl J Med.* 2002; 346(11): 793-801.

6. Gulati M, Black HR, Shaw LJ, et al. The prognostic value of a nomogram for exercise capacity in women. *N Engl J Med.* 2005; 353(5): 468-475.

7. Blair SN, Kampert JB, Kohl HW, 3rd, et al. Influences of cardiorespiratory fitness and other precursors on cardiovascular disease and all-cause mortality in men and women. *Jama.* 1996; 276(3): 205-210.

8. Warburton DE, Nicol CW, Bredin SS. Health benefits of physical activity: The evidence. *CMAJ.* 2006; 174(6): 801-809.

9. Jones LW, Eves ND, Mackey JR, et al. Safety and feasibility of cardiopulmonary exercise testing in patients with advanced cancer. *Lung Cancer.* 2007; 55(2): 225-232.

10. Jones LW, Haykowsky M, Peddle CJ, et al. Cardiovascular risk profile of patients with HER2/neu-positive breast cancer treated with anthracycline-taxane-containing adjuvant chemotherapy and/or trastuzumab. *Cancer Epidemiol Biomarkers Prev.* 2007; 16(5): 1026-1031.

11. Jones LW, Haykowsky M, Pituskin EN, et al. Cardiovascular reserve and risk profile of postmenopausal women after chemoendocrine therapy for hormone receptor-positive operable breast cancer. *Oncologist.* 2007; 12(10): 1156-1164.

12. Brown JK, Byers T, Doyle C, et al. Nutrition and physical activity during and after cancer treatment: An American Cancer Society guide for informed choices. *CA Cancer J Clin.* 2003; 53(5): 268-291.

13. Zachariae R, Paulsen K, Mehlsen M, Jensen AB, Johansson A, von der Maase H. Chemotherapy-induced nausea, vomiting, and fatigue—The role of individual differences related to sensory perception and autonomic reactivity. *Psychother Psychosom.* 2007; 76(6): 376-384.

14. Meinardi MT, van Veldhuisen DJ, Gietema JA, et al. Prospective evaluation of early cardiac damage induced by epirubicin-containing adjuvant chemotherapy and locoregional radiotherapy in breast cancer patients. *J Clin Oncol.* 2001; 19(10): 2746-2753.

15. Morrow GR, Hickok JT, DuBeshter B, Lipshultz SE. Changes in clinical measures of autonomic nervous system function related to cancer chemotherapy-induced nausea. *J Auton Nerv Syst.* 1999; 78(1): 57-63.

CHAPTER 6

Exercise Prescription and Programming Adaptations

Based on Surgery, Treatment, and Side Effects

Kathryn Schmitz, PhD, MPH

Content in this chapter covered in the CET exam outline includes the following:

- Knowledge of current American Cancer Society guidelines for exercise in cancer survivors.

- Knowledge of how common cancer treatments affect the ability of cancer survivors to perform exercise, and how to adjust programs accordingly.

- Ability to describe benefits and risks of exercise training in the cancer survivor.

- Ability to recognize relative and absolute contraindications for starting or resuming an exercise program, and knowledge of when it is necessary to refer participant back to an appropriate care provider.

- Knowledge, skill, and ability to modify exercise prescription/program based on:

  a. current medical condition
  b. time since diagnosis on or off adjuvant treatment
  c. type of current therapies (e.g., no swimming during radiation)

    d. type and recency of surgical procedures (e.g., curative or reconstructive)

    e. range of motion

    f. presence of implants

    g. amputations/fusions

    h. effects of treatment on all elements of fitness (agility, speed, coordination, flexibility, strength, and endurance)

    i. hematologic considerations (e.g., anemia, neutropenia)

    j. presence of a central line (PIC or Port)

    k. current adverse effects of treatment, both acute and chronic

    l. individuals that may be at increased risk for adverse late effects that could increase risks associated with exercise (e.g., heart failure)

- Knowledge of potential for overtraining with the cancer survivor.

- Knowledge of and ability to use appropriate sun protection for outdoor programming.

- Knowledge that cancer treatment may accelerate functional decline associated with aging, particularly in the elderly, and that exercise programming may need to be adjusted accordingly.

- Knowledge of National Lymphedema Network (NLN) 18 risk reduction practices, and exercise guidelines.

- Knowledge of lymphatic, neurological, and immune system factors in cancer survivors that may require further evaluation by medical or allied health professionals before participation in physical activity.

As noted in chapters 2 and 4, the experience of being diagnosed and treated for cancer results in numerous physiological and psychosocial changes. The goal of this chapter is to focus on what those changes mean with regard to exercise prescription. This chapter will help fitness professionals answer the following questions:

- What are the recommendations for exercise prescription for the general public, and how should this be altered for cancer survivors?

- What knowledge about a cancer survivor is needed for individualizing that person's exercise prescription? For example:
  - How does treatment with a cardiotoxic chemotherapy drug alter a person's exercise prescription?
  - How should a fitness professional alter exercise prescriptions for survivors at high risk for bone metastases, osteoporosis, or both?
  - What forms of exercise are recommended, and what should be avoided, for those with peripheral neuropathy secondary to chemotherapy?
  - How should an exercise prescription be modified for those who have had lymph nodes removed and have developed lymphedema as a result?

Throughout this chapter, the terms *physical activity* and *exercise* are used interchangeably. Technically, *physical activity* is a more inclusive term that includes multiple forms of movement, including exercise.

Health Promotion and Risk of Disease Reduction

To modify an exercise program for a specific population, we need to start with something that can be modified: the recommendations for the general public. This section outlines the current guidelines for exercise prescription from the American College of Sports Medicine, issued jointly with the American Heart Association, as well as the exercise guidance from the American Cancer Society and the U.S. Department of Health and Human Services.

The Physical Activity Guidelines for Americans developed by the U.S. Department of Health and Human Services (U.S. DHHS) indicate that when people with chronic conditions—such as cancer—

are unable to meet the stated recommendation based on their health status, they "should be as physically active as their abilities and conditions allow." An explicit recommendation is to "avoid inactivity," and it is clearly stated that "Some exercise is better than none." The key guideline for aerobic activity from the U.S. DHHS focuses on weekly activity of 150 minutes of moderate-intensity exercise, 75 minutes of vigorous-intensity exercise, or some combination of the two. Guidance for strength training is to perform two or three weekly sessions that include exercises for major muscle groups. Flexibility guidelines, from the ACSM/AHA guidelines and in the U.S. DHHS guidelines for older adults, are to stretch major muscle groups and tendons on days that other exercise is performed.[1-3] For further details on the general exercise prescriptions for health for adults, see the sidebars that follow. In addition to these two specific sets of guidelines, the American Cancer Society recommends that adults engage in at least 30 minutes of moderate to vigorous exercise, beyond their usual activities, on five or more days of the week. The ACS guidelines further state that 45 to 60 minutes of intentional exercise five times weekly is even better for cancer prevention than 30 minutes.[4,5] The ACS, ACSM/AHA, and U.S. DHHS exercise recommendations for promoting health in adults have much in common. They also form the basis for any modification in exercise guidance for specific populations such as cancer survivors.

The goals of these recommendations are as follows:

- To promote general health
- To reduce the risk of chronic diseases such as diabetes, cardiovascular disease, osteoporosis, and cancer

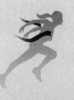

Take-Home Message
Developing exercise prescriptions that are specifically adapted for the unique needs of cancer survivors requires knowledge of exercise prescription guidelines for the general public. The U.S. DHHS and AHA/ACSM exercise prescriptions for the general public form the basis from which any adaptations are made for any special population, including cancer survivors. An important message for all populations is to avoid inactivity.

ACSM/AHA Exercise Prescription for Adults

Aerobic Activity

- Do moderately intense cardiovascular exercise 30 minutes a day, five days a week, *or* do vigorously intense cardiovascular exercise 20 minutes a day, three days a week.
- Moderate-intensity exercise means working hard enough to raise your heart rate and break a sweat while still being able to carry on a conversation.
- It should be noted that to lose weight or maintain weight loss, 60 to 90 minutes of exercise may be necessary.

Strength Training Activity

- Do 8 to 10 strength training exercises, 8 to 12 repetitions of each exercise, twice a week.
- For older adults (65+), the following recommendations are added:
  - If a health professional has told you that you are at risk of falling, perform balance exercises.
  - Have an exercise plan.
  - Both aerobic and muscle-strengthening activities are critical for healthy aging.
  - Moderate-intensity aerobic exercise means working hard at about a level-6 intensity on a scale of 1 to 10 (with 10 being highest intensity).
  - You should still be able to carry on a conversation during exercise.

Adapted from Haskell et al. 2007[2]; M.E. Nelson et al. 2007[3].

U.S. Department of Health and Human Services Physical Activity Guidelines

Adults (aged 18–64)

- Adults should do a minimum of 2 hours and 30 minutes a week of moderate-intensity, or 1 hour and 15 minutes (75 minutes) a week of vigorous-intensity aerobic exercise, or an equivalent combination of moderate- and vigorous-intensity aerobic exercise. Aerobic activity should be performed in episodes of at least 10 minutes, preferably spread throughout the week.

- Additional health benefits are provided by increasing up to 5 hours (300 minutes) a week of moderate-intensity aerobic exercise, or 2 hours and 30 minutes a week of vigorous-intensity exercise, or an equivalent combination of both.

- Adults should also do muscle-strengthening activities that involve all major muscle groups performed on 2 or more days per week.

Older Adults (aged 65 and older)

- Older adults should follow the adult guidelines. If this is not possible due to limiting chronic conditions, older adults should be as physically active as their abilities allow. They should avoid inactivity. Older adults should do exercises that maintain or improve balance if they are at risk of falling.

- For all individuals, some activity is better than none. Exercise is safe for almost everyone, and the health benefits of exercise far outweigh the risks. People without diagnosed chronic conditions (such as diabetes, heart disease, or osteoarthritis) and who do not have symptoms (e.g., chest pain or pressure, dizziness, or joint pain) do not need to consult with a health care provider about exercise.

Adults With Disabilities

- Follow the adult guidelines.

- If this is not possible, these persons should be as physically active as their abilities allow. They should avoid inactivity.

United States Department of Health and Human Services 2008.

- To promote functional independence in older adults
- To improve cardiorespiratory, metabolic, and musculoskeletal fitness

There are many other possible goals for exercise and exercise training. The specifics of an exercise prescription should be established according to the person's baseline health and fitness status as well as the person's goals. For example, the exercise prescription and levels of supervision appropriate for a young, healthy, fit 18-year-old with a goal to run competitively at the collegiate level would be quite different from the exercise prescription for an overweight, sedentary 70-year-old who wishes to return to playing singles tennis after 45 years of sedentary living.

Exercise Prescription Alterations to Address Individual Needs

The definition of *cancer survivor* varies according to the source. The National Cancer Institute defines a cancer survivor as anyone who has had a diagnosis of cancer; the term is used for the remainder of the person's life.[6] This definition is useful for many purposes, but when prescribing exercise for this population, it may be useful to distinguish between cancer patients who are currently receiving treatment and those who have completed treatment.

The U.S. DHHS guidelines to avoid inactivity to improve health and reduce the burden of chronic diseases[1] is likely excellent advice for the cancer survivor, even during treatment. But clearly, more specifics are needed than merely to avoid inactivity. Further, appropriate exercise prescriptive advice likely varies across the cancer experience (e.g., during versus posttreatment).

The first published guidance for exercise among cancer survivors came from the American Cancer Society (ACS) in 2003.[7] This guidance differs somewhat from the ACS guidance for cancer *prevention* presented earlier in this chapter. Briefly, the guidance is for cancer survivors to continue normal daily activities as much as possible throughout treatment, and to return to the recommendations for cancer prevention (presented earlier) as soon as it is safe to do so, even while undergoing adjuvant treatments such as chemotherapy and radiation. However, as noted earlier and in chapter 2, numerous adverse effects associated with a cancer diagnosis, surgery, and treatment might interfere with the ability to be regularly physically active, particularly during active treatment. The published ACS guidelines and advice on the ACS website (www.cancer.org) outline many of the ways cancer treatment can alter what would be appropriate and safe in terms of exercise programming.

Historically, physicians have advised those with any chronic illness (including cancer) to rest, take it easy, and reduce exercise. This is still advisable if movement causes severe pain, rapid heart rate, or shortness of breath. However, it is increasingly recognized that exercise is not only safe and possible during and after cancer treatment, but also can improve physical functioning and quality of life.[8, 9] Further, the risks associated with physical *inactivity* are considerable, including loss of function, strength, and range of motion, as well as negative psychosocial outcomes. Regular exercise is increasingly recognized as an effective way to counteract the negative effects of cancer treatment (e.g., lymphedema, weight gain, fatigue, loss of physical function).[8–10] Some clinical cancer treatment teams urge their patients to keep moving and be active even during treatment.

As with the general population, the goals of an exercise program for someone undergoing cancer treatment will vary according to the person's prediagnosis general health history, fitness and activity levels prior to diagnosis, and fitness and activity goals. For a young athletic person, avoiding loss

of aerobic endurance and preventing long-term cardiotoxicities might be the primary focus of an exercise program during and after cancer treatment. For an older person with multiple health problems, maintaining functional mobility in order to live independently might be the focus. The fact that cancer strikes people of many ages and such a broad variety of health and fitness backgrounds makes creating exercise prescriptions that will be safe, effective, and enjoyable for each survivor challenging. The programming should take the following into account:

- Prior history of exercise
- What the person is physically capable of doing while undergoing and recovering from treatment
- Any physical problems or limits resultant to treatment

The ACS recommends that survivors consult with their physicians to ensure that the exercise program will not interfere with treatment efficacy. Unfortunately, there is very little empirical evidence regarding what specific effects exercise may have on treatment efficacy. As a result, physicians are likely to base their advice on personal opinion and clinical experience, as well as their primary aim of protecting the patient from any possible stresses beyond cancer treatment.

In June 2009, the American College of Sports Medicine convened a roundtable to develop the first-ever ACSM guidance for exercise testing and prescription specifically for cancer survivors.[8] The expert panel conclusions are outlined in the two sidebars on pages 92-95. The process of developing these guidelines started with a review of the scientific peer-reviewed literature, to discern both the safety and effectiveness of exercise and exercise training among survivors during and posttreatment. This evidence is reviewed in chapter 4 and briefly reiterated in the next section of this chapter. Starting with the backdrop of the guidelines reviewed earlier, the panel decided to adopt much of the existing recommendations from both the ACSM/AHA and the U.S. DHHS, particularly these two words: *avoid inactivity.*

The panel generally recommends that survivors follow the age-appropriate ACSM/AHA, U.S. DHHS guidelines for aerobic activity, strength training, balance exercises, and flexibility activities.

The ACSM guidelines for exercise prescription for cancer survivors and the recommended adaptations to the U.S. DHHS physical activity guidelines are presented in the two sidebars on pages 92-95. Numerous adverse effects of cancer treatment will affect the extent to which survivors will be able to adhere to this guidance as well as the safety of each of these recommendations. Later in this chapter we review the many risks to survivors of exercise and how these might result in the need for an altered exercise prescription. In the next section, however, we summarize both the risks and benefits of exercise training to the cancer survivor.

Exercise Prescription for Cancer Survivors

This sidebar is pertinent to survivors of the following types of cancer: Breast, prostate, colon, adult hematologic (no HSCT), adult HSCT, and gynecologic.

Objectives and goals of exercise prescription

1. To regain and improve physical function, aerobic capacity, strength, and flexibility.
2. To improve body image and quality of life.
3. To improve body composition.
4. To improve cardiorespiratory, endocrine, neurological, muscular, cognitive, and psychosocial outcomes.
5. Potentially to reduce or delay recurrence or a second primary cancer.
6. To improve the ability to physically and psychologically withstand the ongoing anxiety regarding recurrence or a second primary cancer.
7. To reduce, attenuate, and prevent long-term and late effects of cancer treatment.
8. To improve the physiologic and psychological ability to withstand any current or future cancer treatments.

General contraindications for starting an exercise program common across all cancer sites

Allow adequate time to heal after surgery. The number of weeks required for surgical recovery may be as high as 8. Do not exercise individuals who are experiencing extreme fatigue, anemia, or ataxia. Follow ACSM Guidelines for exercise prescription with regard to cardiovascular and pulmonary contraindications for starting an exercise program. However, the potential for an adverse cardiopulmonary event might be higher among cancer survivors than age-matched comparisons given the toxicity of radiotherapy and chemotherapy and long-term/late effects of cancer surgery.

Cancer-specific contraindications for starting an exercise program

- Breast: Women with immediate arm or shoulder problems secondary to breast cancer treatment should seek medical care to resolve those issues prior to exercise training with the upper body.
- Prostate: None
- Colon: Physician permission recommended for patients with an ostomy prior to participation in contact sports (risk of blow) and weight training (risk of hernia).
- Adult hematologic (no HSCT): None
- Adult HSCT: None
- Gynecologic: Women with swelling or inflammation in the abdomen, groin, or lower extremity should seek medical care to resolve these issues prior to exercise training with the lower body.

Cancer-specific reasons for stopping an exercise program.

Note: General ACSM guidelines for stopping exercise remain in place for this population.

- Breast: Changes in arm/shoulder symptoms or swelling should result in reductions or avoidance of upper body exercise until after appropriate medical evaluation and treatment resolves the issue.

- Prostate: None

- Colon: Hernia, ostomy-related systemic infection.

- Adult hematologic (no HSCT): None

- Adult HSCT: None

- Gynecologic: Changes in swelling or inflammation of the abdomen, groin, or lower extremities should result in reductions or avoidance of lower body exercise until after appropriate medical evaluation and treatment resolves the issue.

General injury risk issues in common across cancer sites

Patients with bone metastases may need to alter their exercise program with regard to intensity, duration, and mode given increased risk for skeletal fractures. Infection risk is higher for patients who are currently undergoing chemotherapy or radiation treatment or have compromised immune function after treatment. Care should be taken to reduce infection risk in fitness centers frequented by cancer survivors. Patients with known metastatic disease to the bone will require modifications and increased supervision to avoid fractures. Patients with cardiac conditions (secondary to cancer or not) will require modifications and may require increased supervision for safety.

Cancer-specific risk of injury, emergency procedures

- Breast: The arms and shoulders should be exercised, but proactive injury prevention approaches are encouraged, given the high incidence of arm and shoulder morbidity in breast cancer survivors. Women with lymphedema should wear a well-fitting compression garment during exercise. Be aware of risk for fracture among those treated with hormonal therapy, a diagnosis of osteoporosis, or bony metastases.

- Prostate: Be aware of risk for fracture among patients treated with ADT, a diagnosis of osteoporosis, or bony metastases.

- Colon: Advisable to avoid excessive intra-abdominal pressures for patients with ostomies.

- Adult hematologic (no HSCT): Multiple myeloma patients should be treated as if they are osteoporotic.

- Adult HSCT: None

- Gynecologic: The lower body should be exercised, but proactive injury prevention approaches are encouraged, given the potential for lower extremity swelling or inflammation in this population. Women with lymphedema should wear a well-fitting compression garment during exercise. Be aware of risk for fractures among those treated with hormonal therapies, with diagnosed osteoporosis, or with bony metastases.

HSCT = hematopoietic stem cell transplantation.

Adapted, by permission, from K.H. Schmitz et al., 2010, "American College of Sports Medicine roundtable on exercise guidelines for cancer survivors," *Medicine and Science in Sports and Exercise* 42(7): 1409-26.

Review of U.S. DHHS Exercise Guidelines (PAGs) for Americans and Alterations Needed for Cancer Survivors

This sidebar is pertinent to survivors of the following types of cancer: Breast, prostate, colon, adult hematologic (no HSCT), adult HSCT, and gynecologic.

General statement

Avoid inactivity; return to normal daily activities as quickly as possible after surgery. Continue normal daily activities and exercise as much as possible during and after nonsurgical treatments. Individuals with known metastatic bone disease will require modifications to avoid fractures. Individuals with cardiac conditions (secondary to cancer or not) may require modifications and may require greater supervision for safety.

Aerobic exercise training (volume, intensity, progression)

- Breast: Recommendations are the same as age-appropriate guidelines from the PAGs for Americans.
- Prostate: Recommendations are the same as age-appropriate guidelines from the PAGs for Americans.
- Colon: Recommendations are the same as age-appropriate guidelines from the PAGs for Americans.
- Adult hematologic (no HSCT): Recommendations are the same as age-appropriate guidelines from the PAGs for Americans.
- Adult HSCT: Okay to exercise every day, lighter intensity and lower progression of intensity recommended.
- Gynecologic: Recommendations are the same as age-appropriate guidelines from the PAGs for Americans. Morbidly obese women may require additional supervision and altered programming.

Cancer site-specific comments on aerobic exercise training prescriptions

- Breast: Be aware of fracture risk.
- Prostate: Be aware of increased potential for fracture.
- Colon: Physician permission recommended for patients with an ostomy prior to participation in contact sports (risk of blow).
- Adult hematologic (no HSCT): None
- Adult HSCT: Care should be taken to avoid over-training given immune effects of vigorous exercise.
- Gynecologic: If peripheral neuropathy is present, a stationary bike might be preferable over weight-bearing exercise.

Resistance training (volume, intensity, progression)

- Breast: Altered recommendations. See below.
- Prostate: Recommendations same as age-appropriate PAGs.
- Colon: Altered recommendations. See below.
- Adult hematologic (no HSCT): Recommendations same as age-appropriate PAGs.
- Adult HSCT: Recommendations same as age-appropriate PAGs.
- Gynecologic: Altered recommendations. See below.

Cancer site-specific comments on resistance training prescription

- Breast: Start with a supervised program of at least 16 sessions and very low resistance; progress resistance at small increments. No upper limit on the amount of weight to which survivors can progress. Watch for arm and shoulder symptoms, including lymphedema, and reduce resistance or stop specific exercises according to symptom response. If a break is taken, back off the level of resistance by 2 weeks' worth for every week of no exercise (e.g., a 2-week exercise vacation = back off to resistance used 4 weeks ago). Be aware of risk for fracture in this population.

- Prostate: Add pelvic floor exercises for those who undergo radical prostatectomy. Be aware of risk for fracture.

- Colon: Recommendations same as age-appropriate PAGs. For patients with a stoma, start with low resistance and progress resistance slowly to avoid herniation at the stoma.

- Adult hematologic (no HSCT): None

- Adult HSCT: Resistance training might be more important than aerobic exercise in bone marrow transplant patients.

- Gynecologic: There is no data on the safety of resistance training in women with lower limb lymphedema secondary to gynecologic cancer. This condition is very complex to manage. It may not be possible to extrapolate from the findings on upper limb lymphedema. Proceed with caution if the patient has had lymph node removal or radiation to lymph nodes in the groin.

Flexibility training (volume, intensity, progression)

- Breast: Recommendations are the same as age-appropriate PAGs for Americans.

- Prostate: Recommendations are the same as age-appropriate PAGs for Americans.

- Colon: Recommendations same as-age appropriate PAGs, with care to avoid excessive intra-abdominal pressure for patients with ostomies.

- Adult hematologic (no HSCT): Recommendations are the same as age-appropriate PAGs for Americans.

- Adult HSCT: Recommendations are the same as age-appropriate PAGs for Americans.

- Gynecologic: Recommendations are the same as age-appropriate PAGs for Americans.

Exercises with special considerations (e.g., yoga, organized sports, pilates)

- Breast: Yoga appears safe as long as arm and shoulder morbidities are taken into consideration. Dragon boat racing not empirically tested, but the volume of participants provides face validity of safety for this activity. No evidence on organized sport or pilates.

- Prostate: Research gap.

- Colon: If an ostomy is present, modifications will be needed for swimming or contact sports. Research gap

- Adult hematologic (no HSCT): Research gap.

- Adult HSCT: Research gap.

- Gynecologic: Research gap.

HSCT = hematopoietic stem cell transplantation.

Adapted, by permission, from K.H. Schmitz et al., 2010, "American College of Sports Medicine roundtable on exercise guidelines for cancer survivors," *Medicine and Science in Sports and Exercise* 42(7): 1409-26.

Benefits and Risks of Exercise and Exercise Training

Historically, cancer patients were told to rest and take it easy. This advice continues in many places even today as a result of the fear that excessive activity will make a patient who is already not well feel even worse. Given that cancer treatment can result in fragile physiological and psychological states, it is useful to establish, first, that it is safe for survivors to be physically active.

A review of the peer-reviewed scientific literature on exercise interventions in cancer survivors during and after cancer treatment for multiple cancer sites, including breast, colon, prostate, hematological, and gynecological cancers, reveals that exercise is quite safe, with few adverse events reported in the 48 studies evaluated.[8] In many cases, the adverse events were not unique to cancer survivors. For example, in one study, a few breast cancer survivors participating in a walking intervention developed plantar fasciitis.[11] In a study of prostate cancer survivors, an older man experienced a myocardial infarction 15 minutes after completing an exercise session.[12] These events may have occurred in these participants regardless of any cancer history. The overall conclusion of the review panel was that a wide variety of exercise programs are well tolerated, with few adverse effects, even during severe cancer treatments such as stem cell transplantation.[8] Fears that cancer survivors are too fragile to exercise during treatment may be unfounded.[8] In fact, exercise has been shown to be beneficial to cancer survivors during and after treatment, as reviewed next.

The benefits of exercise training during and after cancer treatment were reviewed in greater depth in chapter 4. Table 4.1 on page 51 presents the levels of evidence for specific outcomes within cancer survivorship populations as noted by the recently completed guidelines panel from ACSM. To summarize, considerably more research has been published on breast cancer survivors than on any other diagnostic category among survivors. As a result, sufficient studies exist to warrant the strongest possible evidence rating (evidence level A). Multiple randomized controlled trials demonstrate benefits of exercise both during and following treat-ment for breast cancer, including improvements in aerobic fitness and strength, as well as flexibility, physical function, and safety with regard to risk for lymphedema among survivors who have completed treatment. Studies of prostate cancer survivors have shown evidence of improvements in aerobic fitness, strength, body size and composition, quality of life, energy level, and physical function, with evidence levels of A or B for all of these categories. From there, the number of studies decreases considerably, resulting in few outcomes that provide sufficient evidence to warrant any conclusion of benefit. For example, only four intervention studies have been published to date that have examined the benefits of exercise among adults with hematological malignancies who are not treated with hematopoietic stem cell transplantation (HSCT).

As noted earlier, many factors converge to determine the risks of specific types of exercise for any given survivor. The next section reviews some of the factors that fitness professionals should consider when developing an individualized exercise prescription for a cancer survivor.

Exercise Prescription Individualization

Cancer treatment results in changes that must be considered when individualizing the exercise prescription to a specific survivor. Chapter 2 covered these changes in depth. This section considers those changes in the context of how they alter exercise prescription. As an overview, it might be helpful to think about all of the body systems required to exercise, and then compare those systems to the systems affected by cancer treatments. We need the musculoskeletal, nervous, cardiovascular, respiratory, metabolic, and endocrine hormonal systems to perform exercise. The capacity of each of these systems can be altered by the various treatments used to treat cancer. Other body systems are also altered as a result of exercise training, including cell signaling pathways, the immune system, and reproductive hormonal systems. Exercise prescriptions need to be adapted to the current condition, abilities, and interests of each individual survivor. The safety of the survivor must be foremost in the fitness professional's mind when developing a program.

Take-Home Message
The following physiological systems are affected by exercise:

- Muscles, tendons, ligaments
- Bones
- Nervous system: Cognition, memory, sensory and motor systems
- Cardiovascular system
- Respiratory system
- Hormones (endocrine and metabolic systems)

When developing individualized exercise prescriptions for the cancer survivor, the fitness professional must know the effects of the cancer and its treatments on these systems as well as the relevant medical history of these body systems. Only then can risks be minimized and benefits maximized.

Current Medical Condition

Prior to prescribing exercise for a cancer survivor, the fitness professional must know how the cancer diagnosis, treatment, or both, have affected each of the systems required for and affected by exercise. During active treatment, it is appropriate, though not always necessary, to ask for physician clearance prior to prescribing exercise for a survivor. A request for physician clearance should include details of the exercise mode, frequency, intensity, and session duration. Figure 6.1 is a note survivors can use to request written clearance from their physicians during active cancer treatment. Survivors who have completed cancer treatment can use an adapted version of this form. The note can also be altered to address the unique needs of clients.

Whether a fitness professional chooses to get physician's clearance or not, it is important to know the current medical condition of the client with regard to the following:

- Bone health: Is there any reason to think that this person is at risk for bone fractures?
- Cardiovascular health: Has this person ever been diagnosed with hypertension, conges-

tive heart failure, kidney disease, or any other diseases or events associated with the cardiovascular system?

- Hematological parameters and immune function: Does this person have anemia or reduced blood cell counts that would place him or her at increased risk of infection?
- Respiratory health: Does this person have asthma? Chronic obstructive pulmonary disease? Abnormal respiratory function for any other reason?
- Musculoskeletal health: Do any body parts or joints lack normal functional range of motion, strength, or coordination?
- Nervous system health: Does this person have a normal walking gait? Any loss of sensation, pain, or altered sensation in the feet, hands, or elsewhere?
- Cognitive health: Does this person have normal cognition and memory? Is there any obvious impairment in understanding and following directions or remembering what was discussed at a prior meeting?
- Metabolic and hormonal health: Does this person have diabetes, metabolic syndrome, obesity, thyroid disease, or any other disorder associated with hormones?

Take-Home Message
Those who have a cancer diagnosis are likely to be older adults, a population likely to have other chronic health conditions as well, such as orthopedic issues, cardiopulmonary disease, diabetes, and obesity. A fitness professional prescribing exercise for a cancer survivor needs to consider the person's full medical history and current condition, not just the person's cancer history.

Time Since Diagnosis

Those diagnosed with cancer and receiving treatment experience a variety of physiological and psychological changes over time. Those who have recently been diagnosed and are awaiting treatment

Figure 6.1 Physician's Permission Form

Dear Dr. _____ :

I am interested in participating in an exercise program during my active cancer treatment. I would like you to know what I plan to do and ask you to sign below if you believe that my current medical condition will allow me to participate in this program without compromising my treatment outcomes or general health. Thank you for reviewing this. I am working with a fitness professional who has obtained a certification from the American College of Sports Medicine (ACSM Certified Cancer Exercise Trainer) to work with cancer survivors. My fitness trainer has asked me to have you review this program and obtain your written permission.

Exercise mode: _____
(Examples: Walking program, weight training, tennis lessons, yoga, Pilates, dragon boat racing)

Frequency of activity: _____
(Examples: Once weekly, three times weekly, daily)

Intensity of activity: _____
(Examples: mild intensity—I will not sweat doing this activity; moderate intensity—I will sweat but I will be able to converse while participating; vigorous intensity—I will sweat and breathe hard while doing this activity)

Duration of each activity session: _____
(Examples: 20 minutes, 30 minutes, 60 minutes, 2 hours)

Setting in which this activity will occur: _____

Level of supervision: _____

For physician signature only:

I, _____, have reviewed the above proposed program and approve of my patient _____ participating in the above-described program while undergoing chemotherapy, radiation therapy, or other active cancer treatments. I recommend the follow adaptations to the program above for my patient's safety.

Check one:

___ No adaptations from what is stated above

___ Adaptations as follows: _____

_____

_____

_____

Print Name/Signature/Date

From ACSM, 2012, *ACSM's guide to exercise and cancer survivorship* (Champaign, IL: Human Kinetics).

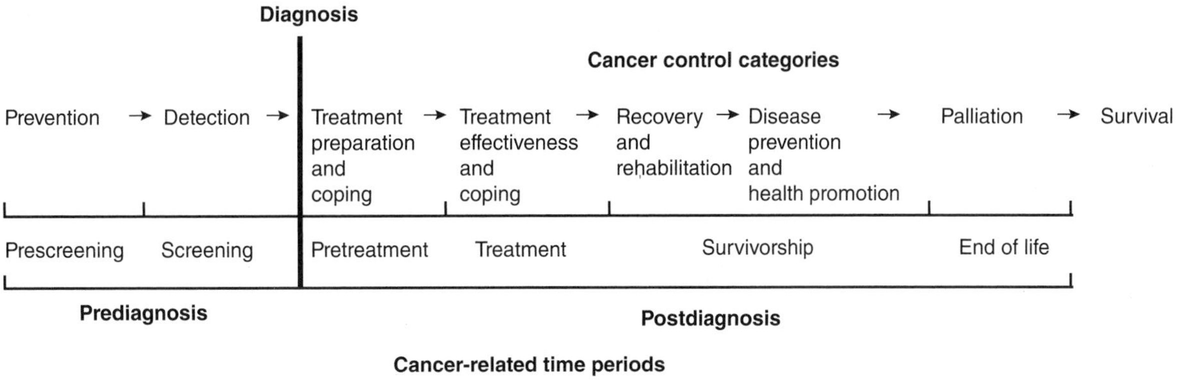

Figure 6.2 Physical activity and cancer control framework.

Reprinted from *Seminars in Oncology Nursing*, Vol. 23(4), K.S. Courneya and C.M. Friedenriech, "Physical activity and cancer control," pgs. 242-252, copyright 2007, with permission from Elsevier.

are different, physically and psychologically, from cancer survivors who are 1, 5, and 15 years out from the end of their curative treatment. Those who have had multiple diagnoses (e.g., second cancers, recurrences) differ from those with a single cancer diagnosis.

This continuum of the cancer experience is depicted in the exercise and cancer control framework in figure 6.2. The goal of this framework is to distinguish among the needs and abilities of survivors based on where they are in the continuum (e.g., currently undergoing treatment, recently completed treatment, or in long-term survivorship and exercising to promote general health and prevent recurrence). The exercise prescription must take into account the time since diagnosis and the appropriate goals for that time frame. Goals of exercise prescriptions range from improving treatment effectiveness and coping with the side effects of treatment (during active treatment) to preventing disease and promoting health (in the years after the end of active treatment).

On or Off Adjuvant Treatment and Timing of Current Treatment

The goals of exercise and the ability of cancer survivors to participate in exercise will change throughout the cancer experience. Therefore, understanding where the client is with regard to the treatment trajectory is crucial. Those who have recently undergone or are currently undergoing systemic treatments (e.g., radiation and chemotherapy) will

be the most physiologically vulnerable. Although treatments can be spread out over several years for some types of cancer, others may take only a few weeks or months. Therefore, even if the client reports being done with treatment, it is a good idea to ask whether any additional follow-up treatment is planned. It is also a good idea to inquire about any lymphatic, neurological, or immune system factors that may require further evaluation by medical or allied health professionals before participation in physical activity.

Some forms of treatment may last five or more years. The most common example is the hormonal therapies provided orally to women with reproductive cancers and to men with prostate cancer. Technically, these medications are considered adjuvant treatment for cancer. However, when most clients report being finished with treatment, they are referring to being finished with appointments that require going to a facility for cancer treatments, such as radiation therapy or intravenous chemotherapy.

Cancer survivors who are undergoing chemotherapy, radiation therapy, or both, may have reduced immune function that may render exercise in a public facility hazardous, because they are susceptible to developing systemic infections with fevers. Knowing whether a client is currently immune compromised is crucial. Fitness professionals should ask clients whether they were told that they are susceptible to infections as a result of their current treatment regimens.

Further, energy levels will be reduced during chemotherapy and radiation treatments. These treatments work by killing rapidly dividing cells. Although treatments are increasingly targeted at the tumor cells themselves, it is still common for both chemotherapy and radiation therapy to result in systemic alterations in the types of healthy body cells that turn over rapidly, such as those that make up skin, hair, nails, the inside of the mouth, and the lining of the digestive tract. Also, these treatments can result in an increase in the number of cells that respond to inflammation (i.e., cytokines). Cytokines also increase when we are sick, such as when we have the flu, and explain, in part, the achy feeling that comes with being sick. Cancer patients with increased cytokine levels in their blood may feel achy and sick all the time.

The side effects of both chemotherapy and radiation treatments are the result of the treatments on nontumor cells that turn over rapidly. One common side effect is a reduced energy level (i.e., cancer-related fatigue). These side effects can be short lived, going away as soon as the treatment is over, or persistent, lasting for years. For example, those who undergo high-dose chemotherapy in association with a stem cell transplant can have reduced immune parameters and increased inflammatory markers for several years after completing treatment. Fitness professionals should also be aware that cancer treatment may accelerate functional decline associated with aging, particularly in the elderly. Exercise programming may need to be adjusted accordingly.

Fitness professionals should ask their clients what treatments they are currently undergoing, have undergone, and still need to complete, as well as the timing of these treatments, to get an idea of the extent to which the side effects of systemic treatments are likely to be an issue. Also of note is the fact that some treatments may cause skin discoloration, skin tightening, dryness, and ulcerations. Thus, the fitness professional should know of, and remind the survivor to use, appropriate sun protection for outdoor exercise.

Type and Recency of Surgical Procedures and Presence of Implants

Surgery for cancer might include both curative and cosmetic or reconstructive procedures. The curative surgeries are intended to remove the cancer cells and immediate surrounding tissue. Sometimes lymph nodes are removed as well, to prevent cancer from spreading to other parts of the body via lymphatic vessels. Breast cancer patients, for example, commonly have at least a few lymph nodes removed to check for cancer cells in that lymphatic tissue. This is a way to determine whether the cancer cells have migrated to distant parts of the body, such as the lungs, bone, or liver. Some cancer patients undergo additional reconstructive surgical procedures. The most common reconstructive surgery in cancer patients is breast reconstruction. Reconstructive or cosmetic surgery is also associated with other cancer types, such as testicular cancer (testicular implants) and head and neck cancers (facial plastic surgery to recreate altered facial features, or improve speech or swallowing function, or both).

Regardless of whether the purpose of the surgery is curative or reconstructive/cosmetic, musculoskeletal tissue is generally severed and altered as a result. This is a traumatic event for the musculature and soft tissue that requires healing time. It may also result in scarring and a change in the function in the soft tissue that has been cut through and sometimes altered as a result of the procedures.

The sidebar Example of Effects of Surgery on Exercise Prescription: Breast Reconstruction With Expanders discusses one type of cancer surgery and how it might affect the choice of upper-body activities. This example illustrates the need to ask about the location of any cancer surgeries that have been performed for curative or reconstructive purposes. Knowing the medical guidelines for returning to normal daily activities (and exercise) for the surgeries experienced by each client is important. (The American Cancer Society website is an outstanding source of information on guidelines for exercise after cancer surgeries of all kinds.) It could be useful to ask the client about changes in sensation, function, strength, and range of motion in the area where surgery was performed prior to developing an individualized prescription or clearing the client for participation in an exercise program that assumes a particular level of ability.

Another relevant issue related to postsurgical guidelines for exercise prescription is the removal of lymph nodes. This is done to investigate whether the cancer has spread to or through the lymph system, or because the cancer has been determined to have spread to or through the lymph system. When lymph nodes are removed, the portion of

> ## Example of Effects of Surgery on Exercise Prescription: Breast Reconstruction With Expanders
>
> Reconstructive surgery for breast cancer might include the use of expanders, which are temporary implants that are surgically inserted under the pectoral muscles. Expanders are inserted flat, with a port to allow gradual filling over one to three months. To increase the size of the expander, saline is injected into it to gradually stretch the soft tissues, skin, and pectoral muscles to allow room for the permanent implants (saline or silicone) that are intended to stay in place for decades. Some expanders are left in place as the permanent implants.
>
> While expanders are in place and for four to six weeks after the final placement of the permanent implants, physicians generally recommend that women avoid overhead lifting or any strenuous exercise. The range of motion possible in the shoulder girdle is reduced, as might be expected when the pectoral muscles are stretched from underneath. This would need to be considered when choosing stretches, weight training exercises, yoga poses, or other activities that require a full range of motion in the shoulder girdle.
>
> Expanders are just one example of a common breast reconstruction surgery. Another involves moving a small piece of muscle from the transverse abdominis or latissimus dorsi with fat from the abdomen or back to recreate a breast from the woman's own tissues. This surgery also would have implications for the safety of certain exercises, at least in the short term.

the body served by those lymph nodes is forever altered with regard to its response to infection, injury, inflammation, and trauma. Exercise training needs to be approached in a rehabilitative manner, rather than a training manner, for the affected body part. For example, after breast cancer surgery that includes the removal of lymph nodes from the armpit (called axillary node dissection), some women find that a simple cut on a finger while gardening results in a systemic bacterial infection that requires antibiotics. This occurs because the removal of lymph nodes disrupts the usual communication through the lymph system that bacteria and cellular debris have entered the body. This can result in the development of a common persistent adverse effect called lymphedema.

Lymphedema is thought to occur in 17 to 42% of breast cancer survivors,[14-16] and approximately 30% of patients who have lymph nodes removed for melanoma or gynecological, bladder, and testicular cancers.[17-19] It is a chronic, incurable condition that is increasingly difficult to manage as it progresses. Therefore, fitness professionals working with cancer survivors must understand this condition and how best to prevent it. The best source of information about lymphedema is the National Lymphedema Network website, which includes a number of printable handouts that can be shared with cancer survivors as well as information on 18 risk reduction practices (www.lymphnet.org).

Range of Motion

As discussed earlier, cancer surgeries cut through soft tissues. This can result in scarring and altered range of motion, particularly when the survivor is encouraged to protect the area after treatment. Further, radiation therapy can result in scarring and trauma to soft tissues as well and may alter range of motion. Prior to developing an individualized exercise prescription or clearing a survivor for a premade program that assumes some particular range of motion in any particular joint, fitness professionals would do well to evaluate the person's current range of motion. Methods for evaluating range of motion prior to exercise prescription are reviewed in chapter 5.

Amputations

One possible outcome of a cancer surgery is amputation of a limb or part of a limb. The need for rehabilitation following an amputation is obvious to the medical community to ensure a return to functional mobility and activities of independent living. Most cancer survivors with limb amputations undergo both physical therapy and occupational therapy to regain basic functions to allow for self-care, the return to occupational activities, and independent living. However, after that, they are on their own for determining a personalized exercise prescription to regain full fitness and health.

Clearly, the exercise prescription and programming needs of those who experience amputation as part of cancer surgery are unique. However, because amputation is not a common outcome in cancer survivors, exercise adaptations for this population are beyond the scope of this book. The ACSM offers a certification to prepare personal trainers to work with people with disabilities. Certified personal trainers and other allied health professionals who plan to work with a cancer survivorship population that includes a high proportion of amputees (such as those who have had sarcomas) are directed to materials specific to that population.

Effects of Treatment on All Elements of Fitness

The elements of fitness include agility, speed, coordination, flexibility, strength, and endurance. Before clearing a cancer survivor for participation in a specific program or developing an individualized exercise prescription for that person, the fitness professional must understand what the exercise program will require of the survivor with regard to each of these elements, and whether the survivor is capable of participating in that component of exercise. For example, if a specific mode of aerobic exercise requires the ability to sustain an intensity level of 7 to 9 METS, but the maximal aerobic capacity of the client is 8 METs, it would not be appropriate to prescribe that particular mode of aerobic exercise. It is important to match the programming with the ability of the client.

One particular challenge in working with the cancer survivorship population is the interaction of aging with cancer. Cancer is more likely to occur in older people. Also, those who are diagnosed with cancer seem to experience an acceleration of functional aging. However, a healthy, fit 70-year-old diagnosed with early-stage cancer that requires minimal surgery, no chemotherapy, and a short round of radiation therapy could be ready to join a masters running club three months after treatment. By contrast, a sedentary, overweight, diabetic 40-year-old diagnosed with stage III colon cancer that requires extensive surgical resection, an external ostomy (e.g., a bag outside the body that stores waste), and a long bout of chemotherapy might need physical therapy just to return to functional mobility and independent living prior to beginning a basic walking and weight training program. The point is to evaluate survivors according to their current abilities and prescribe appropriate exercise programming according to the findings.

Hematological Considerations

Systemic cancer treatments such as chemotherapy and radiation kill rapidly dividing cells, which may include healthy cells as well as cancer cells. Because blood cells are among those that divide rapidly, blood cell counts are depleted during chemotherapy and radiation therapy. This is important to consider when prescribing exercise because red blood cells carry oxygen, and because a low white blood cell count (e.g., as a result of thrombocytopenia, leucopenia, or neutropenia) results in an increased risk for systemic infections with fever.

In prescribing exercise for cancer survivors, fitness professionals should know whether they are currently undergoing or have recently undergone any treatments that would alter blood cell counts, such as chemotherapy or radiation therapy. If so, home exercise might be preferable to programming in public settings. Frequent hand washing and ensuring that exercise equipment is cleaned often would be important as well. Fitness professionals should also be mindful of the inverted J-shaped relationship between exercise and immune function: vigorous-intensity, prolonged aerobic activity suppresses immune function.[20] In contrast, those who are moderately physically active have better immune function than those who are inactive. Survivors who are immune compromised already should avoid high-intensity activity.

A survivor who is fatigued during the weeks or months after completing chemotherapy, radiation therapy, or both, might be anemic or have reduced white blood cell counts. This would need to be assessed by an oncology clinician. A condition called cancer-related fatigue is distinct from anemia, and exercise is the leading nonpharmacological intervention for it.[10] However, the first line of treatment for the drop in energy level experienced by most cancer survivors during adjuvant therapies is to prescribe hematopoietic growth factors that stimulate the bone marrow to produce more blood cells. Erythropoietin is prescribed to improve cancer patients' ability to transport and use oxygen and increase hematocrit and white blood cell counts. One study suggests that aerobic exercise during chemotherapy may result in the need for additional monitoring of the dosage required for these blood product medications, given that aerobic exercise training also increases red blood cell counts.[21]

As noted in earlier sections, the advice is to individualize exercise prescriptions according to the current needs and abilities of the cancer survivor.

Presence of a Central Line or an Ostomy

Survivors receiving intravenous chemotherapy commonly have a catheter inserted just under the skin, usually just below the collarbone, so they don't have to go through a catheter insertion every time they come in for treatment. These PIC lines (also known by the brand name Port-a-Catheter) can be damaged by overstretching the area where they are placed. Asking survivors who are currently undergoing chemotherapy whether they have an indwelling catheter, a PIC, or Port prior to designing an exercise program enables fitness professionals to adapt the activities to avoid overstretching or straining the area of the indwelling catheter. There is no evidence currently available to establish the safety of weight training with an indwelling catheter in the antecubital space (e.g., inner elbow). Therefore, clients with PIC lines in the bicep or elbow area should proceed with caution when undertaking weight training activities.

Some cancer survivors have a stoma, or opening out of the digestive or urinary tract, that allows for waste to be removed from the body after a surgery to remove cancerous tissue from the colon, rectum, or urinary system. An ostomy bag is worn to collect bodily waste. This new hole coming out of the body creates two issues for exercise prescriptions.

First, there is the potential for a hernia at the site of a stoma. This requires prescribing exercise that works the muscles around the stoma without overstraining them. Second, a stoma is a new route through which infection can enter the body. This requires attention to stoma cleanliness on the part of the survivor before, during, and after each exercise session. Cancer survivors with ostomies should review appropriate cleaning procedures for before, during, and after exercise sessions with their medical care teams prior to starting new programs.

Acute and Chronic Adverse Effects of Treatment

A variety of symptoms and side effects occur as a result of cancer treatments. Some are acute, or short-lived, effects that dissipate soon after treatment ends, such as hair loss. Others are chronic, such as peripheral neuropathy in the hands and feet after treatment with one of several classes of chemotherapy drugs called taxanes or platinum-based drugs such as cisplatin. Chapter 2 provides a comprehensive review of the common side effects of cancer treatments. Fitness professionals adapting exercise programs to meet the needs, goals, and abilities of cancer survivors should know which treatments have been received, so they can look at chapter 2 or the American Cancer Society website to determine what the common side effects are and which adverse effects might occur later. They can then ask their clients what they are currently experiencing and adapt their programs accordingly.

Exercise Risks Attributed to Cancer

In addition to learning about the side effects their clients may be currently experiencing, fitness professionals should know what treatments their clients are currently undergoing, given that exercise could be riskier following particular types of cancer treatment. For example, people with multiple myeloma may be at risk for bone fractures at a variety of sites.

To avoid overstressing their bones, these people may want to avoid certain modes of exercise that might result in falls or strain on the skeletal system (e.g., tennis, plyometrics). Following are conditions that may result from certain cancer treatments, which should be considered when planning exercise programming:

- Cardiac arrhythmias, myopathies, or heart failure after some forms of chemotherapy and radiation to the chest wall
- Bone metastases due to disease progression
- Decreased bone strength due to hormonal therapies
- Peripheral neuropathies due to some forms of chemotherapy
- Muscle pain or arthralgia due to treatment with aromatase inhibitors
- Altered memory or coordination due to chemotherapy, surgery, or radiation treatment
- Lymphedema after removal of lymph nodes in the armpit or groin

The level of supervision should be increased for people with these issues, based on their particular needs. Similarly, alterations in exercise programming as a result of these issues will also need to be individualized. Following are some examples:

- A person with cognitive impairment after chemotherapy might not be the best candidate for learning a complicated weightlifting routine that requires excellent biomechanical form and that the person has to remember from session to session.
- A person with severe sensory changes in his hands after platinum-based chemotherapy might be likely to drop dumbbells if he cannot sense where they are in his hands.
- A survivor with bone metastases might prefer a recumbent stationary bike to equipment that requires balance and weight bearing, which might risk a fall.
- A person at risk for arrhythmia and heart failure might need greater monitoring of heart rate, dyspnea, and angina during exercise.
- Progressive weightlifting regimens should start at very low weights and progress in very small increments for survivors with lymphedema secondary to the removal of lymph nodes for cancer treatment.

Contraindications and Knowing When to Refer to Medical Care

Cancer can create a medical condition severe enough that any type of exercise would be inadvisable. Thankfully, this is not a common scenario. Improvements in early screening and the detection of cancer result in the majority of cases being diagnosed at early enough stages that exercise is feasible for most cancer survivors, including those undergoing treatment.

Adverse effects of cancer treatment can also be intense enough to create a medical condition that is incompatible with just about any type of exercise. Again, thankfully, this occurs infrequently, and when it does, it typically resolves within days or weeks, or once treatment is complete. Therefore, the majority of cancer survivors are capable of participating in at least some form of exercise. Many are capable of performing exercise at the levels recommended by the U.S. DHHS for promoting health and preventing disease in healthy adults or older adults.

None of the dozens of well-executed randomized controlled exercise intervention trials conducted in cancer survivors during and after treatment concluded that exercise is unsafe.[9] That said, these trials included volunteers and often recruited only a small proportion of the possible survivors who could have participated at any given cancer treatment center. Therefore, it is possible that the studies are biased because they examined the safety of exercise only among those who were most capable of tolerating the programs prescribed.

Cancer is not a disease to be taken lightly. It does cause significant physiological and psychological challenges. Therefore, fitness professional working with cancer survivors must be aware of the signs and symptoms that indicate the need to delay starting an exercise program. Two items crucial for discerning are whether the survivor is anemic or immune compromised. These conditions are most likely to occur during chemotherapy or radiation therapy and are likely to clear up within weeks or months after the end of these treatments.

Survivors undergoing treatments that result in hematological parameter changes should have written clearance from a physician before starting an exercise program. Further, survivors should be asked whether they have normal blood cell counts according to their physician after completing these treatments. Finally, people who undergo hematopoietic stem cell transplants receive high doses of chemotherapy prior to transplant. White blood cell counts may take longer to recover from HSCT than from typical doses of chemotherapy. Some patients experience suppressed immune function for years after HSCT.

Finally, because cancer can recur and adverse effects of cancer treatment can show up months and years after completing therapy, fitness professionals must know the signs that indicate the need for a referral to a health care professional for further evaluation or treatment. One caveat to presenting this list of signs is that many cancer survivors live in fear of recurrence and take every symptom as a sign that the cancer has returned. In fact, some equate muscle soreness with the pain that is a sign of cancer having metastasized to the bone. Therefore, a delicate balance is required between taking symptoms seriously and recommending that a survivor seek medical attention, and adding to the ongoing fear that the smallest symptom is a sign that the cancer has returned. A key indication that medical attention is warranted is when the signs listed in the sidebar Signs Indicating the Need for Referral to a Health Care Provider cannot be obviously explained as resulting from some other cause. For example, a survivor who develops a fever without any obvious source of infection (e.g., upper respiratory symptoms, bladder symptoms) should seek medical attention.

Take-Home Message

Cancer is a catchall term for more than 200 types of illness. It takes time and experience to understand all the signs and symptoms indicating that a cancer survivor needs to be referred to a health care provider. Establishing a channel of communication with the clinicians who treat the cancer can help to determine the specific issues to watch for, particularly in patients currently undergoing treatment.

Setting Goals

Each cancer survivor will have his or her own goals, and those goals will shift during the cancer experience (e.g., during versus after treatment). The exercise prescription should match those goals. A specific goal (e.g., to climb Mount Rainier someday) can help the fitness professional design a program to prepare the person physiologically to achieve that goal. However, many survivors have very general goals, such as wanting to feel better, look better, or live longer. In this case, the exercise prescription can build from whatever is currently possible to meeting the general guidelines of the U.S. DHHS, the ACSM/AHA, or the ACS.

One thing to watch for carefully in this population is increasing fatigue and symptoms with overtraining. To avoid this, the fitness professional

Signs Indicating the Need for Referral to a Health Care Provider

- Unusual tiredness or unusual weakness
- Fever or infection
- Difficulty maintaining weight, severe diarrhea, or vomiting
- Leg pain or cramps, unusual joint pain or bruising
- Sudden onset of nausea during exercise
- Irregular heartbeat, palpitations, or chest pain

- Flare of lymphedema symptoms
- Change in the appearance or feel of the cancer site
- Lump in the breast or groin, change in skin color or texture
- Significant changes in coordination, vision, hearing

Based on www.ncpad.org/disability/fact_sheet.php?sheet=195&section=1465.

should check in with the client regularly between exercise sessions to find out if any changes in side effects are occurring, including increasing fatigue or reduced energy levels. If there is an increase in fatigue or a worsening of any acute or persistent negative effects of treatment, the exercise dose should be reduced by modifying intensity, session duration, session frequency, or all of these things. Decreasing the intensity and duration rather than the frequency of exercise, however, will promote continued exercise compliance. The sidebar Tips From the American Cancer Society: When You Are Too Tired to Exercise—Fatigue and Cancer provides tips on how to maintain an exercise program during active cancer treatment, given the common challenge of increased fatigue. Monitoring fatigue levels with a standardized survey is a good way to determine whether fatigue levels are changing. Multiple surveys are available for this purpose. Figure 6.3 is one such survey.[22]

In addition, simply asking "How tired are you today on a scale of 0 to 10?" and whether there are any particular reasons for increased fatigue at the beginning of each session might be sufficient for such monitoring. A recent review noted that on a scale of 0 to 10 (0 = no fatigue, 10 = worst fatigue imaginable), a score of 1 to 3 is considered mild, 4 to 6 is moderate, and 7 to 10 is severe.[10]

It is well established that prolonged vigorous exercise may decrease immune system effectiveness and increase the risk of infection[23] as well as injury.[24] Fitness professionals working with cancer survivors—especially those undergoing active treatments—should monitor for signs of overtraining, including the following:

- Increased fatigue
- Insomnia
- Increased irritability
- Increased heart rate at a given exercise intensity
- Poor exercise performance
- Weight loss
- Psychological effects of overtraining (e.g., depression, loss of enthusiasm)
- Excessive muscle soreness
- Injury
- Headaches, dehydration, or both

If any of these occur, exercise dose should be reduced immediately. If the signs of overtraining do not reverse themselves after reducing the exercise dose, the client should seek a medical evaluation and stop exercising until that evaluation is complete.

Tips From the American Cancer Society: When You Are Too Tired to Exercise—Fatigue and Cancer

Many people notice a loss of energy during cancer treatment.

- During chemotherapy and radiation, the majority of patients have fatigue.
- Fatigue may be severe and limit activity.
- Inactivity leads to muscle wasting and loss of function.

An aerobic training program can help break this cycle.

- Regular exercise has been linked to reduced fatigue.
- It is also linked to being able to do normal daily activities without major limitations.
- An aerobic exercise program can be prescribed as treatment for fatigue in cancer survivors during and after treatment.
- Talk with your doctor about this.

Based on American Cancer Society. Available: www.cancer.org/Treatment/SurvivorshipDuringandAfterTreatment/StayingActive/physical-activity-and-the-cancer-patient

Figure 6.3   Fatigue Symptom Inventory

For each of the following, circle the one number that best indicates how that item applies to you.

1. Rate your level of fatigue on the day you felt most fatigued during the past week:

      0   1   2   3   4   5   6   7   8   9   10

   Not at all   As fatigued as
   fatigued   I could be

2. Rate your level of fatigue on the day you felt least fatigued during the past week:

      0   1   2   3   4   5   6   7   8   9   10

   Not at all   As fatigued as
   fatigued   I could be

3. Rate your level of fatigue on the average during the past week:

      0   1   2   3   4   5   6   7   8   9   10

   Not at all   As fatigued as
   fatigued   I could be

4. Rate your level of fatigue right now:

      0   1   2   3   4   5   6   7   8   9   10

   Not at all   As fatigued as
   fatigued   I could be

5. Rate how much, in the past week, fatigue interfered with your general level of activity:

      0   1   2   3   4   5   6   7   8   9   10

   No   Extreme
   interference   interference

6. Rate how much, in the past week, fatigue interfered with your ability to bathe and dress yourself:

      0   1   2   3   4   5   6   7   8   9   10

   No   Extreme
   interference   interference

7. Rate how much, in the past week, fatigue interfered with your normal work activity (includes both work outside the home and housework):

      0   1   2   3   4   5   6   7   8   9   10

   No   Extreme
   interference   interference

8. Rate how much in the past week, fatigue interfered with your ability to concentrate:

      0   1   2   3   4   5   6   7   8   9   10

   No   Extreme
   interference   interference

(continued)

Figure 6.3 Fatigue Symptom Inventory *(continued)*

9. Rate how much, in the past week, fatigue interfered with your relations with other people:

0 1 2 3 4 5 6 7 8 9 10
No   Extreme
interference   interference

10. Rate how much in the past week, fatigue interfered with your enjoyment of life:

0 1 2 3 4 5 6 7 8 9 10
No   Extreme
interference   interference

11. Rate how much, in the past week, fatigue interfered with your mood:

0 1 2 3 4 5 6 7 8 9 10
No   Extreme
interference   interference

12. Indicate how many days, in the past week, you felt fatigued for any part of the day:

0 1 2 3 4 5 6 7
Days   Days

13. Rate how much of the day, on average, you felt fatigued in the past week:

0 1 2 3 4 5 6 7 8 9 10
None of   The entire
The day   day

14. Indicate which of the following best describes the daily pattern of your fatigue in the past week:

0	1	2	3	4
Not at all fatigued	Worse in the morning	Worse in the afternoon	Worse in the evening	No consistent daily pattern of fatigue

From ACSM, 2012, *ACSM's guide to exercise and cancer survivorship* (Champaign, IL: Human Kinetics). With kind permission from Springer Science+Business Media: *Quality of Life Research,* "Measurement of fatigue in cancer patients: Further validation of the Fatigue Symptom Inventory," 9(7), 2000, page 847-854, D.M. Hann, M.M. Denniston and F. Baker, table 1.

Sample Exercise Prescriptions

There is so much to learn about cancer, how it is treated, and how those treatments might affect the survivor. Further, this is layered on top of the need to understand the basics of training for the generally healthy person. Add to this the high likelihood that survivors will also be overweight, be sedentary, and have several cardiovascular risk factors at the point of diagnosis. To top it off, most survivors are over age 60. Put this all together and the complexity of altering exercise prescriptions for cancer survivors becomes readily apparent.

A single text cannot provide a program description for every possible combination of cancer site, treatment, and medical history that a cancer fitness professional will encounter. This section presents sample programs for two survivors as examples of how to synthesize all of the information contained in this book into personalized exercise prescriptions.

Program 1

Client Description

This person is a breast cancer survivor, diagnosed three years ago, who is generally healthy, currently age 65, overweight and sedentary, but with no other comorbidities. Treatment with carboplatin resulted in persistent peripheral neuropathy. She has lymphedema in her left arm as a result of having had six lymph nodes removed. She reports no other lingering adverse effects of treatment. She takes trastuzumab (Herceptin). Her fitness evaluation reveals that she has low muscular strength, poor cardiorespiratory endurance, and limited ability to raise her left arm higher than her shoulder. Balance, agility, and coordination results are within age-matched normative ranges.

Fitness Goals

Her goal is to return to horseback riding. She has not ridden in 20 years, and she has not participated in any regular exercise program in 10 years. Horseback riding will require her to have stamina, agility, coordination, flexibility, and balance, as well as muscular strength and endurance. Therefore, the fitness program should include activities to enhance each of these fitness domains. The intensity level for horseback riding is estimated to be 4 METs, but could be higher, depending on specifics. Muscular strength, cardiorespiratory endurance (stamina), and upper-body stretching are the first domains of fitness that should be emphasized for the client to reach her goal.

Safety Concerns

The client is currently sedentary. The major limitations and concerns for exercise prescription for this person may be her lymphedema; the peripheral neuropathy from her chemotherapy treatment (platinum-based chemotherapy), which may alter her ability to hold weights (if the neuropathy is in her hands); balance and the likelihood of falls (if the neuropathy is in her feet); and her cardiorespiratory response to aerobic exercise (given the cardiotoxicity of several treatments and her poor general conditioning).

Exercise Prescription

The initial prescription for this client could be the following:

Cardiorespiratory Exercise

- Three times weekly for 20 minutes, starting at a comfortable pace
- Modes of aerobic activity can vary from weight-supported aerobic activities to swimming or biking.
- Increase intensity and duration in alternating weeks, and by no more than 10% per week until she reaches the U.S. DHHS guidelines of vigorous-intensity exercise or has increased the number of sessions per week to meet the U.S. DHHS guidelines for moderate-intensity exercise.

Strength Training

- Two times weekly, one set for each major muscle group
- 8 to 10 exercises
- 48 hours between sessions

It is vital that this program be supervised for the first several months and that the client's lymphedema be stable (no recent acute increases in swelling or symptoms that have required treatment by a lymphedema therapist) during any upper-body strength training programming. Further, the client should wear a well-fitted compression garment during these sessions. She should opt for

(continued)

Program 1 *(continued)*

variable resistance machines rather than dumbbells because of the peripheral neuropathy. Lower-body exercise can proceed as with any other client, unless peripheral neuropathy interferes. If so, the program should be altered the same way for the upper and lower body. For the upper body, the client should start with the lightest possible weights and progress by the smallest possible increments after she has had two to four sessions at the same weight that resulted in no change in lymphedema symptoms. The limited range of motion in the left shoulder should be considered when choosing exercises. If the client experiences any changes in lymphedema symptoms, she should stop upper-body strength training and consult a certified lymphedema therapist. The lymphedema therapist must clear the client for upper-body strength training before resuming.

Upper-body exercise training should be started in a supervised setting to ensure that the client learns the proper biomechanics for each exercise. The goal is to avoid increases in inflammation and injury as a result of improper form, because these are likely to exacerbate lymphedema. Therefore, the increments of resistance progression should be small, and attention should be given to avoiding the overuse of smaller muscles to do exercises intended for larger muscles. For example, the woman should *not* finish a seated row (intended for strengthening the large muscles of the back) by curling her wrists, because this will require more work from the small muscles of the wrists than they are able to do and may result in an injury or inflammatory response that would exacerbate her lymphedema.

Regular performance of weight training (two or three times per week) is necessary for ensuring that this mode of exercise is useful and safe. If the client cannot attend regularly because of other life commitments, progressive strength training should not be included in her exercise prescription. For example, if she comes to exercise twice weekly for a month, but then has to go away for several weeks to care for a family member, then returns for three weeks (twice weekly), then has a business trip for a week, then comes twice weekly for two weeks followed by a vacation for two weeks, she should not increase (progress) the weights; rather, she should continue to use the lightest possible resistance. Only those who are able to attend sessions on a regular basis over the course of more than a month should progress resistance. All clients will take "exercise vacations" during illness and when other life events preclude participation. This client with lymphedema, however, should back off on the resistance when she has had a gap in exercise performance of a week or more, to avoid the inflammatory responses that can exacerbate lymphedema.

Stretching

- Stretch all major muscle groups at the end of each exercise session.

- Focus special attention and extra time on gradually increasing range of motion in the left arm and shoulder.

Summary

Advice given to the general public is likely excellent advice for all cancer survivors: Avoid inactivity. It is likely that all but a very small proportion of cancer survivors can build to 150 minutes per week of physical activity, even if on some days during active treatment they will require more rest than they do on other days. Even those undergoing treatments such as intensive chemotherapy for leukemia have been shown to tolerate aerobic exercise.[26] That said, fitness professionals should know the general medical and cancer treatment history of each person for whom they plan to develop an individualized exercise plan. The combined knowledge of cancer treatment history and the recently published ACSM guidelines for exercise in cancer survivors allows for the development of individualized activity prescriptions that will minimize risk while maximizing the benefits of exercise in this growing population.

Program 2

Client Description

This client is a prostate cancer survivor diagnosed one year ago who completed treatment within the past six months. He has cardiovascular disease and is diabetic, age 70, overweight, sedentary, and osteoporotic. He reports no lingering side effects from the treatment, and he takes beta blockers for hypertension. He has not been regularly physically active since college. His fitness evaluation reveals low cardiorespiratory endurance and poor flexibility. Strength testing was not performed.

Fitness Goal

His goal is to continue to live independently and to be able to get himself to the floor and back up so he can play with his grandchildren.

Safety Concerns

This client's history is made up specifically to point out that cancer survivors often have contraindications that are related to other chronic diseases. In this case, the client has cardiovascular disease and diabetes. Therefore, guidance regarding exercise safety for a 70-year-old diabetic, overweight, sedentary man with cardiovascular disease will come from the well-established ACSM Guidelines for Exercise Testing and Prescription.[25] Because he has known cardiovascular disease and low fitness, he is a good candidate for a supervised exercise program.

Exercise Prescription

Based on where the client is starting and given the osteoporosis, it would be appropriate to start with supervised cardiorespiratory exercise on a recumbent cycle ergometer, at an RPE of 6 on a scale of 0 to 10. It would be inappropriate to prescribe exercise according to heart rate, given that the client takes beta blockers, which blunt heart rate response to exercise. Common stretches for general health would be appropriate. Evaluation of the ability to kneel and get to the floor and back up will be needed, and the safety of strength training activity would need to be evaluated given the osteoporosis. Medical clearance prior to initiating strength training or cardiorespiratory exercise would be advisable.

References

1. U.S. Department of Health and Human Services. *Physical Activity Guidelines for Americans.* Washington, DC: U.S. Department of Health and Human Resources; 2008.

2. Haskell WL, Lee IM, Pate RR, Powell KE, Blair SN, Franklin BA, Macera CA, Heath GW, Thompson PD, Bauman A. Physical activity and public health: Updated recommendation for adults from the American College of Sports Medicine and the American Heart Association. *Med Sci Sports Exerc.* 2007 Aug; 39(8): 1423-1434.

3. Nelson ME, Rejeski WJ, Blair SN, Duncan PW, Judge JO, King AC, Macera CA, Castaneda-Sceppa C. Physical activity and public health in older adults: Recommendation from the American College of Sports Medicine and the American Heart Association. *Med Sci Sports Exerc.* 2007 Aug; 39(8): 1435-1445.

4. Doyle C, Kushi LH, Byers T, Courneya KS, Demark-Wahnefried W, Grant B, McTiernan A, Rock CL, Thompson C, Gansler T, Andrews KS. Nutrition and physical activity during and after cancer treatment: An American Cancer Society guide for informed choices. *CA Cancer J Clin.* 2006 Nov-Dec; 56(6): 323-353.

5. Kushi LH, Byers T, Doyle C, Bandera EV, McCullough M, McTiernan A, Gansler T, Andrews KS, Thun MJ. American Cancer Society Guidelines on Nutrition and Physical Activity for cancer prevention: Reducing the risk of cancer with healthy food choices and physical activity. *CA Cancer J Clin.* 2006 Sep-Oct; 56(5): 254-281; quiz 313-314.

6. National Cancer Institute. Estimated US Cancer Prevalence Counts: Definitions. http://dccps.nci.nih.gov/ocs/definitions.html. Accessed June 13, 2011.

7. Brown JK, Byers T, Doyle C, Coumeya KS, Demark-Wahnefried W, Kushi LH, McTieman A, Rock CL,

Aziz N, Bloch AS, Eldridge B, Hamilton K, Katzin C, Koonce A, Main J, Mobley C, Morra ME, Pierce MS, Sawyer KA. Nutrition and physical activity during and after cancer treatment: An American Cancer Society guide for informed choices. *CA Cancer J Clin.* 2003 Sep-Oct; 53(5): 268-291.

8. Schmitz KH, Courneya KS, Matthews C, Demark-Wahnefried W, Galvao DA, Pinto BM, Irwin ML, Wolin KY, Segal RJ, Lucia A, Schneider CM, von Gruenigen VE, Schwartz AL. American College of Sports Medicine roundtable on exercise guidelines for cancer survivors. *Med Sci Sports Exerc.* 2010 Jul; 42(7): 1409-1426.

9. Speck RM, Courneya KS, Masse LC, Duval S, Schmitz KH. An update of controlled physical activity trials in cancer survivors: A systematic review and meta-analysis. *J Cancer Surviv.* 2010 Jun; 4(2): 87-100.

10. Berger AM, Abernethy AP, Atkinson A, Barsevick AM, Breitbart WS, Cella D, Cimprich B, Cleeland C, Eisenberger MA, Escalante CP, Jacobsen PB, Kaldor P, Ligibel JA, Murphy BA, O'Connor T, Pirl WF, Rodler E, Rugo HS, Thomas J, Wagner LI. Cancer-related fatigue. *J Natl Compr Canc Netw.* 2010 Aug; 8(8): 904-931.

11. Irwin ML, Cadmus L, Alvarez-Reeves M, O'Neil M, Mierzejewski E, Latka R, Yu H, Dipietro L, Jones B, Knobf MT, Chung GG, Mayne ST. Recruiting and retaining breast cancer survivors into a randomized controlled exercise trial: The Yale Exercise and Survivorship Study. *Cancer.* 2008 Jun 1; 112(11 Suppl): 2593-2606.

12. Segal RJ, Reid RD, Courneya KS, Sigal RJ, Kenny GP, Prud'Homme DG, Malone SC, Wells GA, Scott CG, Slovinec D'Angelo ME. Randomized controlled trial of resistance or aerobic exercise in men receiving radiation therapy for prostate cancer. *J Clin Oncol.* 2009 Jan 20; 27(3): 344-351.

13. Courneya KS, Friedenreich CM. Physical activity and cancer control. *Semin Oncol Nurs.* 2007 Nov; 23(4): 242-252.

14. Norman SA, Localio AR, Potashnik SL, Simoes Torpey HA, Kallan MJ, Weber AL, Miller LT, Demichele A, Solin LJ. Lymphedema in breast cancer survivors: Incidence, degree, time course, treatment, and symptoms. *J Clin Oncol.* 2009 Jan 20; 27(3): 390-397.

15. Hayes SC, Janda M, Cornish B, Battistutta D, Newman B. Lymphedema after breast cancer: Incidence, risk factors, and effect on upper body function. *J Clin Oncol.* 2008 Jul 20; 26(21): 3536-3542.

16. Francis WP, Abghari P, Du W, Rymal C, Suna M, Kosir MA. Improving surgical outcomes: Standardizing the reporting of incidence and severity of acute lymphedema after sentinel lymph node biopsy and axillary lymph node dissection. *Am J Surg.* 2006 Nov; 192(5): 636-639.

17. Karakousis CP, Driscoll DL. Groin dissection in malignant melanoma. *Br J Surg.* 1994 Dec; 81(12): 1771-1774.

18. Okeke AA, Bates DO, Gillatt DA. Lymphoedema in urological cancer. *Eur Urol.* 2004 Jan; 45(1): 18-25.

19. van Akkooi AC, Bouwhuis MG, van Geel AN, Hoedemaker R, Verhoef C, Grunhagen DJ, Schmitz PI, Eggermont AM, de Wilt JH. Morbidity and prognosis after therapeutic lymph node dissections for malignant melanoma. *Eur J Surg Oncol.* 2007 Feb; 33(1): 102-108.

20. Gleeson M. Immune system adaptation in elite athletes. *Curr Opin Clin Nutr Metab Care.* 2006 Nov; 9(6): 659-665.

21. Courneya KS, Jones LW, Peddle CJ, Sellar CM, Reiman T, Joy AA, Chua N, Tkachuk L, Mackey JR. Effects of aerobic exercise training in anemic cancer patients receiving darbepoetin alfa: A randomized controlled trial. *Oncologist.* 2008 Sep; 13(9): 1012-1020.

22. Mendoza TR, Wang XS, Cleeland CS, Morrissey M, Johnson BA, Wendt JK, Huber SL. The rapid assessment of fatigue severity in cancer patients: Use of the Brief Fatigue Inventory. *Cancer.* 1999 Mar23. Moreira A, Delgado L, Moreira P, Haahtela T. Does exercise increase the risk of upper respiratory tract infections? *Br Med Bull.* 2009; 90: 111-131.

24. Hootman JM, Macera CA, Ainsworth BE, Addy CL, Martin M, Blair SN. Epidemiology of musculoskeletal injuries among sedentary and physically active adults. *Med Sci Sports Exerc.* 2002 May; 34(5): 838-844.

25. American College of Sports Medicine. *Guidelines for Exercise Testing and Prescription.* 8th ed. Philadelphia, PA: Lippincott, Wilkins, and Williams; 2009.

26. Elter T, Stipanov M, Heuser E, von Bergwelt-Baildon M, Bloch W, Hallek M, Baumann F. Is physical exercise possible in patients with critical cytopenia undergoing intensive chemotherapy for acute leukaemia or aggressive lymphoma? *Int J Hematol.* 2009 Sep; 90(2): 199-204.

CHAPTER 7

Nutrition and Weight Management

Stephanie Martch, MS, RD, LD, and Wendy Demark-Wahnefried, PhD, RD

Content in this chapter covered in the CET exam outline includes the following:

- Knowledge of common effects of cancer treatment on energy balance and body composition for individuals with nonmetastatic disease.

- Knowledge of effects of cancer cachexia on energy balance, intake, and activity level among individuals with metastatic disease.

- Knowledge of relationship between body composition as a risk factor for the development of some cancers, and possibly as a risk factor for cancer recurrence.

- Knowledge that many cancer survivors may use complementary and alternative medicine (CAM) approaches, and of the potential for these remedies to influence exercise testing and prescription parameters.

- Ability to identify unintentional weight change that may relate to disease status, and recommend that the client seek appropriate medical attention.

- Knowledge of effect of chemotherapy and radiation on the mouth and gastrointestinal system, and the result of these changes on appetite and food preferences and choices.

- Ability to discern when a participant's nutritional questions or status would be best managed by referral to a registered dietitian.

- Knowledge of current American Cancer Society nutrition guidelines during and after cancer treatment.

- Knowledge of hydration needs specific to cancer patients and survivors.

- Knowledge of safety of weight loss programs for cancer survivors.

From a nutrition perspective, care for cancer patients and survivors can be both simple and complex: simple, in that the nutrient needs and recommended food patterns are often the same as those for the population at large; complex, because disease-related treatments can trigger multiple physiological alterations that inhibit the desire or ability to eat. However, this is also a time when cancer survivors may be highly motivated to make lifestyle changes as a template for healing and to reduce the future risk of not only cancer, but also other comorbid diseases. This chapter addresses the assessment of weight-related problems, provides guidelines for the calculation of energy requirements, and most important, establishes principles for healthy eating for various stages of cancer care and treatment, including recommendations about when to consult a nutrition professional.

Diet in Cancer Prevention, Control, and Overall Health

Whether a person is cancer free or not, the essential nutrients found in foods (carbohydrate, protein, fat, vitamins, minerals, and water) are just that—essential. These nutrients fuel the body and provide the necessary substrate to ensure optimal physiological functioning. A healthy body is about 60% water; 20% protein, carbohydrate, and bone mineral compounds; 20% fat; and less than 1% vitamins and other minerals.[1] We truly are what we eat, and to optimally function, especially while managing the burden of cancer and related treat-

ment, people must make informed and nutritious food choices.

In 1981, Doll and Peto estimated that dietary factors were directly associated with about 30 to 35% of cancer deaths.[2] Although the methods to scientifically pinpoint the exact magnitude of this relative risk still do not exist, this range is nonetheless accepted by the scientific community as a reasonable estimate. This estimate ranges between 10 and 90% depending on the type of cancer and whether it is thought to be relatively unrelated to diet (e.g., hematological malignancies) or shows greater evidence of association (e.g., cancers of the colon, breast, prostate, and endometrium).

Both the American Institute for Cancer Research (AICR), in collaboration with the World Cancer Research Fund (WCRF), and the American Cancer Society (ACS) have issued nutrition-specific guidelines for cancer prevention and control[3-5] (see table 7.1). These recommendations are for cancer survivors and share many similarities with those created to prevent and manage other prevalent chronic diseases (e.g., cardiovascular disease [CVD], diabetes, and osteoporosis), for which cancer survivors, when compared to the general population, are at significantly greater risk.[6-16] (Table 7.2 provides resources for specific nutrition recommendations related to these comorbid diseases.)

More than a decade ago, Brown and colleagues examined more than 1.2 million patient records and found overwhelming evidence that cancer survivors die of noncancer causes at a higher rate than do people in the general population, and almost half of these deaths are due to CVD.[17] Over the ensuing years, several other studies have shown that cancer survivors are at increased risk for second malignan-

Nutrition Professional for Cancer Treatment

Registered dietitians (RDs) are specially trained to translate nutrition research into healthful diets. The RD credential is available to those who obtain a bachelor's degree in nutrition accredited by the American Dietetic Association (ADA), complete an ADA-approved internship, and pass a comprehensive written exam covering all aspects of nutrition therapy. To maintain this credential, RDs must regularly participate in ADA-approved continuing education programs. The ADA also has an advanced-level certification process for RDs specializing in oncology nutrition. To find an RD in their area, fitness professionals should speak with their client's oncologist, or visit the American Dietetic Association's website at www.eatright.org and select "Find a Registered Dietitian."

TABLE 7.1   Nutrition Recommendations for Cancer Prevention

	American Cancer Society	World Cancer Research Fund/ American Institute for Cancer Research
Healthy weight	Achieve and maintain a healthy weight if currently overweight or obese.	Be as lean as possible within the normal range of body weight.
	Avoid excessive weight gain throughout the life cycle.	
	Balance caloric intake with physical activity.	
	Choose foods and beverages in amounts that help achieve and maintain a healthy weight.	Limit consumption of energy-dense foods. Avoid sugary drinks.
Diet (emphasis on plants)	Eat five or more servings of a variety of vegetables and fruits each day.	Eat mostly foods of plant origin.
	Choose whole grains in preference to processed (refined) grains.	
	Limit consumption of processed and red meats.	Limit intake of red meat and avoid processed meat.
Alcohol	Drink no more than one drink per day for women or two drinks per day for men.	Limit alcoholic drinks.
Preservation, processing, preparation		Limit consumption of salt.
Dietary supplements	Consume needed nutrients through food sources.	Aim to meet nutritional needs through diet alone.

Adapted from Doyle et al. 2006[4]; World Cancer Research Fund/American Institute for Cancer Research 2007[5].

TABLE 7.2   National Health Association Professional Statements of Nutrition Recommendations for Comorbid Disease Prevention

Disease or syndrome	Organization	Website
Cardiovascular	American Heart Association	http://circ.ahajournals.org/cgi/reprint/102/18/2284
Diabetes	American Diabetes Association	http://care.diabetesjournals.org/cgi/reprint/31/ Supplement_1/S61
High blood pressure	National Institutes of Health; National Heart, Lung and Blood Institute	www.nhlbi.nih.gov/health/public/heart/hbp/dash/ dash_brief.pdf
Osteoporosis	Centers for Disease Control and Prevention	www.cdc.gov/nutrition/everyone/basics/vitamins/ calcium.html

cies as well as other comorbidities.[18-22] The magnitude of this problem, however, has gained increasing attention as the population of survivors has grown dramatically and cancer survivors now comprise approximately 4% of the U.S. population.[23] In addition, these survivors have almost a twofold increase in functional limitations that threaten their ability to live, work, and function independently, particularly at older ages.[24] Recognizing that many cancer sur-

vivors have unmet needs for adequate health care posttreatment, in 2005 the Institute of Medicine (IOM) issued a report calling for increased efforts targeting the health care needs of this growing population, including efforts to improve nutritional status.[25]

For people with cancer and undergoing cancer treatment, normal nutrition recommendations may no longer suffice. Many cancers create a body state in which problems of nutrient deficiencies, loss of lean body mass, and treatment-induced nutrition-related side effects may compromise the ability to secure optimal nutrition.[4] Certified Cancer Exercise Trainers (CCET) design and implement physical activity programs best suited to patients throughout the weight spectrum. This chapter addresses basic nutritional assessments and provides basic nutritional guidance and reinforcement; it also provides helpful benchmarks for recognizing when a referral to a nutrition professional is warranted.

Weight Status and Body Composition

The prevalence of overweight and underweight in cancer patients often follows a site-specific pattern. Survivors of early-stage prostate and breast cancers frequently are overweight at diagnosis and gain weight during treatment. Those being treated for cancers related to eating (e.g., esophageal, head and neck, and stomach cancer) not surprisingly often experience problems with appetite, ingestion, and absorption that lead to tissue wasting and weight loss, both of which can profoundly affect physical functioning and the ability to tolerate subsequent treatments. Weight and body composition assessments provide baseline data to help fitness professionals monitor the outcomes related to nutrition therapy.

Overweight and Obesity

Obesity contributes to roughly 40,000 U.S. cancer diagnoses annually and plays a significant role in breast (postmenopausal), colon, kidney, endometrial, gallbladder (in women), and upper stomach cancers.[5, 25, 26] Moreover, overweight and obesity may account for 14 to 20% of all cancer-related deaths—including multiple myeloma; non-Hodgkin's lymphoma; and cancers of the uterus, cervix, breast, prostate, colon, rectum, esophagus, stomach, gallbladder, pancreas, and liver.[27–30] Although overweight and obesity contribute to the primary risk of select cancers, their contribution to cancer promotion (i.e., growing the tumor once it is established) is exceptionally important.

The exact mechanisms by which overweight and obesity contribute to cancer initiation and promotion have yet to be firmly established. However,

some hypothesized pathways include increased levels of endogenous hormones or hormone-related factors (e.g., sex steroids, leptin, insulin and insulin-like growth factor-1); decreased levels of binding proteins, which results in higher levels of free circulating hormones; increased availability of substrate such as glucose and free fatty acids; decreased apoptosis via suppressed glucocorticoids; decreased T helper (Th2) factors; and enhanced immune response via various adipokines and eicosanoid-mediated events.[26, 27, 31–33]

Weight gain, which is common during and after treatment for a variety of cancers, reduces quality of life and exacerbates the risk for functional decline and comorbidity.[4, 34–36] Moreover, an overwhelming number of cancer survivors struggle with excess weight, including more than 70% of breast and prostate cancer survivors—the two largest populations of adult cancer survivors in the United States—as well as survivors of acute lymphoblastic leukemia, a prevalent cancer among American children.[28, 37] Although studies exploring the relationship between postdiagnosis weight gain and disease-free survival have been somewhat inconsistent,[4, 35, 36, 38] one of the largest cohort studies found that breast cancer survivors who experienced an increase of at least 0.5 body mass index (BMI) units postdiagnosis had a significantly higher risk of recurrence and all-cause mortality.[35] This accumulating evidence of the adverse effects of obesity in cancer survivors makes weight management a priority for survivorship.[4, 28, 29, 31, 36] Furthermore, the cancer diagnosis may create a teachable moment that may motivate people who have been denying weight gain and delaying action on weight management to participate in health-promoting changes.[4, 5, 39]

Take-Home Message

Patients caring for family members may feel guilty about introducing dietary changes into the family's long-standing way of eating. Fitness professionals can remind these clients that nudging family members toward healthier eating is in fact a caring thing to do, because it can reduce disease risk, particularly for offspring who may be genetically susceptible.

Although the pursuit of a desirable weight can be postponed until primary treatment is complete, fitness professionals should be aware that among patients who are overweight or obese, there are no contraindications to a modest rate of weight loss (no more than 2 lb, or 0.9 kg, per week) during treatment, as long as the oncology care physician approves and it does not interfere with treatment.[4, 34, 36]

The sidebar Nutrient-Dense Eating Strategies for Weight Management offers weight management strategies to recommend for promoting the intake of lower-calorie, nutrient-dense foods. Diets that rely heavily on these foods can aid in weight management, as well as increase the chance of taking in adequate nutrition.

Underweight

On the other end of the scale (literally and figuratively), some patients, such as those with aerodigestive tumors, tend to be underweight at the time of diagnosis. Moreover, these same patients, as well as others, can experience unintended weight loss secondary to treatment-related surgery, chemotherapy, and radiation therapy. In addition, anorexia and cachexia can place some cancer patients at risk for compromised nutritional status.[40–42] In most early-stage cancers, weight loss is fairly rare; however, with more aggressive and later-stage tumors, especially cancers of the lung, gastrointestinal tract, pancreas, head, and neck,

---

Nutrient-Dense Eating Strategies for Weight Management

Eat More

- Fruits and vegetables
  - Slice to make them ready-to-eat while watching TV, for the car trip home, at work.
  - Try homemade fruit smoothies.
- Whole grains
  - Have oatmeal for breakfast.
  - Make sure the first ingredient on your bread or cereal label is a whole grain.
- Broth-based soups
- Foods with high nutrient density (e.g., legumes; dark green, yellow, and orange vegetables; fruits; whole grains; lean meats; nonfat milk products; and, in moderation because of their high fat content, nuts and seeds)

Eat Less (or Fewer)

- Fat (and saturated fat)
  - Trim fat from meats; remove skin from poultry.
  - Broil or bake instead of frying.
  - Choose low-fat dairy products.
  - Ask for salad dressing on the side, and choose low-fat or nonfat dressings.
  - Choose broth- instead of cream-based soups.
  - Use liquid oils (olive and canola oil) instead of solid fat (butter, margarine, shortening, lard).
- Simple sugars
  - Avoid beverages with added sugar or corn syrup. Choose water, unsweetened tea, or diet beverages.
  - Limit added white and brown sugar, honey, molasses, and raw sugar.
  - Limit intake of pies, cakes, candies, and pastries.

Substitute

Legumes and soy meat substitutes for meat and meat products

weight loss is a common and characterizing symptom.[43, 44] The loss of less than 5% of body weight, especially among patients presenting with either a normal or lower BMI, is associated with poorer treatment tolerance and outcomes and poorer quality of life,[44–47] and is a significant predictor of reduced survival rates.[40, 48–50]

Factors that contribute to weight loss, many of which stem from chemotherapy and radiation therapy, include appetite loss, early satiety (feelings of fullness), an altered sense of taste and smell, chewing and swallowing difficulties, nausea, vomiting, diarrhea, and compromised nutrient intake.[4, 41] The sidebar Nutrition Recommendations for Common Symptoms of Cancer Treatment provides recommendations that fitness professionals can propose to address these symptoms among patients, while advising those who experience severe weight loss to seek professional nutritional care.[51] Note: Severe weight loss is indicated by a loss in body weight of >2% per week, >5% per month, >7.5% in three months, or >10% in six months.

Cancer cachexia, most commonly associated with lung and gastrointestinal tract cancers as well as a variety of advanced-staged cancers, differs from typical anorexia-induced starvation.[52] Indeed, the body normally adapts to starvation by triggering metabolic alterations to preserve lean body mass, by shifting toward fat catabolism. With cachexia, however, tumor-induced alterations upset normal tissue repair, wherein cytokines and eicosanoids appear to mediate an inflammatory-like catabolic response in which lean body mass, in addition to stored fat, is lost.[48, 50, 52] Cachexia cannot be reversed by food intake alone,[41, 50, 53] and it becomes imperative to aggressively identify and treat nutrition-related side effects to help stabilize or reverse weight loss.[54] The Nutrition Screening Initiative—a project of the American Academy of Family Physicians, the American Dietetic Association, and the National Council on Aging—devised a brief nutritional screening tool that fitness professionals can use to identify underweight (and overweight) clients requiring intensive professional nutrition therapy (see figure 7.1).

Nutrition Recommendations for Common Symptoms of Cancer Treatment

Anorexia (Loss of Appetite)

- Increase energy- and protein-dense foods such as peanut butter, nuts, milk, cheese, yogurt, eggs, legumes, granola, and dried fruit.
- Eat small, frequent meals, or three small meals plus several snacks.
- Seek out favorite foods and foods that smell good.
- Try bland, unspicy foods.
- Look for foods that smell good.
- Try meal-replacement beverages.

Nausea and Vomiting

- Focus on bland foods.
- Avoid strongly scented foods.
- Take small sips of fluids or suck on ice chips.
- Eat crackers, dry toast, or plain cookies.
- Try beverages such as Gatorade or Pedialyte.
- Rinse mouth before and after eating.

Mucositis or Stomatitis (Mouth Sores)

- Eat foods at room temperature.

- Choose liquids high in nutritional value (milk, 100% juices, meal-replacement drinks); use a straw.

- Cut foods into small pieces.

- Choose soft and soothing foods such as frozen desserts, milkshakes, baby foods, bananas, applesauce, fruit nectars, mashed potatoes, cooked cereals, soft-boiled or scrambled eggs, cottage cheese, macaroni and cheese, puddings, gelatin, pureed foods, and liquid supplements.

- Avoid tomatoes, citrus fruits and juices, salty or spicy foods, raw vegetables and fruits (unless soft and ripe), beverages containing caffeine or alcohol, pickles, vinegar, chocolate, and rough or dry foods (e.g., tortilla chips).

Xerostomia (Dry Mouth)

- Choose foods that are soft and moist, such as hot cereals, soups, tuna or egg salad, smoothies, casseroles, and fruits.

- Drink 8 to 12 cups of fluid per day, suck on ice chips, or try tart foods to stimulate saliva production.

- Avoid
    - Caffeine, alcohol, and alcohol-containing mouthwashes
    - Dry, crumbly foods
    - Salty or spicy foods

Taste and Smell Abnormalities or Food Aversions

- Eat small, frequent meals and snacks.

- Add spices and sauces.

- Eat meats with something sweet.

- Experiment with temperature; cold foods often are acceptable, whereas hot foods may not be.

- Use plastic utensils (if food tastes metallic).

Diarrhea

- Drink 8 to 12 glasses (at least an 8 ounce glass) of fluids, including drinks such as Gatorade or Pedialyte.

- Avoid alcoholic or caffeine-containing beverages.

- Choose eggs, well-cooked; lean meats, poultry, and fish; smooth peanut butter; beans; low-fat milk, yogurt, or cottage cheese; cooked vegetables; fruits without the skin; and desserts low in fat (sorbets, fruit ices, graham crackers).

- Avoid fried or fatty meats; pizza; full-fat milk or cheese; raw vegetables; dried fruits; spicy foods; high-fat desserts or ice creams; candies or gums containing sorbitol, mannitol, or xylitol.

Constipation

Eat more fiber-containing foods (bran, whole grains, fruits, and vegetables).

From American Cancer Society.

Figure 7.1 Determine Your Nutritional Health

The warning signs of poor nutritional health are often overlooked. Use this checklist to find out if you or someone you know is at nutritional risk.

Read the statements below. Circle the number in the yes column for those that apply to you or someone you know. For each yes answer, score the number in the box. Total your nutritional score.

	YES
I have an illness or condition that made me change the kind or amount of food I eat.	2
I eat fewer than two meals per day.	3
I eat few fruits, vegetables, or dairy products.	2
I have three or more drinks of beer, liquor, or wine almost every day.	2
I have tooth or mouth problems that make it hard for me to eat.	2
I don't always have enough money to buy the food I need.	4
I eat alone most of the time.	1
I take three or more different prescribed or over-the-counter drugs a day.	1
Without wanting to, I have lost or gained 10 pounds in the last six months.	2
I am not always physically able to shop, cook, or feed myself.	2
TOTAL	_____

Total your nutritional score. If it's—

0-2   Good! Recheck your nutritional score in six months.

3-5   You are at moderate nutritional risk. See what can be done to improve your eating habits and lifestyle. Your office on aging, senior nutrition program, senior citizens center, or health department can help. Recheck your nutritional score in three months.

6 or more   You are at high nutritional risk. Bring this checklist the next time you see your doctor, dietitian, or other qualified health or social service professional. Talk with them about any problems you may have. Ask for help to improve your nutritional health.

Remember that warning signs suggest risk, but do not represent diagnosis of any condition.

The Nutrition Checklist is based on the warning signs described below. Use the word DETERMINE to remind you of the warning signs.

Disease

Any disease, illness, or chronic condition that causes you to change the way you eat, or makes it hard for you to eat, puts your nutritional health at risk. Four out of five adults have chronic diseases that are affected by diet. Confusion or memory loss that keeps getting worse is estimated to affect one out of five or more of older adults. This can make it hard to remember what, when, or if you've eaten. Feeling sad or depressed, which happens to about one in eight older adults, can cause big changes in appetite, digestion, energy level, weight, and well-being.

Eating Poorly

Eating too little and eating too much both lead to poor health. Eating the same foods day after day or not eating fruit, vegetables, and milk products daily will also cause poor nutritional health. One in five adults skips meals daily. Only 13% of adults eat the minimum amount of fruits and vegetables needed. One in four older adults drinks too much alcohol. Many health problems become worse if you drink more than one or two alcoholic beverages per day.

Tooth Loss or Mouth Pain

A healthy mouth, teeth, and gums are needed to eat. Missing, loose, or rotten teeth or dentures that don't fit well or cause mouth sores make it hard to eat.

Economic Hardship

As many as 40% of older Americans have incomes of less than $6,000 per year. Having less—or choosing to spend less—than $25 to $30 per week for food makes it very hard to get the foods you need to stay healthy.

Reduced Social Contact

One third of all older people live alone. Being with people daily has a positive effect on morale, well-being, and eating.

Multiple Medicines

Many older Americans must take medicines for health problems. Almost one half of older Americans take multiple medicines daily. Growing old may change the way we respond to drugs. The more medicines you take, the greater the chance for side effects such as increased or decreased appetite, change in taste, constipation, weakness, drowsiness, diarrhea, or nausea. Vitamins or minerals when taken in large doses act like drugs and can cause harm. Alert your doctor to everything you take.

Involuntary Weight Loss or Gain

Losing or gaining a lot of weight when you are not trying to do so is an important warning sign that must not be ignored. Being overweight or underweight also increases your chance of poor health.

Needs Assistance in Self-Care

Although most older people are able to eat, one of every five has trouble walking, shopping, buying, and cooking food, especially as they get older.

Elder Years Above Age 80

Most older people lead full and productive lives. But as age increases, risk of frailty and health problems increase. Checking your nutritional health regularly makes good sense.

From ACSM, 2012, *ACSM's guide to exercise and cancer survivorship* (Champaign, IL: Human Kinetics). Reprinted from B. Bagely, 1998, "Nutrition and health," *American Family Physician* (57)5:933-934. American Academy of Family Physicians. Available online at: http://www.aafp.org/afp/980301ap/edits.html

Weight and Height Assessment

Weight status may be the fitness professional's most valuable and accessible tool in assessing cancer-related health status. Even small changes in weight, particularly when unintentional, can be difficult to overcome if not immediately addressed. Because weight changes are common along the cancer continuum from diagnosis and treatment to recovery and survivorship, it is good practice to record a precancer weight as a reference point, and to use this to calculate weight change at each visit.

Weight Change Calculation

$$\frac{\text{Current weight (lbs)} - \text{Precancer weight (lbs)}}{\text{Precancer weight (lbs)}} \times 100 = \text{Percent weight change}$$

Calculating a reasonable body weight can be helpful for setting goals for both the under- and overweight. The Hamwi method is preferred by many clinicians because of its ease of use and commitment to memory:[55]

Hamwi Estimation for Reasonable Body Weight

Women: 100 lb (45 kg) + 5 lb (2.3 kg) for each inch (2.5 cm) in height over 60 in. (152 cm)

Men: 106 lb (48 kg) + 6 lb (2.7 kg) for each inch (2.5 cm) in height over 60 (152 cm)

The fitness professional may wish to adjust for height by adding or subtracting 10% from the resulting value if a person's height is significantly taller

or shorter than average. See table 7.3 for concepts related to weight management in cancer treatment.

People being measured for height should be standing straight, without shoes, heels together, shoulders back, and head level; height is recorded after they have taken and are holding a deep breath. If height cannot be measured because of illness, arm span measurement can serve as a surrogate for height.[56] To be measured this way, the person extends her arms out to her sides, parallel to the floor, with palms facing forward.[57] The distance from one middle fingertip to the other middle fingertip across the shoulders at the clavicle level is measured (in inches) (see figure 7.2). Height can then be calculated using the following formula:[56]

TABLE 7.3   Summary of Weight Management in Cancer Treatment*

Weight status	Definition	Health risks	Goals	Suggested strategies*
Normal weight	BMI = 18.5–24.9**		Optimize nutrient intake; maintain weight.	Visit www.choosemyplate.gov for food group recommendations for desired weight by age, height, and gender.
Underweight Mild underweight Moderate underweight Severe underweight	BMI = <18.5 BMI = 17.0–18.49 BMI = 16.0–16.9 BMI = <16***	Malnutrition, poor prognosis	Stabilize weight; prevent loss of lean body mass; prevent or treat nutrient deficiencies; minimize nutrition-related side effects.	• Eat small, frequent meals (6-8 times a day). • Keep snacks handy. • Eat energy-dense foods when experiencing poor appetite (e.g., dried fruit, sauces and gravies, ice cream). • Consider liquid meal replacements. • Address eating-related symptoms.
Overweight Obese Class I Class II Class III	BMI = 25.0–29.9 BMI = 30 or more 30.0–34.9 35.0–39.9 ≥40.0***	Functional decline; comorbidities (diabetes and cardiovascular disease); cancers of the breast (postmenopausal), colon, kidney, endometrium, gallbladder, pancreas, and gastric cardia (upper stomach); progressive disease	Lose up to 2 lb (0.9 kg) per week (secure doctor's approval if currently receiving primary cancer treatment); increase physical activity and reduce energy intake.	Reduce energy density of diet by doing the following: • Increase fruit and vegetable intake. • Increase the intake of foods that have high fluid or high fiber contents (e.g., broth-based soups, sugar-free gelatin, unbuttered popcorn). • Limit the intake of fat and simple sugar. • Limit the portion sizes of energy-dense foods.

*Combine dietary and physical activity strategies (see chapter 6) to achieve energy deficits.

**A BMI between 18.5 and 22.9 is recommended by WCRF/AICR for optimal health.[5]

***Refer these patients to a registered dietitian.

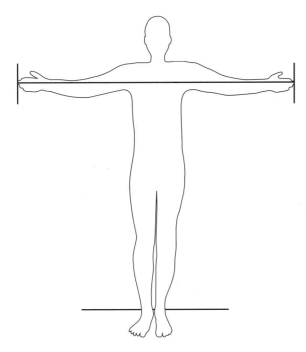

Figure 7.2 Arm span measurement.

Height Calculation (Arm Span Method):

Height (inches) = (0.87 × arm span [inches]) + 20.54

Adiposity and Body Composition

It is important to use caution when evaluating the weight status of cancer patients. Fluid retention from ascites or edema coexisting with lean body mass loss can present a picture of weight stability. Normal weight gain involves increases in both lean and adipose tissue, whereas a distinct form of weight gain, sarcopenic obesity, refers to a weight gain largely composed of fat, but not lean tissue.[58] This phenomenon has been reported in 50 to 90% of breast cancer patients during the time of adjuvant chemotherapy; it has also has been reported with hormonal therapies, as well as in those being treated for solid tumors of the respiratory and gastrointestinal tracts.[59–67] Certain aromatase inhibitors may protect against the development of sarcopenic weight gain, although results are conflicting.[65] Physical activity, particularly resistance training, is currently the cornerstone for both the prevention and treatment of this type of obesity.[58] Fitness professionals are obviously well qualified to play a major role in managing this syndrome.

Also of concern is weight gain secondary to hypothyroidism—found commonly in 15 to 48% of head and neck cancer patients receiving treatments targeting the thyroid gland, but also occurring in people with other cancers as well.[68, 69] Regular examination with periodic thyroid function tests may be warranted in these cancer survivors, because hypothyroidism may go unrecognized, and subsequently, untreated.[68, 69] Be aware that certain symptoms common with hypothyroidism—edema, fatigue, weakness, muscle pain, dry skin—mimic those often stemming from the cancer itself or its treatment.[68]

Adiposity and Body Composition Assessment

Although the use of BMI, or the Quetelet Index, has become a standard assessment technique for estimating obesity of populations, because of the ease of collecting weight and height measurements (see the sidebar BMI Calculation), caution must be used with this approach.[70, 71] Simple weight and height measurements do not distinguish between lean and fat tissue. In fact, because BMI is an assessment of heaviness, it can be abnormally high in those with ascites, edema, a well-developed musculature, or a large, dense skeleton; or abnormally low as a result of muscle wasting or osteoporosis.[72] As such, BMI should be viewed as a proxy for assessing body fatness, and is best used as a screening measure for disease risk:[71, 73]

<18.5 = Underweight

18.5–24.9 = Normal weight

25.0–29.9 = Overweight

30.0–34.9 = Moderate obesity

35.0–39.9 = Severe obesity

≥40 = Very severe or morbid obesity

Within the "normal weight" category, and to maximize health potential, the WCRF/AICR guidelines endorse an even stricter BMI goal range of 18.5 to 22.9 kg/m².[5]

BMI Calculation

Metric: Weight (kg) / height (m)²
U.S. units: Weight (lb) × 703 / height (in)²

Waist circumference (WC) serves as a fairly reliable measure of abdominal fat and has been associated with abnormal blood lipid levels, hypertension, insulin resistance, and diabetes.[70,74] Established indicators of high risk are the WC cut-points >102 cm (>40 in.) for men and >88 cm (>35 in.) for women.[75] In years that predated the U.S. National Institutes of Health consensus report on the identification, evaluation, and treatment of overweight and obesity in adults,[71] the use of a waist-to-hip ratio to assess health risk was common; however, it is used less frequently today, because WC alone is considered a more reliable measure.[74]

The two most commonly used WC assessment techniques are as follows: (1) place the tape at the natural waist, halfway between the lowest rib and the iliac crest (mark the bony protuberances on both sides and then mark the halfway point between the two measures; ensure that your tape covers both halfway marks—see figure 7.3); or (2) place the tape at the umbilicus level (often chosen for obese subjects, because bony protuberances can

be difficult to locate).[76] The tape should be horizontal to the floor, and the patient should exhale slowly prior to the reading, which is observed by pulling the tape so that it is snug, but without compressing the skin. Ideally, nonstretch tape measures with tension-control features (often used in research studies) should be used to obtain the most accurate readings. More important, however is the use of consistent technique across all waist assessments.

Other methods to assess body fat levels (skinfold thickness measurements, dual-energy X-ray absorptiometry [DXA], whole body air-displacement plethysmography [BOD POD], hydrodensitometry [underwater weighing], and bioelectrical impedance) require assessment by a skilled technician using regularly calibrated, and often costly, equipment.[74,77,78] Of note is the fact that although bioelectrical impedance devices are frequently available to the public, consumer models often forgo the standard pretest regimens for hydration, physical activity, and food and beverage consumption; furthermore, they omit the standardization of ambient air and skin temperatures and body electrode positioning (hand + foot) necessary for accurate clinical measurements.[74,79] Another method, near infrared interactance—frequently used in fitness and athletic facilities to estimate body fat—involves sending an electromagnetic signal into the biceps of the nondominant arm.[72] This signal, based on the water, protein, and fat composition of the subject, is scattered and reflected back for measurement. Reference standards for this technique have not yet been validated in humans, and variability of values is fairly broad. Thus, its limitations appear to outweigh its advantages, such as ease of use.[72] In contrast, DXA is increasingly recognized as a gold standard for assessing body composition, and also is able to discern lean and adipose tissue distribution in various body regions. However, as stated earlier, its use may be limited to research endeavors.[74]

To assess muscle mass changes, a measure of mid-arm muscle circumference (MAMC) can be made using a nonstretch, tension-controlled tape.[74] The measure is taken at the midpoint of the upper arm between the acromion process and the tip of the olecranon while the arm hangs naturally by the side with palm facing forward (see figure 7.4). The tape should not compress the skin. Fitness professionals should keep in mind that, at least among

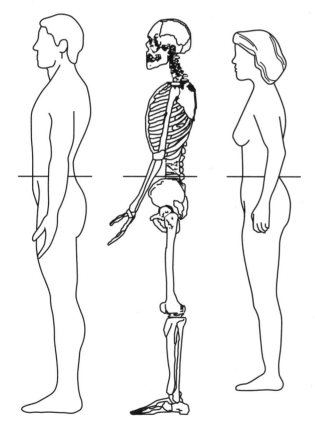

Figure 7.3 Tape placement for waist circumference measurement.

Reprinted from National Heart and Lung Institute 1998. Available: www.nhlbi.nih.gov/guidelines/obesity/e_txtbk/txgd/4142.htm

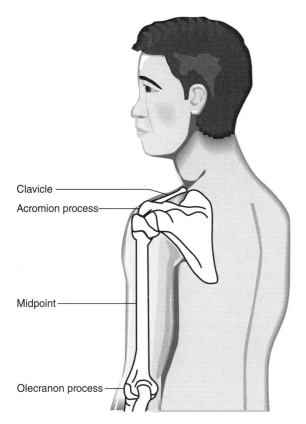

Clavicle

Acromion process

Midpoint

Olecranon process

Figure 7.4 Measure mid-upper-arm circumference by placing the tape at the midpoint.

From ROLFES/PINNA/WHITNEY, *Understanding Normal and Clinical Nutrition*, 8E. © 2009 Brooks/Cole, a part of Cengage Learning, Inc. Reproduced by permission. www.cengage.com/permissions.

Americans, arm fat deposition varies substantially, and the inconsistencies in muscle mass changes identified with this technique may make it less useful for interindividual comparisons.[74]

Energy Consumption and Cancer

In laboratory animals, restricting energy consumption by 60 to 80% of normal slows tumor growth and extends the life span by upwards of 25%.[80, 81] Although it may be difficult to pursue randomized controlled trials of energy restriction in humans, observational data on women undergoing puberty during World War II–imposed food shortages show a reduced lifetime risk of breast cancer when compared against younger and older cohorts.[82] On the other hand, recent results from a large study ($n = 28,098$) conducted over 16 years found that a (self-reported) low calorie intake did not protect against cancer, but this population's level of energy restriction was of lesser magnitude than that found to slow tumor growth in animal models.[83]

To avoid weight gain, energy intake (measured in calories) must be balanced against energy expenditure. Ingestion of 3,500 calories in excess of what is needed—for body metabolism, processing of food, and physical activity—results in approximately 1 pound (0.5 kg) of weight gain. To lose 1 to 2 pounds (0.5 to 1 kg) per week, a person must have a daily deficit of 500 to 1,000 calories (either as reduced intake, increased expenditure, or a combination of both). Trends in population-based data suggest that Americans, in fact, are eating more and exercising less. From 1971 to 2000, calorie intakes increased by 7% in men and 22% in women, while chosen portions, particularly of high-energy dense foods, got larger.[84, 85] At the same time, more time was spent on sedentary work-related activities in lieu of leisure activities. Less physically exerting activities, such as driving a car, office work, and television viewing, became the top three means of energy expenditure, even though these activities burn relatively few calories per hour.[86] Cancer type and stage can alter metabolic rates by 50 to 175% of predicted levels, affecting both energy balance and weight status.[87, 88] An awareness of these associations prepares fitness professionals to work with nutrition professionals to adjust diet and exercise prescriptions to help patients meet their weight goals.

Take-Home Message

Why do most people choose the foods they do? *Because they taste good* is the primary reason. Fitness professionals should discuss with their patients how they can begin to alter their food-related thought processes. Can they begin to eat for health instead? How would that change their food choices?

Total energy needs are comprised of fuel expended (1) at rest (resting metabolic rate [RMR]), (2) during the digestion and absorption of food (approximately 10% of energy intake), (3) during physical activity, and (4) to meet the metabolic demands of compromised health status (e.g., infection, recovery from physical injury or surgery, or disease-related trauma).[72] In most cases, RMR is the primary contributor to energy needs (it accounts for 60 to 75% of the total) and far overshadows energy needs for physical activity.[72] Of note, RMR is largely driven by two factors: external temperature (any deviation from 78 °F, or 26 °C, requires increased energy use) and lean body or muscle mass (i.e., tissue that is metabolically quite active).[72] Exercise can therefore indirectly influence energy needs through its effect on muscle mass—mass that may be diminishing as a result of cancer treatment or the normal aging process, both of which exercise can ameliorate. As stated earlier, cancer also can influence energy needs dramatically—large increases over basal levels may be anticipated if tumor burden is high and/or if the cancer is situated in highly metabolic tissues or in those that directly influence energy balance (e.g., the thyroid gland).

Total energy needs can be measured via direct calorimetry, which requires an overnight stay in a highly sophisticated chamber capable of measuring the amount of heat (directly related to energy use) released by the body.[74] Because this technique is impractical in most clinical settings, other methods have been developed to assess energy needs. The indirect calorimeter determines resting energy needs by measuring oxygen intake and carbon dioxide output with a portable device. This value is then added to energy estimations for food processing, physical activity, and health status. For those without access to an indirect calorimeter, a standard formula to estimate RMR may be used. The Mifflin-St. Jeor equation was deemed most likely to yield results comparable to those obtained with calorimetry:[89]

Men: Resting energy calorie needs =
(9.99 × weight [kg]) + (6.25 × height [cm])
− (4.92 × age [yr]) + 5

Women: Resting energy calorie needs =
(9.99 × weight [kg]) + (6.25 × height [cm])
− (4.92 × age [yr]) − 161

Perhaps more simply, fitness professionals can estimate *total* energy needs for cancer patients and survivors using one of the following formulas:[90, 91]

Obese patients   21–25 calories/kg
Sedentary adults 25–30 calories/kg

Underweight adults   30–35 calories/kg
Severely stressed adults* ≥35 calories/kg

Stress refers to a metabolic derangement common in cancer treatment wherein normal corrective metabolic adaptations do not occur. The oncologist or registered dietitian assesses symptoms and laboratory values to determine the level of stress.

Take-Home Message
When talking about what to eat, patients often are interested in knowing an exact calorie prescription. Fitness professionals should let them know that, without expensive equipment, such calculations are gross estimates at best. It's far better to focus on improving the nutrient density of food choices by reducing fats and sugars and eating more fruits, vegetables, and whole grains. In addition, portion control is also important. Behavioral strategies, such as keeping a journal of the foods consumed, eating slowly and deliberately, and reducing exposure to food also are key strategies for weight management.

The ACS guidelines recommend referral to a registered dietitian of all cancer patients who are having trouble eating or gaining weight.[4] By the same token, a referral often is indicated for patients who require guidance on weight loss diets. If weight loss is indicated, the dietitian will formulate plans that ensure the intake of adequate nutrients, and adjust the patient's energy level to ensure a weight loss of no more than 2 pounds (0.9 kg) per week, because more rapid weight loss is apt to have adverse effects on muscle mass.[58]

Diet Composition and Nutrition Status

The importance of good nutrition to cancer treatment was highlighted in a length-of-stay study that revealed that the average hospital stay of well-nourished patients' was 5.8 days, whereas malnourished patients stayed an average of 13.4 days.[92] Not surprisingly, poorly nourished patients face diminished quality of life and less tolerance of therapy, which may result in lower survival rates.[42] Being overweight or obese does not offer protection from poor nutrition, especially when high-energy but nutrient-devoid diets, which focus on chips, sodas, cakes, and pastries, are consumed consistently.[93, 94]

Fitness professionals can guide food choices based on the ACS and WCRF/AICR guidelines, thereby increasing the likelihood of adequate nutrient intake. One of the easiest ways to encourage the adoption of a healthy diet (i.e., low fat and nutrient dense) is to recommend a plant-based diet. In general, plants (fruits, vegetables, whole grains, nuts, seeds, herbs, and spices) are high in vitamins, minerals, fiber, and phytochemicals; low in fat, cholesterol, sodium, and calories; and associated with a reduced incidence of many types of cancers and diseases common to cancer survivors.[4, 5]

Carbohydrate, Protein, and Fat

Macronutrients—the protein, carbohydrate, and fat components of diet—are essential dietary constituents that provide fuel or energy. (One other dietary component—the alcohol in alcoholic products—provides calories; however, alcoholic beverages have little nutritional value and also may stimulate appetite). Weight gains or losses result from consuming too many or too few calories, but maintenance of a weight within the healthy range does not uniquely indicate optimal nutrition status. A woman needing 1,450 calories to support a desirable weight of 125 pounds (57 kg) could consume those calories as sugar (carbohydrate), gelatin (protein), and butter (fat) to maintain that weight. Then again, with that diet, her micronutrient (vitamin and mineral) profile, and thus her health status, would be quite poor. Indeed, a diet that derives macronutrients from fruits, vegetables, and whole grain breads and cereals (carbohydrate); lean meat, poultry, and fish (protein); and nuts, seeds, avocados, and olive or canola oil (fat) also would include necessary micronutrients and would thus be far superior.

Eating a wide variety of nutrient-dense foods allows all nutrients to work synergistically to help prevent cancer development, disease recurrence, and the occurrence of comorbidities, and

may enhance treatment efficacy. As such, the IOM endorses dietary reference intakes (DRIs) for macronutrients, which directs dietary intake toward decreasing the risk of developing chronic disease.[95] Current IOM recommendations endorse 45 to 65% of energy from carbohydrate, 10 to 35% from protein, and 20 to 35% from fat.

Carbohydrate provides glucose—the body's primary fuel source and the preferred fuel for brain, peripheral nerve, and red blood cell energy. Adequate dietary carbohydrate conserves functional body protein, which is burned as an energy source when dietary carbohydrate is low. One class of dietary carbohydrate, fiber, is largely indigestible, and as such, helps lower the risk of heart disease (by increasing the excretion of cholesterol); it is also associated with improved bowel function.[4] When carbohydrate sources are refined to produce micronutrient-deficient sugars (e.g., white and brown sugars and corn sweeteners), these are often consumed in lieu of more nutritious choices. Food products made with refined sugars, particularly soft drinks and other sugar-sweetened beverages, can add substantially to a diet's energy level, promoting weight gain and thus adversely affecting the outcomes of many cancers.[4] Recommended nutrient-dense foods rich in carbohydrate include fruits, vegetables, whole grains, and low-fat milk (the latter three are sources of both carbohydrate and protein, with low-fat dairy products serving as the richest protein source of the three).

Protein plays fundamental structural and functional roles in all body cells. It acts in cellular signaling, drives reaction response rates, and plays key roles in immune and cellular function, affecting

Take-Home Message

Fitness professionals can use an empty carbonated beverage can to demonstrate how sugar can add up: a 12-ounce (360 ml) drink containing 39 grams (or 9.3 teaspoons) of sugar also contains 156 calories. Over a year, this adds up to 56,940 calories—enough fuel to support 16 pounds (7.3 kg) of body weight. They can ask their patients: Is this a healthy (nutrient-dense) way to fuel those tissues?

both normal and cancer cells. Because many high-protein foods contain large amounts of saturated fat, cancer patients should select lower-saturated-fat protein-rich foods (e.g., lean meat, fish, low-fat milk products, eggs, legumes, nuts, and seeds) to best achieve a heart-healthy diet. Adequate protein intake becomes critical for the cancer patient experiencing tissue destruction as a result of surgery, chemotherapy, or radiation therapy, particularly when these treatments are complicated by diarrhea or malabsorption.[4] The following guidelines can help estimate protein requirements for cancer patients:[91]

Normal or maintenance needs	0.8–1.0 g/kg of body weight
Nonstressed cancer patients	1.0–1.2 g/kg of body weight
Severely stressed cancer patients	1.5–2.5 g/kg of body weight

Inconclusive evidence highlighted by the recent completion of two large clinical trials suggests that total fat consumption affects cancer outcomes. The Women's Healthy Eating and Living (WHEL) study tested a diet low in fat and high in fruits, vegetables, and fiber against usual care in breast cancer survivors followed over seven years.[96] No differences were observed in either disease-free or overall survival; however, these findings have been attributed to high baseline fruit and vegetable intakes in both study arms, as well as an absence of weight loss, despite following the low-energy diet.[97] In contrast, findings of the Women's Intervention Nutrition Study (WINS) differ markedly. In this trial of 2,437 breast cancer survivors followed for five years, the dietary intervention was focused solely on dietary fat restriction (≤15% of energy) and tested against a healthy diet.[98] A significantly reduced risk of recurrence, which was of even greater magnitude in women with estrogen-receptor-negative breast cancer, was observed in the low-fat group. However, the findings may have been confounded by the 6-pound (2.7 kg) weight loss observed within this same group over the course of the study (reinforcing the importance of weight control as a key lifestyle factor in cancer survivors).[97]

Preliminary data suggest that foods high in omega-3 fatty acids (e.g., fish and walnuts) may help with cachexia and enhance the effects of some treatments, and are associated with a reduced risk

for CVD and a lower overall mortality rate.[4] High intakes of omega-6 fatty acids (food sources include corn, cottonseed, and safflower oils, as well as products containing these oils, such as cookies, crackers, snack foods, and salad dressings) interfere with the conversion of plant-based omega-3 fatty acids into their more active forms (eicosapentaenoic acid and docosahexaenoic acid), as well as the overall metabolism of these fats. It is believed that humans evolved on a diet containing a 1:1 ratio of omega-6 to omega-3 essential fatty acids, whereas the U.S. current ratio is between 15:1 and 16.7:1.[99] Thus, there is concern about the potential health risks of the present-day dietary pattern.

Current IOM recommendations for fat intake include limits on saturated fats (<10% of energy) and the elimination of trans fats (i.e., fats that are formed during the hydrogenation process of unsaturated vegetable oils, so as to improve shelf life, transform liquid oils into solid margarines and shortenings, or enhance the texture of baked products).[95, 100] Healthy fat-containing food choices include nuts, seeds, wheat germ, avocados, olive oil, and fatty fish. However, patients may need to be advised that although these foods provide essential nutrients, they also provide many calories; therefore, judicious use is recommended.

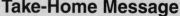

Take-Home Message

Fitness professionals should teach their clients a simple way to choose healthier fats. They should reduce saturated fat intake by limiting animal-based fats (e.g., those found in meats, milk, cheeses) and solid fats, and eat moderate amounts of monounsaturated fats by choosing plant-based fats that, when purified, are typically liquids or oils. Canola and olive oils are good choices.

Fad Diets

Carbohydrate restriction, as proposed by the Atkins diet and other spin-offs in the popular press, may promote weight loss at least in the short term, but their long-term effects are unknown, particularly in cancer survivors.[101] The best available data on successful and long-term weight loss indicate that a relatively low-fat, low-calorie diet is the optimal approach to healthy weight management and should be, of course, combined with regular exercise and behavior modification.[28,102,103] This prescription for weight management is currently endorsed by every U.S. health organization, including the American Cancer Society, American Institute for Cancer Research, World Cancer Research Fund, American Dietetics Association, American Heart Association, Centers for Disease Control, and American Diabetes Association.

Fruits and Vegetables

Because fruits and vegetables are loaded with both fiber and water, they enhance satiety, are low in calories, and may promote healthy weight management. Fruits and vegetables contain multiple nutrients and phytochemicals related to cancer reduction, and although it is not yet known which combination provides the best protection, the U.S. Centers for Disease Control and Prevention, along with the Department of Health and Human Services and the National Cancer Institute, recommend at least seven daily servings for women and nine for men.[104]

Fresh, frozen, and canned fruits and vegetables can all be nutrient-dense food choices. Fresh produce typically has the greatest nutritional value, but long periods in transit, in grocery stores, and on home shelves all contribute to nutrient loss. For this reason, produce frozen immediately after harvest may contain more nutrients than some fresh produce. Canning and drying processes reduce heat-sensitive and water-soluble nutrient content, although foods preserved with these methods may pose less of an infection risk for patients undergoing immunosuppressive cancer treatment.[4] Immunosuppressed patients also should avoid eating unpeeled raw fruits or vegetables because they may contain pathogens, which are destroyed in the cooking process. In terms of cooking methods, microwaving and steaming, instead of boiling, avoids nutrient losses that occur when nutrients leach into cooking water that is then discarded.

Juicing provides a means for increasing fruit and vegetable intake, particularly for those who have difficulty chewing or swallowing. For those concerned about overeating, however, juices do not match the satiety value of whole fruits and vegetables; additionally, when large juice servings are consumed, excess calories can contribute to weight gain. Only 100% juices should be chosen—added sugars detract from the nutrient density of any beverage.

Pesticides

The use of pesticides and herbicides has increased tremendously since the 1940s, and although many have been phased out, their residues may still be in foods eaten today.[5] There is no epidemiological evidence that current exposure levels cause cancer,[5] but for those interested in a cautionary approach, fruits and vegetables may be peeled or washed in lemon juice or vinegar baths to reduce residual surface pesticides. The Environmental Working Group (EWG), a research and advocacy organization based in Washington, D.C., has identified "Dirty Dozen" fruits and vegetables (pears, apples, bell peppers, celery, nectarines, strawberries, cherries, kale, lettuce, and imported grapes and carrots), which may have comparatively higher pesticide residues than other fruits and vegetables; as a result, consumers are advised to buy those raised organically. In contrast, they deem the "Clean 15" (onions, avocados, sweet corn, pineapples, mangos, asparagus, sweet peas, kiwi, cabbage, eggplant, papaya, watermelon, broccoli, tomatoes, and sweet potatoes) to be relatively free of pesticide residues. Given shifting patterns in agriculture and large-scale buying in the free market, it is unknown whether these categorizations will be useful to those seeking to minimize their exposure to pesticides over the long term.

Organic Foods

The term *organic* commonly refers to plant foods grown without pesticides or genetic modifications, or to meat, poultry, and dairy products from animals raised without antibiotics or growth hormones.[4] The FDA sets limits for produce exposure to agricultural chemicals, but as stated previously, it is unknown whether the choice of organic versus inorganic foods influences cancer incidence, recurrence, or progression.[4] With regard to nutrient quality, a recent 50-year systematic literature review found no difference between organically and conventionally produced foodstuffs.[105]

Whole Grains

Whole grains, rich in antioxidants and biologically active compounds, may reduce the risk and progression of cancer.[106] In refined grains both the bran and germ are removed during the milling process, along with other key nutrients, which lessens their protective qualities. In the United State most refined grains are enriched to ensure that certain B vitamins and iron are added back after milling (a legal requirement). Unfortunately, most of the lost nutrients are not replenished through enrichment, nor is fiber.[107] For this reason, people should choose products whose first label ingredient is a whole grain (e.g., brown rice, bulgur, wheat germ, graham flour, whole grain corn, oatmeal, popcorn, pearl barley, whole oats, whole rye, or whole wheat). Note that color alone can be misleading, because many grain products add caramel coloring to mimic the appearance of whole grain products.

Meats and Meat Substitutes

Lean meats provide valuable nutrients, particularly protein, zinc, iron, and vitamins B_6 and B_{12}. Although the iron from red meat (beef, lamb, goat, and pork) is absorbed more readily than the iron from plant sources or supplements, eating red meat may increase the formation of *N*-nitroso compounds that are linked to the development of colon cancer.[5] Carcinogens, such as heterocyclic amines and polycyclic aromatic hydrocarbons, can be generated by cooking meats at high temperatures or by broiling or charbroiling over a direct flame.[5] Processed

meats (those preserved by smoking, curing, salting, or adding preservatives) have been convincingly linked to colorectal cancers.[5]

Compared to animal protein sources, plant-based sources (beans, lentils, peas) have low-saturated-fat and high-phytochemical profiles. There is one caveat, however: Soybean products contain notable concentrations of phytoestrogens, which can mimic biological hormones; their effect on female cancers is still under debate. For this reason, experts recommend that people consume soy in moderate amounts only—no more than three daily servings.[4]

Food Safety

Certain cancer treatment regimens, especially those involving chemotherapy, can induce immunosuppression, which makes people susceptible to infections. For this reason, food safety is of particular concern. All surfaces and implements (including hands) used in food preparation should be thoroughly cleaned, with particular care given to washing surfaces, tools, and sponges that come in contact with raw meats. Cancer patients should cook meats and eggs thoroughly and store all foods promptly at low temperatures to minimize bacterial growth. In restaurants, foods that may be contaminated with bacteria (e.g., sushi, undercooked meats, food in salad bars) should be avoided, especially during times of active treatment.

Nutrition Biomarkers

Biomarkers are substances identified and monitored in body fluids or tissues that allow an assessment of the incidence or biological behavior of a disease, or the health status of the person.[108–110] Registered dietitians evaluate a host of nutrition-related biomarkers, including the following:

- Creatinine height index, nitrogen balance, and albumin and pre-albumin levels as markers of protein status
- C-reactive protein as an indicator of inflammation and increased stress-related nutrition risk
- Delayed cutaneous hypersensitivity and total lymphocyte count to evaluate immunocompetence
- Hematocrit, hemoglobin, and mean corpuscular volume as determinants of vitamin and mineral status

Take-Home Message
Although large meat portions are commonly consumed in the United States and other industrialized nations, an ample protein amount for most adults is two 2- to 3-ounce (60 to 90 g) meat servings per day. A one-finger-sized portion of meat is equivalent to 1 ounce (30 g). Using this rule of thumb to monitor meat intake is a good way to monitor exposure to meat carcinogens. A vegan diet offers another avenue for reducing exposure to the carcinogens contained in meat.

- Serum vitamin D or vitamin B_{12} levels to examine respective vitamin status

Although laboratory tests are available for assessing most vitamins and mineral levels in a person, many of these tests are cost prohibitive and not routinely performed in the clinical setting.[72] Commercial laboratories advertise nutritional assessment via hair, saliva, or toenail analysis; however, with few exceptions (e.g., certain metals in toenails), these compounds are not substantiated indicators of nutritional status. Clinical Laboratory Improvement Amendment (CLIA)-certified facilities are reliable resources for nutrient assessments.

Water and Hydration

Body water content declines with age as a result of both reduced activity and reduced lean body mass. Dehydration can easily occur among cancer patients undergoing chemotherapy or radiation treatments—particularly those who have suffered damage to the esophagus, stomach, or intestines. Drinking sufficient fluids becomes difficult when radiation to the head or neck elicits pain and inflammation in the mouth, throat, and esophagus.[72] Other common cancer treatment–related side effects associated with inadequate hydration are fatigue, light-headedness, and nausea.[4] The thirst mechanism is not always a reliable indicator of fluid needs, particularly in the elderly, who comprise the majority of cancer patients (60% of people with cancer are at least 65 years old).[16] For this reason, fitness professionals should regularly inquire after their clients for signs of dehydration (e.g., dark yellow urine, reduced urination, dry mouth, or rapid weight loss). The following guidelines can help clients estimate their fluid needs:[72, 91]

Maintenance: 30–35 ml/kg of body weight

During cancer treatment: 1 ml fluid per calorie of estimated energy needs

Calcium, Vitamin D, and Osteoporosis

Osteoporosis commonly affects healthy adults over age 50 (one third of American women, one fourth of American men); thus, it should not be surprising that a substantial number of cancer patients have osteoporosis at the time of diagnosis.[111, 112] Various cancer treatments further compromise bone

loss (e.g., hormonal therapies such as glucocorticoids; gonadotropin-releasing hormone agonists; androgen deprivation therapy for prostate cancer; certain chemotherapies such as methotrexate, cyclophosphamide, and fluorouracil for breast cancer; thyroid-stimulating hormone suppressive therapy).[113–115] As a result, osteopenia, osteoporosis, and increased fracture rate have been found in survivors of a wide range of cancer: breast, prostate, testicular, thyroid, gastric, and central nervous system cancers, as well as non-Hodgkin's lymphoma, many hematologic malignancies, and childhood cancers.[115–120]

The goals for patient care include early identification of those at high risk for osteoporosis, as well as prevention of fractures in patients with documented bone deterioration. To address these goals, the American Society of Clinical Oncology advises baseline bone density assessment with continued monitoring and pharmacological treatment based on bone density findings.[121] Fitness professionals can take a proactive stance in reducing bone loss, not only by advocating weight bearing and resistance training exercise, but also by being aware of risk factors: smoking, excessive alcohol intake, low BMI, and poor diet.[122–124] Although the importance of adequate calcium (800 to 1,500 mg/day) and vitamin D (400 to 600 IU/day) in bone formation is well established, a nutrient-dense diet (of which low-fat dairy products are only one part) offers other important contributors to bone health.[125, 126] Excessive caffeine, sodium, protein, or supplemental vitamin A intake may negatively affect calcium absorption and bone turnover.[122, 125]

Take-Home Message
The percentage of fat noted on milk labels can be misleading. Although "2% milk" may imply a small amount of fat, this number refers to the percentage of weight that comprises fat. Practitioners should let their patients know that 2% milk derives 36% of its *calories* from fat, whereas 1% milk derives 21% of its calories from fat. Nonfat milk is the real 2% milk—only 2% of its calories are from fat. Also, because milk fat is an animal fat, it's best to reduce the amount consumed.

Establishing recommendations for vitamin D intake is complicated for the following reasons:

- Exposure to sunlight, not dietary intake, is the major source of vitamin D for most people,[127] and the ability to differentiate oral vitamin D intake from that made endogenously (25-hydroxyvitamin D [25(OH)D]) is limited.[128]

- Food and supplement database values used to assess dietary intakes show excessive variability causing difficulties in quantifying current intakes.[128-130]

- Dose–response relationships are difficult to measure due to variations in serum 25(OH)D assessment techniques compounded by fluctuations in serum levels with respect to study locations (i.e., latitude) and time (seasonality affects the amount of sunlight received).[128]

- Most available data looking at intake dose–response and serum 25(OH)D concentration were drawn from studies designed to measure a single outcome in a specific population (i.e., bone health in white postmenopausal women).[128]

Symptoms of overt vitamin D deficiency (i.e., deep bone and muscle pain) are seen with serum 25(OH)D values <20 nmol/L, whereas subclinical deficiency levels (i.e., those affecting general cellular function but not bone mineralization) are highly controversial, with suggested levels ranging from 27.5 to 100 nmol/L.[131] Serum 25(OH)D levels >75 nmol/L have been proposed to maximize health benefits.[127, 132] Dietary recommendations for adults 31 to 50 years of age are 200 IU per day (for 51 to 70 years, 400 IU; >70 years, 600 IU).[133] Until further evidence is available, high-dosage supplements are not recommended unless blood tests indicate an inadequacy.

Complementary Alternative Medicine and Functional Foods

Complementary and alternative medicine (CAM) refers to the various medical, health, and lifestyle practices and therapies not traditionally part of conventional medicine.[134, 135] Approximately 90% of cancer patients and up to two thirds of adult cancer survivors use some form of CAM therapy, with 69% reporting a belief that such therapies will prevent recurrence and 25% holding the conviction that they will offer cure.[134-136] Nutritional CAM therapies include dietary modification; herbal preparations; vitamin and mineral therapy; and metabolic treatments for detoxification, fasting, and rejuvenation.[134, 136] Little solid data exist to support these methods as cancer treatments. Nevertheless, it is important to recognize that CAM treatments may meet emotional, social, or spiritual needs that remain unaddressed in conventional clinical practices.[72] By the same token, some forms of CAM treatments may be associated with significant side effects. Fitness professionals should openly discuss CAM treatments with their patients and point them to reputable sources of information (e.g., the U.S. National Institutes of Health's Office of Complementary and Alternative Medicine at http://nccam.nih.gov).

Functional Foods

Functional foods include conventional foods and modified foods (i.e., fortified, enriched, or enhanced) that may reduce disease risk, promote optimal health, or both.[137] Tomatoes and tomato products are examples of conventional foods that have been linked to reduced risk for prostate, ovarian, gastric, and pancreatic cancers; and consuming orange juice that has been functionally modified with the addition of calcium may reduce the risk for colorectal cancer.[5, 138]

Manufacturers determine how their functional food products will be regulated (i.e., as a conventional food, food additive, dietary supplement, drug, medical food, or special dietary food) when they write package label claims. These claims determine the quantity and quality of science needed to support their purported health benefits, which can lead to confusion over which products are truly of value.[137] Although research on myriad functional foods is ongoing, and definitive findings and consensus are likely decades away, fitness professionals can play it safe by recommending a diet that contains a variety of conventional plant foods that tend to be rich sources of a variety of anticancer constituents, such as salicylates, phytosterols, saponins, glucosinolates, polyphenols, protease inhibitors, phytoestrogens, sulphides, terpenes, and lectins.[5]

Alternative Dietary Therapies

The belief that specific diets can cure cancer has led to the growth of alternative dietary therapies, typically consisting of vegetable-based or "natural" diets shored up with dietary supplements of mostly unproven value.[139, 140] Of these, the macrobiotic diet is most commonly chosen for cancer treatment, although the Gerson diet also is popular among adult cancer patients.[4, 140] The macrobiotic diet was originally proposed as a Zen-related spiritual climb culminating in a brown rice and water therapy promoted as a cancer cure.[141] In the 1960s, Michio Kushi popularized the diet in the United States and adapted it to include mostly whole cereal grains and vegetables, supplemented with smaller amounts of bean products and sea vegetables, while recommending avoidance of conventional therapy.[141] Although a well-planned macrobiotic diet may be able to meet nutritional needs, special attention is needed to ensure that protein, vitamin B_{12}, calcium, and fluid requirements are met, especially during times of treatment when nutrient needs may be increased.[139, 141]

The Gerson diet was first proposed by a German physician to treat tuberculosis, and he later administered it as a treatment for cancer and other diseases.[139, 141] The diet purports to "detoxify" the body with sodium and fat restrictions, enemas, and potassium supplements, as well as hourly consumptions of raw vegetable-based foods, and supplements of iodine, vitamin B_{12}, thyroid extracts, and pancreatic enzymes.[139-141] Many proponents of the Gerson diet advocate its use in lieu of other scientifically established cancer therapies, which causes obvious concern. Reviews by both the National Cancer Institute and the American Cancer Society have found no evidence that the Gerson diet is of benefit in controlling cancer; in fact, it is associated with several nutritional problems.[4, 139-141]

Dietary Supplements

Limits to the U.S. Food and Drug Administration (FDA)'s ability to regulate dietary supplements (e.g., vitamins, minerals, amino acids, herbs) were established in 1994 with the passage of the Dietary Supplement Health and Education Act.[142] This act allows concentrated nutrient and herbal doses (e.g., pills or powders) to be classified as foods rather than drugs, which effectively frees manufacturers from having to demonstrate product safety or effectiveness. Little evidence suggests that supplements are beneficial for cancer treatment or survival, and a growing number of studies demonstrate harm.[143-148]

Certainly, supplements are warranted when specific risks or deficiencies have been medically identified; unfortunately, problems can arise when patients choose to self-medicate with vitamins or minerals. For example, for the prevention of neural tube defects in offspring, folic acid supplements are prophylactically recommended for women of childbearing age; however, these same supplements are contraindicated for patients receiving certain folate antagonist chemotherapies (e.g., capecitabine, 5-fluorouracil, and methotrexate).[149, 150] Although low-dose multivitamins are generally considered to pose minimal risk, cancer patients should avoid high-dose supplements until the related effects on chemo- or radiation therapies have been medically evaluated.

In light of these data, it is important to reiterate that both the ACS and the WCRF/AICR recommend foods rather than supplements as sources of nutrients. Thus, fitness professionals can provide much-needed guidance in pointing clients to foods that are safer, and perhaps more effective, sources of nutrients (see table 7.4). This is a considerable task given that the majority of cancer survivors (60 to 80%) report supplement use.

Alcohol

Alcohol intake increases the risk for cancers of the mouth, pharynx, larynx, esophagus, liver, and breast; and beer is linked to colon cancer.[4] During treatment for head and neck cancer, continued alcohol consumption is related to higher rates of complication and poorer survival rates; alcohol also exacerbates treatment-related oral mucositis in a variety of patient subgroups. A recent epidemiological review of alcohol intake in more than 1 million women suggests that low to moderate consumption increases the risk of certain cancers (i.e., breast, mouth, pharynx, larynx, esophagus, rectum, and liver), but decreases the risk of others (thyroid and renal cell cancer, and non-Hodgkin's lymphoma).[151]

From a nutritional standpoint, alcohol is a nutrient-poor, calorie-dense beverage that potentially

TABLE 7.4 Nutrient-Dense Food Sources for Selected Food Components

Examples of nutrient-dense food sources	
Nutrients	
Macronutrients	
Carbohydrate	Fruits, vegetables, low-fat milk products, whole grains
Protein	Lean meats and poultry, low-fat milk and milk products, legumes (beans, peas), nuts
Fat	Avocados, nuts, seeds, wheat germ, cold water fish (salmon, mackerel, etc.)
Vitamins	
Vitamin C	Citrus fruits, broccoli, strawberries, tomatoes, dark leafy greens, papayas, peppers
Vitamin D	Fish, fortified milk or ready-to-eat cereal, eggs, mushrooms
Vitamin E	Almonds, pistachios, sunflower seeds, hazelnuts, peanuts, broccoli, spinach
Folate/folic acid	Dark leafy greens, fruits, dried beans and peas, fortified grain products (including ready-to-eat cereals)
Minerals	
Selenium	Brazil nuts, tuna, beef, cod, turkey, enriched pasta, eggs, brown rice
Calcium	Low-fat milk, cheese, and yogurt; dark leafy greens; sardines
Magnesium	Nuts and seeds (pumpkin seeds, almonds, soy nuts, cashews, peanuts, etc.), tofu, beans, oatmeal, spinach, dairy foods
Iron	Clams, meats, legumes, lentils, spinach, ready-to-eat cereals, enriched grain products, raisins and other dried fruit
Potassium	Bananas, oranges, avocados, apricots, sweet potatoes
Fiber	
	Bran, beans, peas, whole grains, strawberries, pears, dark leafy greens
Phytochemicals	
Isothiocyanates	Cabbage, broccoli, cauliflower, kale
Isoflavones	Soy products
Lutein	Yellow and orange fruits and vegetables, dark leafy greens
Lycopene	Tomatoes, tomato products, watermelons, pink grapefruits, apricots, guavas
Phenolic acids	Tomatoes, citrus fruits, strawberries, raspberries, carrots, whole grains, nuts
Polyphenols	Green tea, grapes, wine
Quercetin	Apples, green and black tea, onions, raspberries, red grapes, citrus fruits, dark leafy greens, cherries, broccoli
Terpenes	Cherries, citrus fruit peel

Compiled from information in Whitney and Rolfes[1], 2007, and WCRF/AICR.[5]

contributes to weight management problems and may increase the burden on the liver because it necessitates metabolism via detoxification pathways. On the other hand, when consumed in moderation, alcohol's cardioprotective effects could benefit some cancer survivors, particularly those who are at high risk for CVD (e.g., men with prostate cancer). Certainly, cancer survivors should not be encouraged to initiate alcohol intake if they do not already drink; however, for those free from alcohol-associated cancers, recommendations suggest limiting intake to fewer than two drinks per day for men and one drink per day for women.[4, 5, 152] Fitness professionals should advise clients to consult with their physicians for guidance related to the appropriateness of alcohol use.

Summary

Being adequately nourished is important for everyone, but it is even more important for patients who are undergoing active cancer treatment and for survivors who seek optimal health and well-being after diagnosis and treatment. Fitness professionals can play a key role in detecting nutritional issues, intervening as appropriate, and referring clients needing more specialized care to registered dietitians. In addition, they also can play a key role in reinforcing appropriate nutritional recommendations and motivating clients to adhere to guidelines. Given the interaction and synergy between exercise and diet in governing key issues such as energy balance and overall health, fitness professionals can play an important role in providing sound dietary guidance.

References

1. Whitney E, Rolfes SR. *Understanding Nutrition*. 11th ed. Belmont, CA: Thomson/Wadsworth; 2007.

2. Doll R, Peto R. The causes of cancer: Quantitative estimates of avoidable risks of cancer in the United States today. *J Natl Cancer Inst.* 1981; 66: 1191-1308.

3. Kushi LH, Byers T, Doyle C, Bandera EV, McCullough M, McTiernan A, Gansler T, Andrews KS, Thun MJ, and the American Cancer Society 2006 Nutrition and Physical Activity Guidelines Advisory Committee. American Cancer Society Guidelines on Nutrition and Physical Activity for cancer prevention: Reducing the risk of cancer with healthy food choices and physical activity. *CA Cancer J Clin.* 2006; 56: 254-281.

4. Doyle C, Kushi LH, Byers T, Courneya KS, Demark-Wahnefried W, Grant B, McTiernan A, Rock CL, Thompson C, Gansler T, Andrews KS. Nutrition and physical activity during and after cancer treatment: An American Cancer Society guide for informed choices. *CA Cancer J Clin.* 2006; 56: 323-353.

5. World Cancer Research Fund/American Institute for Cancer Research (AICR). *Food, Nutrition, Physical Activity, and the Prevention of Cancer: A Global Perspective.* Washington DC: AICR; 2007.

6. Aziz NM. Cancer survivorship research: State of knowledge, challenges and opportunities. *Acta Oncol.* 2007; 46: 417-432.

7. Chen Z, Maricic M, Bassford TL, Pettinger M, Ritenbaugh C, Lopez AM, Barad DH, Gass M, Leboff MS. Fracture risk among breast cancer survivors: Results from the Women's Health Initiative Observational Study. *Arch Intl Med.* 2005; 165: 552-558.

8. Chen Z, Maricic M, Pettinger M, Ritenbaugh C, Lopez AM, Barad DH, Gass M, Leboff MS, Bassford TL. Osteoporosis and rate of bone loss among postmenopausal survivors of breast cancer. *Cancer.* 2005; 104: 1520-1530.

9. Fouad MN, Mayo CP, Funkhouser EM, Irene Hall H, Urban DA, Kiefe CI. Comorbidity independently predicted death in older prostate cancer patients, more of whom died with than from their disease. *J Clin Epidemiol.* 2004; 57: 721-729.

10. Herman DR, Ganz PA, Petersen L, Greendale GA. Obesity and cardiovascular risk factors in younger breast cancer survivors: The Cancer and Menopause Study (CAMS). *Breast Cancer Res Treat.* 2005; 93: 13-23.

11. Jemal A, Clegg LX, Ward E, Ries LA, Wu X, Jamison PM, Wingo PA, Howe HL, Anderson RN, Edwards BK. Annual report to the nation on the status of cancer, 1875-2001, with a special feature regarding survival. *Cancer.* 2004; 101: 3-27.

12. Ketchandji M, Kuo Y-F, Shahinian VB, Goodwin, JS. Cause of death in older men after the diagnosis of prostate cancer. *J Am Getriatr Soc.* 2009; 57: 24-30.

13. Michaelson MD, Cotter SE, Gargollo PC, Zietman AL, Dahl DM, Smith MR. Management of complications of prostate cancer treatment. *CA Cancer J Clin.* 2008; 58: 196-213.

14. Ng AK, Travis LB. Second primary cancers: An overview. *Hematol Oncol Clin North Am.* 2008; 22: 271-289.

15. Oeffinger KC, Nathan PC, Kremer LC. Challenges after curative treatment for childhood cancer and long-term follow up of survivors. *Pediatr Clin North Am.* 2008; 55: 251-273.

16. Rowland J, Mariotto A, Aziz N, Tesauro G, Feuer EJ, Blackman D, Thompson P, Pollack LA. Cancer survivorship—United States. 1971-2001. *MMWR.* 2004; 53: 526-529.

17. Brown ML, Riley GF, Potosky AL, Etzioni RD. Obtaining long-term disease specific costs of care: Application to Medicare enrollees diagnosed with colorectal cancer. *Med Care.* 1999; 37: 1249-1259.

18. Chang S, Long SR, Kutikova L, Bowman L, Finley D, Crown WH, Bennett CL. Estimating the cost of cancer: Results on the basis of claims data analyses for cancer patients diagnosed with seven types of cancer during 1999 to 2000. *J Clin Oncol.* 2004; 22: 3524-3530.

19. Ramsey SD, Berry K, Etzioni R. Lifetime cancer-attributable cost of care for long term survivors of colorectal cancer. *Am J Gastroenterol.* 2002; 97: 440-445.

20. Schultz PN, Beck ML, Stava C, Vassilopoulou-Sellin R. Health profiles in 5836 long-term cancer survivors. *Intl J Cancer.* 2003; 104: 488-495.

21. Stokes ME, Thompson D, Montoya EL, Weinstein MC, Winer EP, Earle CC. Ten-year survival and cost following breast cancer recurrence: Estimates from SEER-medicare data. *Value Health.* 2008; 11: 213-220.

22. Yabroff KR, Lawrence WF, Clauser S, Davis WW, Brown ML. Burden of illness in cancer survivors: Findings from a population-based national sample. *J Natl Cancer Inst.* 2004; 96: 1322-1330.

23. Fairley TL, Pollack LA, Moore AR, Smith JL. Addressing cancer survivorship through public health: An update from the Centers for Disease Control and Prevention. *J Women's Health.* 2009; 18: 1525-1531.

24. Hewitt M, Rowland JH, Yancik R. Cancer survivors in the United States: Age, health, and disability. *J Gerontol A Biol Sci Med Sci.* 2003; 58: 82-91.

25. Hewitt M, Greenfield S, Stovall EL. *Institute of Medicine and National Research Council: From Cancer Patient to Cancer Survivors: Lost in Transition.* Washington, DC: National Academies Press; 2005.

26. American Society of Clinical Oncology. *ASCO Curriculum: Cancer Prevention.* Alexandria, VA: American Society of Clinical Oncology; 2007.

27. Calle EE, Rodriguez C, Walker-Thurmond K, and Thun MJ. Overweight, obesity, and mortality from cancer in a prospectively studied cohort of U.S. adults. *N Eng J Med.* 2003; 348(17): 1625-1638.

28. Demark-Wahnefried W, Jones LW. Promoting a healthy lifestyle among cancer survivors. *Hematol Oncol Clin North Am.* 2008; 22(2): 319-342.

29. Irwin ML, Mayne ST. Impact of nutrition and exercise on cancer survival. *Cancer J.* 2008; 14: 435-441.

30. Wolin KY, Colditz GA. Can weight loss prevent cancer? *Br J Cancer.* 2008; 99: 995-999.

31. Chlebowski RT, Aiello E, McTiernan A. Weight loss in breast cancer patient management. *J Clin Oncol.* 2002; 20: 1128-1143.

32. Irwin ML, McTiernan A, Bernstein L, Gilliland FD, Baumgartner R, Baumgartner K, Ballard-Barbash R. Relationship of obesity and physical activity with C-peptide, leptin, and insulin-like growth factors in breast cancer survivors. *Cancer Epidemiol Biomarkers Prev.* 2005; 14(12): 2881-2888.

33. McTiernan A. Obesity and cancer: The risks, science, and potential management strategies. *Oncology.* 2005; 19(7): 871-881.

34. Brown JK, Byers T, Doyle C, et al. Nutrition and physical activity during and after cancer treatment: An American Cancer Society guide for informed choices. *CA Cancer J Clin.* 2003; 53: 268-291.

35. Kroenke CH, Chen WY, Rosner B, Holmes MD. Weight, weight gain, and survival after breast cancer diagnosis. *J Clin Oncol.* 2005; 23: 1370-1378.

36. Rock CL, Demark-Wahnefried W. Nutrition and survival after the diagnosis of breast cancer: A review of the evidence. *J Clin Oncol.* 2002; 20: 3302-3316.

37. Demark-Wahnefried W, Peterson B, McBride C, Lipkus I, Clipp E. Current health behaviors and readiness to pursue lifestyle changes among men and women diagnosed with early stage prostate and breast carcinomas. *Cancer.* 2000; 88: 674-684.

38. Caan B, Sternfeld B, Gunderson E, Coates A, Quesenberry C, Slattery ML. Life After Cancer Epidemiology (LACE) Study: A cohort of early stage breast cancer survivors (United States). *Cancer Causes Control.* 2005; 16: 545-556.

39. Demark-Wahnefried W, Aziz NM, Rowland JH, Pinto BM. Riding the crest of the teachable moment: Promoting long-term health after the diagnosis of cancer. *J Clin Oncol.* 2005; 23(24): 5814-5830.

40. Duguet A, Bachmann P, Lallemand Y, Blanc-Vincent MP. Summary report of the standards, options and recommendations for malnutrition and nutritional assessment in patients with cancer (1999). *Br J Cancer.* 2003; 89(Supp 1): S92-S97.

41. Smith JL, Malinauskas BM, Garner KJ, Barber-Heidal K. Factors contributing to weight loss, nutrition-related concerns and advice received by adults undergoing cancer treatment. *Adv Med Sci.* 2008; 53. doi:10.2478/v10039-008-0019-7

42. Wilkes G. Nutrition: The forgotten ingredient in cancer care. *Am J Nurs.* 2000; 100(4): 46-51.

43. Huhmann MB, August DA. Review of American Society for Parenteral and Enteral Nutrition (A.S.P.E.N.) clinical guidelines for nutrition support in cancer patients: Nutrition screening and assessment. *Nutr Clin Pract.* 2008; 23: 182-188.

44. Capuano GG, Gentile PC, Bianciardi F, Tosti M, Palladino A, Di Palma M. Prevalence and influence of malnutrition on quality of life and performance status in patients with locally advanced head and neck cancer before treatment. *Support Care Cancer.* 2009. doi: 10.1007/s00520-009-0681-8

45. Gupta DD, Lis CG, Granick J, Grutsch JF, Vashi PG, Lammersfeld CA. Malnutrition was associated with poor quality of life in colorectal cancer: A retrospective analysis. *J Clin Epidemiol.* 2006; 59: 704-709.

46. Ravasco P, Monteiro GI, Marques VP, Camilo ME. Nutritional deterioration in cancer: The role of disease and diet. *Clin Oncol.* 2003; 15: 443-450.

47. Ravasco P, Monteiro Grillo I, Marques Vidal P, Camilo ME. Cancer disease and nutrition are keys determinants of patients' quality of life. *Support Care Cancer.* 2004; 12: 246-252.

48. Bosaeus I, Daneryd P, Lundholm K. Dietary intake, resting energy expenditure, weight loss and survival in cancer patients. *J Nutr.* 2002; 132: 3465S-3466S.

49. Bozzetti F and the SCRINIO Working Group. Screening the nutritional status in oncology: A preliminary report on 1,000 participants. *Support Care Cancer.* 2008. doi: 10.1007/s00520-008-0476-3

50. Hopkinson JB, Wright DNM, Foster C. Management of weight loss and anorexia. *Ann Oncol.* 2008; 19(Suppl 7): vii289-vii293.

51. Blackburn GL, Bistrian BR, Maini BS, et al. Nutritional and metabolic assessment of the hospitalized patient. *J Parenter Enteral Nutr.* 1977; 1(1): 11-22.

52. Tisdale MJ. Cachexia in cancer patients. *Nat Rev.* 2002; 2: 862-871.

53. Finley, JP. Management of cancer cachexia. *AACN Clinical Issues: Advanced Practice in Acute & Critical Care.* 2000; 11(4): 590-603.

54. Ottery FD, Kasenic S, DeBolt S, Rodgers K. Volunteer network accrues >1900 patients in 6 months to validate standardized nutritional triage. *Proceedings of ASCO.* 1998; 17: abstract 282.

55. Hamwi GJ. Changing dietary concepts. In: Donowski TS, ed. *Diabetes Mellitus: Diagnosis and Treatment.* New York: American Diabetes Association; 1964: 74.

56. Brown JK, Whittemore KT, Knapp TR. Is arm span an accurate measure of height in young and middle aged adults? *Clin Nurs Res.* 2000; 9: 84-94.

57. McMahon K, Brown JK. Nutritional screening and assessment. *Seminar Oncol Nurs.* 2000; 16(2): 106-112.

58. Heber D, Ingles S, Ashley JM, et al. Clinical detection of sarcopenic obesity by bioelectrical impedance analysis. *Amer J Clin Nutr.* 1996; 64: 472S-477S.

59. Demark-Wahnefried W, Peterson BL, Winer EP, et al. Changes in weight, body composition and factors influencing energy balance among premenopausal breast cancer patients receiving adjuvant chemotherapy. *J Clin Oncol.* 2001; 19(9): 2367-2369.

60. Ali PA, al-Ghorabie FH, Evans CJ, el-Sharkawi AM, Hancock DA. Body composition measurements using DXA and other techniques in tamoxifen-treated patients. *Appl Radiat Isot.* 1998; 49(5-6): 643-645.

61. Aslani A, Smith RC, Allen BJ, et al. Changes in body composition during breast cancer chemotherapy with the CMF-regimen. *Breast Cancer Res Treat.* 1999; 57: 285-290.

62. Demark-Wahnefried W, Hars V, Conaway MR, et al. Reduced rates of metabolism and decreased physical activity in breast cancer patients receiving adjuvant chemotherapy. *Amer J Clin Nutr.* 1997; 65: 1495-1501.

63. Demark-Wahnefried W, Rimer BK, Winer EP. Weight gain in women diagnosed with breast cancer. *J Am Diet Assoc.* 1997; 97: 519-529.

64. Francini G, Petrioli R, Montagnani A, Cadirni A, Campagna S, Francini E, Gonnelli S. Exemestane after tamoxifen as adjuvant hormonal therapy in postmenopausal women with breast cancer: Effects on body composition and lipids. *Br J Cancer.* 2006; 95: 153-158.

65. Goodwin PJ, Ennis M, Pritchard KI, McCready D, Koo J, Sidlofsky S, Trudeau M, Hood N, Redwood S. Adjuvant treatment and onset of menopause predict weight gain after breast cancer diagnosis. *J Clin Oncol.* 1999; 17: 120-129.

66. Kutynec Cl, McCargar L, Barr SI, et al. Energy balance in women with breast cancer during adjuvant chemotherapy. *J Amer Diet Assoc.* 1999; 99: 1222-1227.

67. Prado CMM, Lieffers JR, McCargar LJ, Reiman T, Sawyer MB, Martin L, Baracos VE. Prevalence and clinical implications of sarcopenic obesity in patients with solid tumours of the respiratory and gastrointestinal tracts: A population-based study. *Lancet Oncol.* 2008; 9: 629-635.

68. Miller MC, Agrawal A. Hypothyroidism in postradiation head and neck cancer patients: Incidence, complications, and management. *Curr Opin Otolaryng Head Neck Surg.* 2009; 17: 111-115.

69. Tell R, Lundell GO, Nilsson B, Odin HSJ, Lewin F, Lewensohn R. Long-term incidence of hypothyroidism after radiotherapy in patients with head and neck cancer. *Int J Radiation Oncol Biol Phys.* 2004; 60: 395-400.

70. Expert Panel on the Identification, Evaluation, and Treatment of Overweight in Adults. Clinical guidelines on the identification, evaluation, and treatment of overweight and obesity in adults: Executive summary. *Am J Clin Nutr.* 1998; 68: 899-917.

71. National Institutes of Health. *Clinical Guidelines on the Identification, Evaluation, and Treatment of Overweight and Obesity in Adults.* 1998; NIH Publication 98-4083.

72. Nelms M, Sucher K, Long S. *Nutrition Therapy and Pathophysiology.* Belmont, CA: Thomson Brooks/ Cole; 2007.

73. World Health Organization. BMI classification. http://apps.who.int/bmi/index/jsp?introPage=intro_3.html. Accessed December 23, 2009.

74. Gibson RS. *Principles of Nutritional Assessment.* 2nd ed. New York: Oxford University Press; 2005.

75. Lean MEJ, Han TS, Morrison CE. Waist circumference as a measure for indicating need for weight management. *BMJ.* 1995; 311: 158-161.

76. Lohman TG, Roche AF, Martorell R. *Anthropometric Standardization Reference Manual.* Champaign, IL: Human Kinetics; 1988.

77. Clasey JL, Bouchard C, Teates CD, Riblett JE, Thorner MO, Hartman ML, Weltman A. The use of anthropometric and dual-energy X-ray absorptiometry (DXA) measures to estimate total abdominal and abdominal visceral fat in men and women. *Obesity Research.* 1999; 7(3): 256.

78. Fields DA, Hunter GR, and Goran MI. Validation of the BOD POD with hydrostatic weighing: Influence of body clothing. *Intl J Obes.* 2000; 24: 200-205.

79. Buzzell PR, Pintauro SJ. Bioelectrical impedance analysis (tutorial). University of Vermont, Department of Nutrition and Food Sciences. http://nutrition.uvm.edu/bodycomp/bia. Accessed September 21, 2009.

80. Berrigan D, Perkins SN, Haines DC, et al. Adult-onset calorie restriction and fasting delay spontaneous tumorigenesis in p53-deficient mice. *Carcinogenesis*. 2002; 23: 817-822.

81. Hursting SD, Lavigne JA, Berrigan D, et al. Calorie restriction, aging, and cancer prevention: Mechanisms of action and applicability to humans. *Ann Rev Med*. 2003; 54: 131-152.

82. Tretli S, Gaard M. Lifestyle changes during adolescence and risk of breast cancer: An ecologic study of the effect of World War II in Norway. *Cancer Causes Control*. 1996; 7: 507-583. Leosdottir M, Nilsson P, Nilsson JA, et al. The association between total energy intake and early mortality: Data from the Malmo Diet and Cancer Study. *J Intern Med*. 2004; 256: 499-509.

84. Centers for Disease Control and Prevention. Overweight and obesity. www.cdc.gov/obesity/data/index.html. Accessed November 2, 2009.

85. National Heart, Lung, and Blood Institute. Obesity Education Initiative (OEI) Slide Sets. http://hin.nhlbi.nih.gov/oei_ss/menu.htm#sl2. Accessed November 2, 2009.

86. Centers for Disease Control and Prevention. Behavioral Risk Factor Surveillance System. www.cdc.gov/BRFSS. Accessed November 2, 2009.

87. Knox LS, Crosby LO, Feurer ID, et al. Energy expenditure in malnourished cancer patients. *Ann Surg*. 1983; 197: 152-161.

88. Pi-Sunyer FX. Overnutrition and undernutrition as modifiers of metabolic processes in disease states. *Am J Clin Nutr*. 2000; 72: 533S-537S.

89. Frankenfield D, Roth-Yousey L, Compher C. Comparison of predictive equations for resting metabolic rate in healthy nonobese and obese adults: A systematic review. *J Am Diet Assoc*. 2005; 105(5): 775-789.

90. Martin C. Calorie, protein, fluid and micronutrient requirements. In: MacCallum PD, Polisena CG, editors. *The Clinical Guide to Oncology Nutrition*. Chicago: American Dietetic Association; 2000: 45.

91. Hurst JD, Gallagher AL. Energy, macronutrient, micronutrient, and fluid requirements. In: Elliott L, Molseed LL, McCallum PD, eds. *The Clinical Guide to Oncology Nutrition*. 2nd ed. Chicago: The American Dietetic Association; 2006.

92. Ottery FD. Definition of standardized nutritional assessment and interventional pathways in oncology. *Nutr*. 1996; 12(1): S15-S19.

93. Caballero B. A nutrition paradox—Underweight and obesity in developing countries. *N Eng J Med*. 2005; 352: 1514-1516.

94. Markovic TP, Natoli SJ. Paradoxical nutritional deficiency in overweight and obesity: The importance of nutrient density. *Med J Aust*. 2009; 190(3): 149-151.

95. Institute of Medicine. *Dietary Reference Intakes for Energy, Carbohydrate, Fiber, Fat, Fatty Acids, Cholesterol, Protein, and Amino Acids (Macronutrients)*. Washington, DC: National Academy Press; 2002.

96. Pierce JP, Natarajan L, Caan BJ, et al. Influence of a diet very high in vegetables, fruit, and fiber and low in fat on prognosis following treatment for breast cancer: The Women's Healthy Eating and Living (WHEL) randomized trial. *JAMA*. 2007; 298: 289-298.

97. Gapstur SM, Khan S. Fat, fruits, vegetables, and breast cancer survivorship. *JAMA*. 2007; 298(3): 335-336.

98. Chlebowski RT, Blackburn GL, Thomson CA, et al. Dietary fat reduction and breast cancer outcome: Interim efficacy results from the Women's Intervention Nutrition Study. *J Natl Cancer Inst*. 2006; 98(24): 1767-1776.

99. Simopoulos AP. The importance of the omega-6/omega-3 fatty acid ratio in cardiovascular disease and other chronic diseases. *Exp Biol Med*. 2008; 233: 674-688.

100. Lopez-Garcia E, Schulze MB, Meigs JB, Manson JE, Rifai N, Stampfer MJ, Willett WC, Hu FB. Consumption of trans fatty acids is related to plasma biomarkers of inflammation and endothelial dysfunction. *J Nutr*. 2005; 135(3): 562-566.

101. Katz DL. Pandemic obesity and the contagion of nutritional nonsense. *Public Health Rev*. 2003; 31: 33-44.

102. Katz DL. Competing dietary claims for weight loss: Finding the forest through truculent trees. *Ann Rev Public Health*. 2005; 26: 61-88.

103. Freedman MR, King J, Kennedy E. Popular diets: A scientific review. *Obes Res*. 2001; 9(Suppl 1): 1S-40S.

104. Centers for Disease Control and Prevention, the Department of Health and Human Services, and the National Cancer Institute. Eat a variety of fruits & vegetables every day. www.fruitsandveggiesmatter.gov. Accessed December 3, 2009.

105. Dangour AD, Dodhia SK, Hayter A, Allen E, Lock K, Uauy R. Nutritional quality of organic foods: a systematic review. *Am J Clin Nutr*. 2009. doi: 10.3945/ajcn.2009.28041

106. Slavin J. Why whole grains are protective: Biological mechanisms. *Proc Nutr Soc*. 2003; 62: 129-134.

107. Weaver G. A miller's perspective on the impact of health claims. *Nutr Today*. 2001; 36(3): 115-119.

108. Branca F, Hanley AB, Pool-Zobel B, Verhagen H. Biomarkers in disease and health. *Br J Nutr*. 2001; 85: S55-S92.

109. Crews H, Alink G, Andersen R, Braesco V, Holst B, Maiani G, Ovesen L, Scotter M, Solfrizzo M, van den Berg R, Verhagen H, Williamson G. A critical assessment of some biomarker approaches linked with dietary intake. *Br J Nutr*. 2001; 86: S5-S35.

110. Davis CD, Milner JA. Biomarkers for diet and cancer prevention research: Potentials and challenges. *Acta Pharmacol Sin.* 2007; 28(9): 1262-1273.

111. Nelson RL, Turyk M, Kim J, et al. Bone mineral density and the subsequent risk of cancer in the NHANES I follow-up cohort. *BMC Cancer.* 2002; 2(1): 22.

112. Twiss JJ, Waltman N, Ott CD, et al. Bone mineral density in postmenopausal breast cancer survivors. *J Am Acad Nurse Pract.* 2001; 13: 276-284.

113. Chlebowski RT. Bone health in women with early-stage breast cancer. *Clin Breast Cancer.* 2005; 5 Suppl: S35-S40.

114. Krupski TL, Smith MR, Lee WC, Pashos CL, Brandman J, Wang Q, Botteman M, Litwin MS. Natural history of bone complications in men with prostate carcinoma initiating androgen deprivation therapy. *Cancer.* 2004; 101: 541-549.

115. Mackey JR, Joy AA. Skeletal health in postmenopausal survivors of early breast cancer. *Int J Cancer.* 2005; 114: 1010-1015.

116. Arikoski P, Voutilainen R, Kroger H. Bone mineral density in long-term survivors of childhood cancer. *J Pediatr Endocrinol Metab.* 2003; 16 Suppl 2: 343-353.

117. Greenspan SL, Coates P, Sereika SM, et al. Bone loss after initiation of androgen deprivation therapy in patients with prostate cancer. *J Clin Endocrinol Metab.* 2005; 90: 6410-6417.

118. Kelly J, Damron T, Grant W, et al. Cross-sectional study of bone mineral density in adult survivors of solid pediatric cancers. *J Pediatr Hematol Oncol.* 2005; 27: 248-253.

119. Lee H, McGovern K, Finkelstein JS, et al. Changes in bone mineral density and body composition during initial and long-term gonadotropin-releasing hormone agonist treatment for prostate carcinoma. *Cancer.* 2005; 104: 1633-1637.

120. Smith MR. Therapy insight: Osteoporosis during hormone therapy for prostate cancer. *Nat Clin Pract Urol.* 2005; 2: 608-615.

121. Hillner BE, Ingle JN, Chlebowski RT, et al. American Society of Clinical Oncology 2003 update on the role of bisphosphonates and bone health issues in women with breast cancer. *J Clin Oncol.* 2003; 21: 4042-4057.

122. Davison KS, Kendler DL, Ammann P, Bauer DC, Dempster DW, Dian L, Hanley DA, Harris ST, McClung MR, Olszynski WP, Yuen CK. Assessing fracture risk and effects of osteoporosis drugs: Bone mineral density and beyond. *Am J Med.* 2009; 122: 992-997.

123. Gass M, Dawson-Hughes B. Preventing osteoporosis-related fractures: An overview. *Am J Med.* 2006; 119: S3-S11.

124. National Osteoporosis Foundation. Prevention. www.nof.org. Accessed October 27, 2009.

125. Cashman KD. Diet, nutrition, and bone health. *J Nutr.* 2007; 137: 2507S-2512S.

126. Prynne CJ, Mishra GD, O'Connell MA, Muniz G, Laskey MA, Yan L, Prentice A, Ginty F. Fruit and vegetable intakes and bone mineral status: A cross-sectional study in 5 age and sex cohorts. *Am J Clin Nutr.* 2006; 83: 1420-1428.

127. Holick MF, Chen TC. Vitamin D deficiency: A worldwide problem with health consequences. *Am J Clin Nutr.* 2008; 87(Suppl): 1080S-1086S.

128. Chung M, Balk EM, Brendel M, Ip S, Lau J, Lee J, Lichtenstein A, Patel K, Raman G, Tatsioni A, Terasawa T, Trikalinos TA. Vitamin D and Calcium: *A Systematic Review of Health Outcomes.* Evidence Report No. 183. AHRQ Publication No. 09-E015. Rockville, MD: Agency for Healthcare Research and Quality; 2009.

129. Holden JM, Lemar LE, Exler J. Vitamin D in foods: Development of the US Department of Agriculture database. *Am J Clin Nutr.* 2008; 87(Suppl): 1092S-1096S.

130. Yetley EA, Brule D, Cheney MC, et al. Dietary Reference Intakes for vitamin D: Justification for a review of the 1997 values. *Am J Clin Nutr.* 2009; 89: 719-727.

131. Calvo MS, Whiting SJ. Prevalence of vitamin D insufficiency in Canada and the United States: Importance to health status and efficacy of current food fortification and dietary supplement use. *Nutr Rev.* 2003; 61(3): 107-113.

132. Vieth R, Bischoff-Ferrari H, Boucher BJ, et al. The urgent need to recommend an intake of vitamin D that is effective (editorial). *Am J Clin Nutr.* 2007; 85: 649-650.

133. Institute of Medicine. *Dietary Reference Intakes for Calcium, Phosphorus, Magnesium, Vitamin D, and Fluoride.* Washington DC: National Academy Press; 1997.

134. Molseed LL. Complementary and alternative medicine. In: Elliott L, Molseed LL, McCallum, Grant B, eds. *The Clinical Guide to Oncology Nutrition.* 2nd ed. Chicago: American Dietetic Association; 2006.

135. Hann DM, Baker F, Roberts CS, et al. Use of complementary therapies among breast and prostate cancer patients during treatment: A multisite study. *Integr Cancer Ther.* 2005; 4: 294-300.

136. Yates JS, Mustian KM, Morrow GR, Gillies LJ, Padmanaban D, Atkins JN, Issell B, Kirshner JJ, Colman LK. Prevalence of complementary and alternative medicine use in cancer patients during treatment. *Support Care Cancer.* 2005; 13: 806-811.

137. American Dietetic Association. Position of the American Dietetic Association: Functional foods. *J Am Diet Assn.* 2009; 109: 735-746.

138. Kavanaugh CJ, Trumbo PR, Ellwood KC. The U.S. Food and Drug Administration's evidence-based

review for qualified health claims: Tomatoes, lycopene, and cancer. *J Natl Cancer Inst*. 2007; 99: 1074-1085.

139. Maritess C, Small S, Waltz-Hill M. Alternative nutrition therapies in cancer patients. *Semin Oncol Nurs*. 2005; 21(3): 173-176.

140. Weitzman S. Complementary and alternative (CAM) dietary therapies for cancer. *Pediatr Blood Cancer*. 2008; 50: 494-497.

141. American Cancer Society. Questionable methods of cancer management: 'Nutritional' therapies. *CA Cancer J Clin*. 1993; 43: 309-319.

142. ADA. Position of the American Dietetic Association: Nutrient supplementation. *J Am Diet Assn*. 2009; 109: 2073-2085.

143. The Alpha-Tocopherol, Beta Carotene Cancer Prevention Study Group. The effect of vitamin E and beta carotene on the incidence of lung cancer and other cancers in male smokers. *N Eng J Med*. 1994; 330: 1029-1035.

144. Bjelakovic G, Nikolova D, Gluud LL, Simonetti RG, Gluud C. Mortality in randomized trials of antioxidant supplements for primary and secondary prevention: Systematic review and meta-analysis. *JAMA*. 2007; 297: 842-857.

145. Cole BF, Baron JA, Sandler RS, Haile RW, Ahnen DJ, Bresalier RS, McKeown-Eyssen G, Summers RW, Rothstein RI, Burke CA, Snover DC, Church TR, Allen JI, Robertson DJ, Beck GJ, Bond JH, Byers T, Mandel JS, Mott LA, Pearson LH, Barry EL, Rees JR, Marcon N, Saibil F, Ueland PM, Greenberg ER, and the Polyp Prevention Study Group. Folic acid for the prevention of colorectal adenomas: A randomized clinical trial. *JAMA*. 2007; 297: 2351-2359.

146. Forman D, Alttman D. Vitamins to prevent cancer: Supplementary problems. *Lancet*. 2004; 364: 1193-1194.

147. Lawson KA, Wright ME, Subar A, Mouw T, Hollenbeck A, Schatzkin A, et al. Multivitamin use and risk of prostate cancer in the national institutes of health-AARP diet and health study. *Natl Cancer Inst*. 2007; 99: 754-764.

148. Lippman SM, Klein EA, Goodman PJ, Lucia MS, Thompson IM, Ford LG, Parnes HL, Minasian LM, Gaziano JM, Hartline JA, Parsons JK, Bearden JD 3rd, Crawford ED, Goodman GE, Claudio J, Winquist E, Cook ED, Karp DD, Walther P, Lieber MM, Kristal AR, Darke AK, Arnold KB, Ganz PA, Santella RM, Albanes D, Taylor PR, Probstfield JL, Jagpal TJ, Crowley JJ, Meyskens FL Jr, Baker LH, Coltman CA Jr. Effect of selenium and vitamin E on risk of prostate cancer and other cancers: The Selenium and Vitamin E Cancer Prevention Trial (SELECT). *JAMA*. 2009; 301: 39-51.

149. De Mattia E, Toffoli G. C677T and A1298C MTHFR polymorphisms, a challenge for antifolate and fluoropyrimidine-based therapy personalisation. *Eur J Cancer*. 2009; 45(8): 1333-1351.

150. Sharma R, Rivory L, Beale P, Ong S, Horvath L, Clarke SJ. A phase II study of fixed-dose capecitabine and assessment of predictors of toxicity in patients with advanced/metastatic colorectal cancer. *Br J Cancer*. 2006; 94(7): 964-968.

151. Allen NE, Beral V, Casabonne D, Kan SW, Reeves GK, Brown A, Green J, and the Million Women Study Collaborators. Moderate alcohol intake and cancer incidence in women. *J Natl Cancer Inst*. 2009; 101: 296-305.

152. American Heart Association. Alcohol, wine, and cardiovascular disease. www.americanheart.org/presenter.jhtml?identifier=4422. Accessed October 6, 2009.

CHAPTER 8

Health Behavior Change Counseling

Karen Basen-Engquist, PhD, MPH, Heidi Perkins, PhD, and Daniel C. Hughes, PhD

Content in this chapter covered in the CET exam outline includes the following:

- Knowledge to identify a teachable moment for cancer survivors and ability to use that time to provide appropriate information and education about resuming or adopting an exercise program.

- General knowledge of psycho-social problems common to cancer survivors, such as depression, anxiety, fear of recurrence, sleep disturbances, body image, sexual dysfunction, and work and marital difficulties.

- Knowledge of behavioral strategies that can enhance motivation and adherence (e.g., goal setting, exercise logs, planning).

- Knowledge of the impact of cancer diagnosis and treatment on quality of life (QOL), and the potential for exercise to enhance a range of QOL outcomes for survivors (e.g., sleep, fatigue, and other factors).

- Knowledge of and ability to determine effectiveness of group exercise programming vs. individual exercise to meet client's needs.

- Knowledge of how cancer and cancer treatment relate to ability and readiness to start an exercise program.

- Ability to facilitate the social support needs that are cancer specific including connections to websites and local support groups.

Evidence of the benefits of exercise for cancer survivors is growing. Nevertheless, many cancer survivors are not physically active, or they embark on an exercise program but lapse back into a sedentary lifestyle. Cancer survivors may have unique barriers to adopting an exercise program because of disease- or treatment-related side effects and sequelae. However, research on exercise adoption and maintenance shows that the use of behavioral theory and individually tailored messages can increase the probability that cancer survivors will increase their activity and stay active. This chapter describes the psychological and behavioral effects of cancer diagnosis and treatment, and how they affect a client's willingness to begin exercise along with long-term adherence to an exercise program.

Effect of Cancer on Readiness to Exercise

Despite the benefits of exercise for cancer survivors, aspects of the cancer experience may stand in the way of starting an exercise program or resuming exercise after a cancer diagnosis. This section describes common sequelae of cancer that can interfere with survivors' ability or motivation to exercise. Fatigue, diminished cognitive function, sleep dysfunction, psychological distress, and fear of lymphedema have all been cited as barriers to exercise.

Fatigue is a common side effect of several cancer treatment modalities, and for many survivors fatigue continues after treatment ends. Studies estimate that 30 to 60% of cancer survivors have lingering moderate to severe fatigue after treatment.[1] Not only is fatigue common, but it seems to have a larger effect than other symptoms on patient and survivor quality of life.[2, 3] The causes of fatigue are multidimensional, but physical deconditioning and increased levels of proinflammatory cytokines are both potential mechanisms.

Exercise can ameliorate cancer-related fatigue,[4] but motivating people with fatigue to exercise is problematic. Helpful strategies with this population may include choosing activity that is highly valued by the client, starting with brief bouts of exercise done throughout the day, scheduling exercise during times of the day when people are the

least fatigued, and emphasizing the benefits. Often, encouraging participants to focus on simply starting a scheduled session instead of how long they need to exercise promotes increased activity. For clients with fatigue, fitness professionals should acknowledge that the first minute is always the hardest, but just getting started is the most important thing.[5, 6]

Cancer patients and survivors, particularly those who have received chemotherapy or immune-modulating treatments such as interferon, often report that the treatment has interfered with cognitive function. Survivors often refer to this as chemo-brain and liken it to being in a mental fog. Most frequently, the severity of these deficits are mild,[7] and except in the case of people who have had radical treatments to the central nervous system, these cognitive problems are unlikely to affect the physical ability to exercise. Studies of exercise in the elderly, which provide evidence for associations between physical activity and cognitive function,[8] have led other researchers to speculate that exercise may ameliorate cognitive dysfunction related to cancer treatment as well. This topic has not been well studied, nor has the effect of cancer patients' and survivors' cognitive function on exercise adherence. It is possible that clients with cognitive problems may have more difficulty making time for exercise, because their other daily tasks take longer or they have more difficulty in organizing their time. They may also have difficulty remembering exercise recommendations and prescriptions. Assisting such clients with time management, and providing written and pictorial instructions for all exercises, may support their exercise adherence. In addition, it may be important to focus on the enjoyment of an activity versus detailed goal setting or progression plans.

Sleep dysfunction is one of the most common problems reported by cancer patients and survivors, particularly those who are in active treatment. Symptoms and side effects such as pain and anxiety may exacerbate the sleep problems. In particular, survivors on hormonal therapy or whose treatment has interfered with hormonal functioning often experience vasomotor symptoms (hot flashes) that interfere with sleep.[9–11] Sleep problems can affect multiple dimensions of a person's life, and may exacerbate cognitive functioning problems, fatigue, and psychological distress. Clients reporting symptoms of a sleep disorder such as sleep apnea (symptoms are loud snoring, pauses in snoring followed by gasping or choking noises, daytime tiredness), should see a physician for a referral to a sleep specialist. Those with problems with insomnia should exercise early in the day, avoid naps, pass up caffeine late in the day, and consider some restorative mind–body activity before bed, such as gentle yoga.

Take-Home Message

Cancer patients and survivors may have specific barriers to beginning and maintaining an exercise program that are less common in people who have not had cancer. They may experience fatigue, distress, or difficulties with cognitive functioning and sleep. Such problems may require adaptations to the exercise program or the teaching approach, such as doing exercise in multiple short bouts if fatigue is an issue.

The diagnosis of cancer and the continuum of the cancer experience can be extremely distressing. Psychological distress tends to be highest shortly after diagnosis and in the early phases of treatment, with gradual improvement over time. Approximately 24 to 33% of oncology outpatients screen positive for psychological distress,[12] but studies comparing long-term cancer survivors with the general population often show no increased risk of psychological distress, particularly at clinical levels, in cancer survivors.[13] Although much of the distress associated with cancer seems to dissipate over time, some times, events, and specific areas of distress may be more salient for cancer survivors. For example, fear and anxiety about recurrence is particularly common, and is usually most prominent preceding medical appointments. Fitness professionals should be sensitive to clients in times of heightened distress, and practice active listening skills (see the sidebar Active Listening Skills for Fitness Professionals) rather than reassure clients that "everything will be all right." In addition, clients should be encouraged to continue their exercise program during these times, given that moderate activity is associated with reduced anxiety and improved perceived energy,[5, 6, 14] and may relieve depressive symptoms.[15, 16]

Distress related to appearance changes is also common, both for patients under active treatment and for survivors. Most chemotherapy patients lose their hair, not just on their heads, but also eyebrows, eyelashes, hair on the arms and legs, and pubic hair. Other appearance issues include surgeries that cause disfigurement (e.g., mastectomy, limb amputations, facial surgeries or radiation), chemotherapy agents that cause rashes, and weight loss or gain. Some patients are very self-conscious about the appearance changes and may be uncomfortable exercising in public, particularly when wearing revealing clothing. These participants may be more comfortable exercising in private settings until they feel more comfortable.

Fitness professionals can also promote a positive body image by encouraging clients to talk with people they trust about their feelings and experiences with regard to physical changes. They can help them understand that distress about appearance changes is normal, but that withdrawing from others is not a healthy response. Clients can be

Active Listening Skills for Fitness Professionals

- Watch for the verbal and nonverbal content of the client's message.
- Demonstrate interest through nonverbal behaviors such as facing the client, maintaining eye contact, nodding, and maintaining an open posture.
- Avoid thinking about a response while the client is talking; attend carefully to what he is saying.
- Ask questions to allow the client to express her feelings. Listen rather than interpret or evaluate what the client is saying.
- Paraphrase what the client has said to verify the content of the message.

encouraged to reflect on aspects of their appearance that they like and enjoy, rather than focusing on the negatives. The cancer experience may make some participants want to work out in more private settings, whereas others will want to exercise in group settings because they are seeking the social connection. Either approach can be effective. Feelings will vary among clients and may also change over time for any given client.

Survivors who have had treatment (e.g., lymph node removal, radiotherapy) that puts them at risk for lymphedema may be very fearful about this side effect, which can interfere with their exercise. Exercise recommendations for survivors at risk for lymphedema are provided in chapter 6, but what bears mention here is that data on causes and mechanisms of lymphedema are just beginning to emerge. Although survivors have often received (and may continue to receive) medical advice to avoid exerting the affected limb to prevent potential injury and increasing the risk of lymphedema, this recommendation is not solidly backed by evidence. We are now learning that exercise, properly executed, may even decrease flare-ups in women with breast cancer who have lymphedema.[17] The key is *properly executed* exercise. Nevertheless, many survivors harbor fears about lymphedema, and these fears may interfere with their exercise adherence. Fitness professionals should follow the recommendations in chapter 6 and be cognizant of participants' apprehension about exercise.

Although a cancer diagnosis and its consequences may pose barriers to engaging in exercise, they may also serve as teachable moments—survivors are interested in taking action to improve their

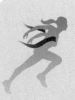
Take-Home Message
Exercise can ameliorate many of the symptoms and side effects related to cancer and cancer treatment. Information on the benefits of exercise for cancer patients and survivors can motivate them to begin or continue an exercise program, particularly those who are reluctant to start a program or are showing signs of discontinuing their exercise program.

health and may be open to making changes such as adopting an exercise program. Surveys of cancer survivors reveal that approximately one quarter to one third report increases in physical activity following a cancer diagnosis.[18-20] Recognizing the potential for increased motivation for behavior change after a cancer diagnosis can help fitness professionals keep clients focused on exercise goals.

Theory-Based Methods and Exercise

There are several advantages to understanding and applying behavioral theory when promoting exercise in cancer patients and survivors. In the general population, programs to increase physical activity or exercise behavior have been shown to be more effective when grounded in behavioral theory. Furthermore, knowledge of these theories helps fitness professionals encourage clients to start and maintain their exercise programs. Three theories, or models, that have been successfully applied to exercise settings are social cognitive theory, the theory of planned behavior, and the transtheoretical model.

Social Cognitive Theory

Social cognitive theory (SCT; see figure 8.1),[21, 22] which is frequently used as a basis for behavior change interventions, suggests that we acquire skills and perform new behaviors by observing others, as well as by enacting the behaviors ourselves and being reinforced for our performance. Furthermore, our behavior is influenced by our expectations about the behavior formed through both direct and observed experiences. These include expectations that we will be able to perform the behavior successfully (self-efficacy) and that the consequences of the behavior (outcome expectations) are predictable and desirable.

Self-efficacy about performing a particular behavior has been linked to a range of health behaviors, including exercise. It appears to have its most potent influence on exercise adherence at times when the exerciser faces new challenges such as beginning a new exercise program[23-25] and continuing exercise after a structured program ends.[25, 26]

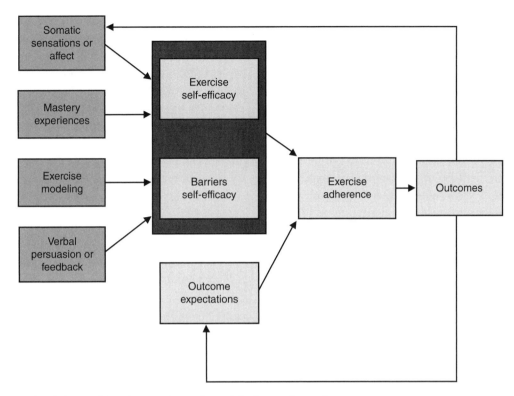

Figure 8.1   Social cognitive theory–based model of exercise adherence.

Adapted from *Psychology of Sport and Exercise*, Vol. 12, K. Engquist et al., "Design of the steps to health study of physical activity in survivors of endometrial cancer: Testing a social cognitive theory model," pgs. 27-35, copyright 2011, with permission from Elsevier.

Changes in self-efficacy among participants in exercise interventions are related to exercise adherence,[27] but a person's self-efficacy at the start of an exercise program is also relevant and has been shown to predict exercise adherence in a range of populations, including cardiac rehabilitation patients,[28, 29] overweight sedentary primary care patients,[30] elderly people,[31, 32] and women at midlife.[33]

Self-efficacy also is related to exercise behavior in cancer survivors. In a survey of breast cancer survivors, self-efficacy about being able to exercise and overcome barriers to maintaining exercise over time was associated with higher daily energy expenditure.[34] Self-efficacy at the beginning of an exercise program for breast cancer survivors predicted how much exercise (minutes of exercise, pedometer steps, and percentage of goal met) they did in the 12-week program.[35] A study of an exercise and diet intervention for breast, prostate, and colon cancer survivors found that self-efficacy at the end of the program was associated with exercise duration.[36]

A person's perception of the outcomes that will result from exercise (outcome expectations) are related first to the initiation of an exercise routine. Whether the person's expectations are met can affect long-term behavior change. In particular, studies have shown that the realization of expected outcomes, such as improved fitness, is related to long-term exercise adherence,[37] and that participants who do not achieve outcomes are more likely to drop out than those who do.[38, 39] Outcome expectations may also play a role in cancer survivors' exercise patterns. Cross-sectional surveys of breast cancer survivors showed that specific positive psychological and physical outcomes, such as experiencing less depression and building muscle strength, as well as general positive expectations scores, were associated with physical activity.[34, 40] Higher negative expectation scores were associated with less physical activity.[34]

Programs that apply SCT to increasing adherence to exercise often use one or more of the four types of experiences or information that affect self-efficacy: *mastery experiences*, or successful experiences with exercise; *modeling*, or observing others engage successfully in exercise; *verbal persuasion*, which can take the form of social support for exercise as well as feedback on performance; and *physiological states and affect* during exercise, such as the experience and interpretation of somatic sensations such as increased heart rate and respiration, muscle soreness, and fatigue.[21, 22] Fitness professionals can help clients increase their self-efficacy and exercise program adherence by providing successful experiences in a supportive context, providing supportive yet realistic feedback on performance, exposing them to examples of other cancer survivors who exercise, and helping them distinguish somatic sensations that are normal for exercise from those that indicate a problem. In addition, helping clients to set positive and realistic expectations about the outcomes of exercise should encourage long-term adherence.

Theory of Planned Behavior

Briefly, the theory of planned behavior (TPB) states that behavior is a function of the intention to perform a behavior and the person's perceived behavioral control over the behavior (a construct similar to self-efficacy). Intention is formed by the attitudes held toward the behavior, the subjective norm (i.e., the perception of how others want the person to act), and perceived behavioral control. Attitudes are formed by beliefs about the outcomes of the behavior weighted by how the person values the outcomes. Similarly, norms are formed by the beliefs of those in the person's social network about whether she should engage in the behavior, and are weighted by the person's motivation to comply with social network members.[41]

Researchers have applied TPB to explaining physical activity in people with breast,[42-44] colorectal,[45-47] and prostate cancer,[44] as well as in mixed cancer samples[48] and bone marrow transplant patients.[49] These studies demonstrate that models of exercise behavior for cancer survivors differ somewhat from those for healthy people,[50] particularly with regard to the beliefs about outcomes that are hypothesized to create attitudes about exercise.[42, 45] Studies vary in the extent to which attitude, subjective norm, or perceived behavioral control predict the intention to exercise, so it is not possible to say which variable makes the most important contribution in forming intentions to exercise. However, intention has been consistently associated with

future exercise behavior.[47-49] Vallance and colleagues[51] tested a physical activity intervention for breast cancer survivors using print material based on TPB. The group that received the TPB print material had a greater improvement in attitudes, intentions, and planning (i.e., making specific plans to start exercising). The effect of the intervention on physical activity was explained in part by the changes it produced in participants' physical activity intentions and planning.

Research on TPB enhances our understanding of some of the factors associated with the adoption of physical activity and helps identify appropriate intervention messages for particular populations.[52] For example, messages about the benefits of exercise may need to be different for cancer survivors than for other clients, focusing on distraction from cancer, coping with the stress of cancer, recovery, and getting back to normal after a cancer diagnosis. Additionally, the strong relationship between intentions and exercise highlights the importance of having clients develop specific goals, as well as plans for achieving them.

Transtheoretical Model

The transtheoretical model (TTM) incorporates variables from a range of theories. It was originally developed to describe the process of smoking cessation and the psychological variables important to the process. It has since been applied to other health behaviors, including exercise. Probably the most well-known concept from the TTM is stages of change. According to TTM, people do not make changes all at once, such as going from being a couch potato to being a committed exerciser overnight. Rather, they go through a series of stages in their decision and commitment to change their behavior. The stages, which range from precontemplation to maintenance, are described in figure 8.2. People in the precontemplation stage are inactive and not even considering changing. Those in the contemplation stage are beginning to think about being active and may be researching or seeking information to weigh the pros and cons of exercising. In the preparation stage people often make an investment in exercise (e.g., purchasing exercise clothes or shoes, making concrete plans to exercise) and have started being active but are not yet doing regular exercise at recommended levels.

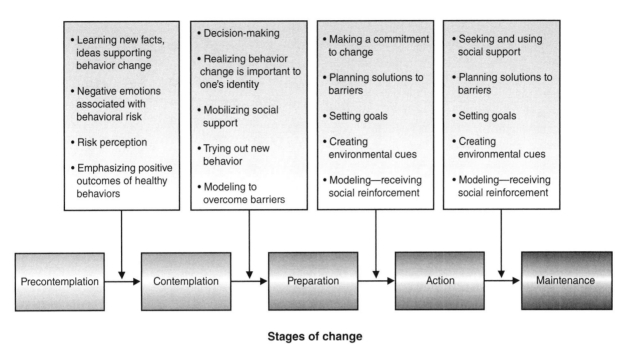

Figure 8.2 Transtheoretical model.

Adapted from Bartholomew et al. 2001. *Intervention Mapping: Designing Theory- and Evidence-Based Health Promotion Programs*. Mountain View, CA: Mayfield.

The action stage includes people who exercise at recommended levels, but have done so regularly for less than six months. Those in the maintenance phase have been exercising regularly for longer than six months.

People adopting an exercise program can move forward and backward among the stages, depending on their experiences and beliefs about exercise. Different strategies to encourage exercise adherence are called for at different stages.[53] For example, a person in the contemplation stage might benefit more from receiving information about the benefits of exercise than specific information on what exercises to do. On the other hand, a person in the preparation or action stage will benefit from activities to increase skill and self-efficacy in exercise. It is important to note that movement through the stages is not necessarily linear and may require several attempts to move from one stage to another. Clients use a variety of behavioral and cognitive processes to move across the stages, employing more cognitive processes (e.g., information gathering) at the earlier stages and more behavioral strategies (e.g., rewards) at the later stages.[54, 55] Therefore, different strategies should be employed at different stages.

Translating Theory Into Practice

Behavioral theory is useful for helping clients adopt and maintain exercise as part of their lifestyle. The first step to incorporate theoretical tools in work with clients is to find out about their interests, preferences, and lifestyles. Fitness professionals should actively involve clients in the planning process to tailor the exercise program to their needs and interests, taking into account their exercise goals and preferences for exercise type (i.e., group versus individual, or a combination), timing, and intensity.

Fitness professionals should consider their clients' stage of readiness when helping to change exercise habits (see figure 8.3 for a form to help evaluate stage of readiness), addressing the barriers clients face to becoming more active, stressing the benefits of being more physically active, and helping them become more confident about their ability to be active. For example, when a client is just starting to think about becoming more active, the fitness professional can explore the benefits of exercise and how these match with the client's own values. For instance, exercise may increase her energy level, which will help her be able to spend more time playing with her grand-children. Additionally, the fitness professional can address health issues or other factors that pose barriers to exercise and discuss strategies to overcome those barriers. At this stage raising awareness of the benefits of and barriers to exercise and exploring potential strategies are appropriate. Expressing confidence in the client's ability to become active builds confidence in the client. Pointing out the success of other cancer survivors makes use of modeling and can also promote confidence in the ability to exercise and overcome barriers.

At a later stage of change, when a client is doing some activity but wants to increase his activity levels or work toward long-term maintenance, additional behavioral theory may be used to promote achievement of goals. Problem solving about how to overcome barriers to exercise is appropriate. Discussions about goal setting, self-monitoring (i.e., use of exercise logs), and rewards are also important.

Take-Home Message

Fitness professionals should consider the client's stage of readiness when helping to change exercise habits. When a client or potential client is just starting to think about becoming more active, exploring the benefits of exercise and discussing how these match with the client's values can be helpful. How will exercise help him achieve his life goals or participate in valued activities? Once a client has made the commitment to start exercise, building skills and self-efficacy is important.

To increase clients' self-efficacy for exercise, fitness professionals should consider the four sources of information that affect self-efficacy: mastery

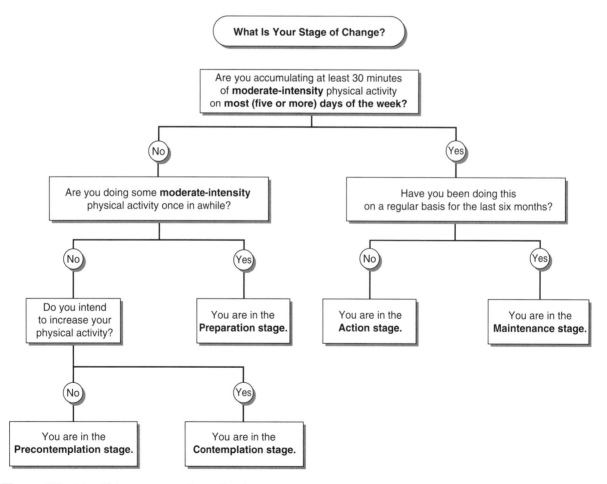

Figure 8.3 Identifying your readiness to change.

Adapted, by permission, from S.N. Blair et al., 2001, *Active living every day: 20 weeks to lifelong vitality* (Champaign, IL: Human Kinetics), 9.

experiences, modeling, verbal persuasion and feedback, and physiological and affective states. The first step is developing a plan for exercise that will enable the client to experience success. The fitness professional and client should develop the exercise plan together, and the fitness professional should guide the client to successful completion of the activity, whether the activity is 10 minutes of walking or a series of stretches or strength exercises. Another way to build confidence is to identify role models similar in age and ability to the client who have succeeded with exercise programs. Clients can also identify people in their own social networks who may encourage them to exercise. This may involve developing a plan for asking a spouse or friend to exercise with them or who can provide moral or logistic support. Pointing out recent success in being active and providing verbal encouragement for recent efforts can increase confidence at this stage.

Appropriate goal setting can motivate clients to exercise (see figure 8.4 for a goal-setting form). Setting and reaching a goal can help clients stay on track with their exercise plans. To be effective, goals should be selected by the client and should be specific, measurable, realistic, and attainable in a fairly short time period. When discussing the benefits of exercise, fitness professionals should determine what the client hopes to gain from exercise and help the client develop goals based on those interests. Although it is important to aim high when setting goals, aiming too high may result in discouragement if the client doesn't reach the goal in the time anticipated. Fitness professionals should be ready to help their clients adjust their goals, if necessary, based on changing circumstances, and to develop more attainable goals as steps to reaching longer-term goals.

Finally, some clients have cancer-related concerns that are outside of the fitness professional's

---

Figure 8.4   **Ready? Set Goals!**

Setting realistic, achievable goals is a key to success.

Are You Doing Any Exercise?

Set a goal to increase the duration or frequency of your activity. Remember to be specific. Think about times in your day you might be able to fit more activity in.

What is your long-term goal? (Make sure it is specific and realistic.)

_____

_____

What is a realistic short-term goal for you for the next week? (Make sure it is specific and realistic.)

_____

_____

How are you going to monitor your progress?

_____

_____

How will you reward yourself when you reach your goal?

_____

_____

From ACSM, 2012, *ACSM's guide to exercise and cancer survivorship* (Champaign, IL: Human Kinetics).

Take-Home Message

An appropriately tailored exercise program and goals can improve self-efficacy. Starting with an accessible exercise program and achievable individualized goals gives clients a feeling of success that builds self-efficacy. Verbal encouragement and normalizing the physical sensations they may experience with exercise may also boost self-efficacy, as does seeing others in a similar situation accomplish their exercise goals.

area of expertise. Fitness professionals should be familiar with support groups and other services in the community for people with cancer, so they can refer clients having undue difficulties such as psychological distress, severe fatigue, or lymphedema. The local chapter of the American Cancer Society can be a good source of this type of information. Its website lists services such as support groups and health education in a person's local area (www.cancer.org/asp/search/crd_global.asp).

Take-Home Message

Fitness professionals should recognize that some of the concerns and problems their clients are experiencing may be beyond their area of expertise. By familiarizing themselves with resources for cancer survivors in the community, such as the American Cancer Society, they will be in a position to refer clients to these groups, if necessary, and seek additional information themselves.

Summary

Cancer patients and survivors face barriers to exercise not experienced by people who have not had the experience of cancer. Cancer and its treatment may have effects such as fatigue, cognitive functioning difficulties, and fear of lymphedema, which can interfere with the motivation to exercise and maintain an exercise program. However, because a regular exercise program can ameliorate many of these issues, cancer patients and survivors should be encouraged to avoid inactivity and engage in regular exercise as much as possible. For example, several studies have shown that exercise lessens feelings of fatigue, improves physical functioning and quality of life, and lessens psychological distress. Evidence is also emerging to indicate that exercise may decrease the risk of developing lymphedema, and among women who have lymphedema, exercise may improve it. Evidence is also emerging to indicate that exercise may improve body image. Studies in noncancer populations have also shown a relationship between exercise and improved cognitive functioning and better sleep quality. These benefits should be emphasized in working with this population, particularly with clients experiencing these difficulties. Using theory-based approaches can optimize the effectiveness of exercise programming for cancer patients and survivors; these approaches include tailoring messages to clients' readiness to change, increasing self-efficacy, and helping clients set goals and identify rewards.

References

1. Bower, JE. Behavioral symptoms in patients with breast cancer and survivors. *J Clin Oncol.* 2008; 26: 768-777.

2. Arndt V, Stegmaier C, Ziegler H, Brenner H. A population-based study of the impact of specific symptoms on quality of life in women with breast cancer 1 year after diagnosis. *Cancer.* 2006; 107: 2496-2503.

3. Meeske K, Smith AW, Alfano CM, McGregor BA, McTiernan A, Baumgartner KB, Malone KE, Reeve BB, Ballard-Barbash R, Bernstein L. Fatigue in breast cancer survivors two to five years post diagnosis: A HEAL Study report. *Qual Life Res*; 2007; 16: 947-960.

4. Cramp F, Daniel J. Exercise for the management of cancer-related fatigue in adults. *Cochrane Database Syst Rev.* 2008: CD006145.

5. Ekkekakis P, Hall EE, VanLanduyt LM, Petruzzello SJ. Walking in (affective) circles: Can short walks enhance affect? *J Behav Med.* 2000; 23: 245-275.

6. Petruzzello SJ, Landers DM, Hatfield BD, Kubitz KA, Salazar W. A meta analysis on the anxiety-reducing effects of acute and chronic exercise. *Sports Med.* 1991; 11: 143-182.

7. Falleti MG, Sanfilippo A, Maruff P, Weih L, Phillips KA. The nature and severity of cognitive impairment associated with adjuvant chemotherapy in women with breast cancer: A meta-analysis of the current literature. *Brain Cogn.* 2005; 59: 60-70.

8. Yaffe K, Fiocco AJ, Lindquist K, Vittinghoff E, Simonsick EM, Newman AB, Satterfield S, Rosano C, Rubin SM, Ayonayon HN, Harris TB. Predictors of maintaining cognitive function in older adults: The Health ABC study. *Neurology.* 2009; 72: 2029-2035.

9. Couzi RJ, Helzlsouer KJ, Fetting JH. Prevalence of menopausal symptoms among women with a history of breast cancer and attitudes toward estrogen replacement therapy. *J Clin Oncol.* 1995; 13: 2737-2744.

10. Carpenter JS, Elam JL, Ridner SH, Carney PH, Cherry, GJ Cucullu, HL. Sleep, fatigue, and depressive symptoms in breast cancer survivors and matched healthy women experiencing hot flashes. *Oncol Nurs Forum.* 2004; 31: 5591-5598.

11. Savard J, Davidson JR, Ivers H, Quesnel C, Rioux D, Dupere V, Lasnier M, Simard S, Morin CM. The association between nocturnal hot flashes and sleep in breast cancer survivors. *J Pain Symptom Manage.* 2004; 27: 513-522.

12. Jacobsen PB, Donovan KA, Trask PC, Fleishman SB, Zabora J, Baker F, Holland JC. Screening for psychologic distress in ambulatory cancer patients. *Cancer.* 2005; 103, 1494-1502.

13. Ganz PA, Desmond KA, Leedham B, Rowland JH, Meyerowitz BE, Belin TR. Quality of life in long-term, disease-free survivors of breast cancer: A follow up study. *J Natl Cancer Inst.* 2005; 94: 39-49.

14. Thayer R. *The Biopsychology of Mood and Arousal.* 1st ed. New York: Oxford University Press; 1989.

15. Dunn AL, Trivedi MH, Kampert JB, Clark CG, Chambliss HO. Exercise treatment for depression: Efficacy and dose response. *Am J Prev Med.* 2005; 28: 1-8.

16. Daley A. Exercise and depression: A review of reviews. *J Clin Psychol Med Settings.* 2008; 15: 140-147.

17. Schmitz KH, Ahmed RL, Troxel A, Cheville A, Smith R, Lewis-Grant L, Bryan CJ, Williams-Smith CT, Greene QP. Weight lifting in women with breast-cancer-related lymphedema. *N Engl J Med.* 2009; 361: 664-673.

18. Alfano CM, Day JM, Katz ML, Herndon JE, Bittoni MA, Oliveri JM, Donohue K, Paskett ED. Exercise and dietary change after diagnosis and cancer-related symptoms in long-term survivors of breast cancer: CALGB 79804. *Psycho-Oncology.* 2009; 18: 128-133.

19. Humpel N, Magee C, Jones SC. The impact of a cancer diagnosis on the health behaviors of cancer survivors and their family and friends. *Support Care Cancer.* 2007; 15: 621-630.

20. Hawkins NA, Smith T, Zhao L, Rodriguez J, Berkowitz Z, Stein KD. Health-related behavior change after cancer: Results of the American cancer society's studies of cancer survivors (SCS). *J Cancer Surviv.* 2010; 4: 20-32.

21. Bandura A. *Social Foundations of Thought and Action: A Social-Cognitive Theory.* Englewood Cliffs, NJ: Prentice Hall; 1986.

22. Bandura A. *Self-Efficacy: The Exercise of Control.* New York: W. H. Freeman; 1997.

23. McAuley E. The role of efficacy cognitions in the prediction of exercise behavior in middle-aged adults. *J Behav Med.* 1992; 15: 65-87.

24. McAuley E, Courneya KS, Rudolph DL, Lox CL. Enhancing exercise adherence in middle-aged males and females. *Prev Med.* 1994; 23: 498-506.

25. Oman RF, King AC. Predicting the adoption and maintenance of exercise participation using self-efficacy and previous exercise participation rates. *Am J Health Promot.* 1998; 12: 154-161.

26. McAuley E. Self-efficacy and the maintenance of exercise participation in older adults. *J Behav Med.* 1993; 16: 103-113.

27. Miller YD, Trost SG, Brown WJ. Mediators of physical activity behavior change among women with young children. *Am J Prev Med.* 2002; 23: 98-103.

28. Moore SM, Dolansky MA, Ruland CM, Pashkow FJ, Blackburn GG. Predictors of women's exercise maintenance after cardiac rehabilitation. *J Cardiopulm Rehabil.* 2003; 23: 40-49.

29. Carlson JJ, Norman GJ, Feltz DL, Franklin BA, Johnson JA, Locke SK. Self-efficacy, psychosocial factors, and exercise behavior in traditional versus modified cardiac rehabilitation. *J Cardiopulm Rehabil.* 2001; 21: 363-373.

30. Steptoe A, Rink E, Kerry S. Psychosocial predictors of changes in physical activity in overweight sedentary adults following counseling in primary care. *Prev Med.* 2000; 31: 183-194.

31. Rhodes RE, Martin AD, Taunton JE. Temporal relationships of self-efficacy and social support as predictors of adherence in a 6-month strength-training program for older women. *Percept Mot Skills.* 2001; 93: 693-703.

32. Garcia AW, King AC. Predicting long-term adherence to aerobic exercise: A comparison of two models. *J Sport & Exerc Psychol.* 1991; 13: 394-410.

33. Wilbur J, Miller AM, Chandler P, McDevitt J. Determinants and physical activity and adherence to a 24-week home-based walking program in African American and Caucasian women. *Res Nurs Health.* 2003; 26: 213-224.

34. Rogers LQ, Shah P, Dunnington G, Greive A, Shanmugham A, Dawson B, Courneya KS. Social cognitive theory and physical activity during breast cancer treatment. *Oncol Nurs Forum.* 2005; 32: 807-815.

35. Pinto, BM, Rabin C, Dunsiger S. Home-based exercise among cancer survivors: Adherence and its predictors. *Psycho-Oncology.* 2009; 18: 369-376.

36. Mosher CE, Fuemmeler BF, Sloane R, Kraus W, Lobach D, Snyder D, Demark-Wahnefried W. Change in self-efficacy partially mediates the effects of the FRESH START Intervention on Cancer Survivors' Dietary Outcomes. *Psycho-Oncology.* 2008; 17: 1014-1023.

37. Brassington GS, Atienza AA, Perczek RE, DiLorenzo TM, King AC. Intervention-related cognitive versus social mediators of exercise adherence in the elderly. *Am J Prev Med.* 2002; 23: 80-86.

38. Sears SR, Stanton AL. Expectancy-value constructs and expectancy violation as predictors of exercise adherence in previously sedentary women. *Health Psychol.* 2001; 20: 326-333.

39. Desharnais R, Bouillon J, Gaston G. Self-efficacy and outcome expectations as determinants of exercise adherence. *Psychological Reports.* 1986; 59: 1155-1159.

40. Rogers LQ, Courneya KS, Shah P, Dunnington G, Hopkins-Price P. Exercise stage of change, barriers, expectations, values and preferences among breast cancer patients during treatment: A pilot study. *Eur J Cancer Care (Engl).* 2007; 16: 55-66.

41. Ajzen I. The Theory of Planned Behavior. *Orgl Beh and Hum Dec Proc.* 1991; 50: 1-33.

42. Courneya KS, Friedenreich CM. Utility of the theory of planned behavior for understanding exercise during breast cancer treatment. *Psycho-Oncology.* 1991; 8: 112-122.

43. Courneya KS, Blanchard CM, Laing DM. Exercise adherence in breast cancer survivors training for a dragon boat race competition: A preliminary investigation. *Psycho-Oncology.* 2001; 10: 444-452.

44. Blanchard C, Courneya KS, Rodgers WM, Murnaghan DM. Determinants of exercise intention and behavior in survivors of breast and prostate cancer: An application of the Theory of Planned Behavior. *Cancer Nurs.* 2002; 25: 88-95.

45. Courneya, KS, Friedenreich CM. Determinants of exercise during colorectal cancer treatment: An application of the theory of planned behavior. *Oncol Nurs Forum.* 1997; 24: 1715-1717.

46. Courneya KS, Friedenreich C, Arthur K, Bobick TM. *Determinants of exercise in postsurgical colorectal cancer patients.* Paper presented at the Society of Behavioral Medicine, San Diego, California, March 3-6, 1999.

47. Courneya KS, Friedenreich CM, Arthur K, Bobick TM. Understanding exercise motivation in colorectal cancer patients: A prospective study using the Theory of Planned Behavior. *Rehabilitation Psychology.* 1999; 44: 68-84.

48. Courneya, KS, Friedenreich CM, Sela RA, Quinney HA, Rhodes RE. Correlates of adherence and contamination in a randomized controlled trial of exercise in cancer survivors: An application of the Theory of Planned Behavior and the five factor model of personality. *Ann Behav Med.* 2002; 24: 257-268.

49. Courneya KS, Keats MR, Turner AR. Social cognitive determinants of hospital-based exercise in cancer patients following high-dose chemotherapy and bone marrow transplantation. *Int J Behav Med.* 2000; 7: 189-203.

50. Rhodes RE, Courneya KS. Investigating multiple components of attitude, subjective norm, and perceived control: An examination of the Theory of Planned Behaviour in the exercise domain. *Br J Soc Psychol.* 2003; 42: 129-146.

51. Vallance JK, Courneya KS, Plotnikoff RC, Mackey, JR. Analyzing theoretical mechanisms of physical activity behavior change in breast cancer survivors: Results from the activity promotion (ACTION) trial. *Ann Behav Med.* 2008; 35: 150-158.

52. Bartholomew, LK, Parcel GS, Kok G, Gottlieb NH. Intervention mapping: Designing theory- and evidence-based health promotion programs. *Health Educ Behav.* 1998; 25: 545-563.

53. Marcus, BH, Bock BC, Pinto BM, Forsyth LH, Roberts MB, Traficante RM. Efficacy of an individualized, motivationally-tailored physical activity intervention. *Ann Behav Med.* 1998; 20: 174-180.

54. Marcus BH, Rossi JS, Selby VC, Niaura RS, Abrams DB. The stages and processes of exercise adoption and maintenance in a worksite sample. *Health Psychol.* 1992; 11: 386-395.

55. Marshall SJ, Biddle SJ. The transtheoretical model of behavior change: A meta-analysis of applications to physical activity and exercise. *Ann Behav Med.* 2001; 23: 229-246.

56. Basen-Engquist K, Carmack C, Perkins H, Hughes D, Serice S, Scruggs S, Pinto BM, Waters AJ. Design of the Steps to Health study of physical activity in survivors of endometrial cancer: Testing a social cognitive theory model. *Psychol Sport Exerc.* 2011; 12: 27-35.

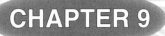

CHAPTER 9

Safety, Injury Prevention, and Emergency Procedures

Anna L. Schwartz, PhD, FNP, FAAN

Content in this chapter covered in the CET exam outline includes the following:

- Knowledge of and ability to recognize and respond to cancer-specific safety issues, such as susceptibility to infection, musculoskeletal and orthopedic changes, unilateral edema, fatigue, lymphedema, neurological changes, osteoporosis, cognitive decline associated with treatment.

- Knowledge of and ability to respond to cancer specific emergencies, including: sudden loss of limb function, fever in immune-incompetent patient, and mental status changes.

- Knowledge of and ability to respond to the signs and symptoms of new-onset and major life-threatening complications of cancer, such as superior vena cava syndrome (SVCS), sepsis or infection, and spinal cord compression.

- Knowledge of and ability to write up incident documentation related to cancer specific adverse events.

Safety, injury prevention, and emergency proce-dures are critically important when working with cancer survivors. All the safety and injury preven-tion strategies that are used with healthy exercisers must be observed, but additional considerations and precautions must be heeded with this popula-tion. This chapter discusses cancer-specific safety considerations, emergency procedures, and incident report documentation related to functional changes of the immune, neurological, and musculoskeletal systems.

Cancer-Specific Safety Considerations

Fitness professionals should be familiar with and aware of several important cancer-specific safety considerations. These include changes in immune, neurological, and musculoskeletal functions. Also, emergency procedures should be in place to ensure quick responses and the clear and accurate docu-mentation of incidents.

Immune Changes

The cause of infection in cancer patients is multifac-torial and can be from the disease itself or treatment-related.[1] Infections that arise from the disease occur when the bone marrow becomes infiltrated with cancer cells from cancers such as leukemia, multiple myeloma, and lymphoma. Infection in an immune-compromised cancer survivor can be a medical emergency; the immune-compromised cancer survivor with a fever can quickly develop sepsis if the infection is left untreated.

Treatment-related infection can be caused by a variety of therapies including myelosuppressive chemotherapy, which includes drugs that cause a decrease in the production of cell lines (red blood cells, white blood cells, and platelets), radiation therapy, and corticosteroids.[2, 3] Chemotherapy can decrease the number and function of white blood cells, red blood cells, and platelets. Radiation to sites of active bone marrow production, such as the sternum, pelvis, and long bones, may reduce hematopoiesis (the formation and development of blood cells). Corticosteroids suppress immune function by reducing the number of white blood cells and their function. The combination of reduced

hematopoiesis, myelosuppression, and impaired cell function increases the risk of infection.

Fever is the cardinal symptom of infection in cancer survivors with low white blood cell counts. Fever is defined as three consecutive oral tempera-tures of >38 °C or 100.4 °F in a 23-hour period, or one temperature >38.5 °C or 101.3 °F. However, fever may be suppressed in cancer survivors who are actively receiving treatment and have extremely low white blood cell counts; these people may not have an adequate immune function to mount an immune response.

Prevention of infection is critical, especially when a cancer survivor is actively receiving treatment. Strategies to reduce risks for infection include good hand washing and avoiding sick people and crowds. If a cancer survivor develops an infection, medical treatment focuses on antibiotic therapy until the infection resolves. Untreated infections can develop into sepsis, or septic shock—a seri-ous systemic infection. Septic shock can cause multisystem failure including cardiovascular func-tion, microvascular perfusion, and oxygenation of tissues. The mortality rate from septic shock is between 30 and 50%.[4]

> ## Take-Home Message
> Fitness professionals should re-mind clients to wash their hands and faces after exercise. This is an easy way to reduce the risk for infection.

A fitness professional who encounters a cancer survivor with fever should focus on helping the person seek medical care before the fever escalates to a serious infection or sepsis. It is vital that the professional recognize the signs of infection and period of risk and refer the cancer survivor to her health care team immediately. The survivor should not exercise at this time. Documentation should include information related to the presentation of the fever or infection, how long the person has reported the symptoms, and where the person was referred for treatment. Before the client returns to exercise, the fitness professional should confer with the survivor and her health care team to learn about

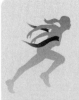

Take-Home Message
Chemotherapy can increase clients' risk for infection. Clients receiving chemotherapy should be asked whether they are having any fevers or chills. They should talk with their medical team if they are feeling sick in the days following chemotherapy administration.

any physical limitations that need to be accommodated. Obtaining medical clearance for the client to resume exercise may be prudent for the fitness professional.

A clean facility can go a long way in ensuring that clients have a healthy exercise experience. Documenting a cleaning regime is a good way to provide this clean environment (see figure 9.1).

Neurological Changes

Neurological symptoms can be profoundly disabling, both physically and psychologically, and may be a complication of cancer or its treatment. Symptoms may occur at any point along the disease trajectory and range from subtle anxiety to expressive aphasia. Aphasia results from brain damage and causes people to have trouble using and even understanding words and sentences. Symptoms range from almost imperceptible to acute, and the severity can range from insignificant to severely disabling and life threatening. Brain tumors and metastasis to the central nervous system and brain can cause neurological changes related to cancer. Treatment-related neurological changes include peripheral neuropathy (numbness in the fingers, toes, or both) and cerebellar dysfunction, and are commonly related to treatment with agents such as paclitaxel, cisplatin, and high-dose cytosine arabinoside. Central nervous system infection and sepsis can also cause neurological disturbances.

Spinal cord compression is a medical emergency. Prompt medical intervention can reduce the risk of permanent neurological disability including sensory and motor deficits and paralysis.[5,9] Back pain, motor weakness, and decreased sensation are early symptoms of spinal cord compression that usually occur over months or within days or hours, depending on how aggressively the tumor or tumors are growing. Symptoms vary, but cancer survivors may complain of heaviness and stiffness in their arms or legs, or tingling or numbness in their fingers and toes. Late symptoms include motor loss, sensory loss, loss of proprioception, and autonomic dysfunction. Proprioception is the unconscious awareness of movement and spatial orientation.

Figure 9.1 Twice-Daily Facility Cleaning Checklist

Task	Date	Initials/time	Date	Initials/time
Soap dispensers filled				
Soap dispensers work				
Antibacterial dispensers filled				
Antibacterial spray bottles filled				
Paper towel dispensers filled				
Clean towels available				
All counters cleaned				
Exercise equipment cleaned				
Showers cleaned and disinfected				
Toilets cleaned and disinfected				
Trash cans emptied				
Soiled linen emptied				

From ACSM, 2012, *ACSM's guide to exercise and cancer survivorship* (Champaign, IL: Human Kinetics).

Personal trainers need to be aware of cancer survivors at risk and quickly recognize neurological changes that may occur. Cognitive declines (e.g., changes in memory, attention, or decision making) or changes in mental status may herald neurological changes that need prompt attention. Clients who appear disoriented, restless, drowsy, or unsteady, or who have marked weakness in their legs or a change in their gait, need to promptly seek medical care. Unfortunately, treatment for spinal cord compression can only limit or ameliorate the symptoms to prevent further disability.

Peripheral neuropathy is caused by inflammation and injury to the peripheral nerve fibers and occurs most commonly in the fingers and toes, but may also extend centrally.[6] Peripheral neuropathy is a common side effect of many chemotherapeutic agents and can significantly threaten personal independence and quality of life. This side effect is often described as a feeling of "pins and needles" in the hands or feet. It can be painful and can make simple, everyday tasks, such as picking up a coin or buttoning a shirt or blouse, difficult, if not impossible. Severe peripheral neuropathy can cause loss of fine motor control, and foot and wrist drop.

The risk of injury from peripheral neuropathy is related to decreased sensitivity to temperature, gait disturbance, and reduced proprioception. The fitness professional needs to be aware of cancer survivors with peripheral neuropathy and make accommodations to the exercises they perform and the equipment they use. A survivor with peripheral neuropathy in his hands may not be able to hold dumbbells and should be advised to use stationary equipment that he cannot drop or sustain an injury from. Peripheral neuropathy in the toes and feet may affect balance and may require program modifications to reduce the risk of falls. Fitness professional may want to consider working on a client's balance and coordination.

The superior vena cava (SVC) can easily be compressed by mediastinal (chest) tumors.[7, 8] Obstruction of the superior vena cava causes pleural effusions and facial, arm, and tracheal edema. When superior vena cava syndrome (SVCS) becomes severe, brain edema and dampened cardiac filling may impair consciousness and neurological function. Symptoms depend on the extent and rapidity of the SVC compression. Only a small percentage of patients with rapid-onset SVCS are at risk for life-threatening complications. Although SVCS can be a medical emergency, it most commonly presents with the gradual onset of symptoms that need to be evaluated and treated promptly.[9, 10]

Musculoskeletal Changes

Musculoskeletal changes can range from weakness and atrophy to actual loss of limb or limb function. Musculoskeletal symptoms vary according to whether the change is a result of surgery, disuse, or disease. Limb amputation from a cancer such as a sarcoma causes sudden, life-changing alterations in mobility and strength. Surgery that disrupts muscle fibers, lymph nodes, and nerves can significantly alter range of motion and muscle function. Muscle weakness and atrophy from disuse may be the most common cause of musculoskeletal changes in cancer survivors and can render a fully functioning person weak and debilitated. Bone density and structure can be negatively affected by metastatic cancer, bone cancer, or chemotherapy. Metastatic bone cancer can change the architecture of the affected bones increasing the risk for fracture. Certain chemotherapy agents and corticosteroids cause bone wasting and also increase a cancer survivor's risk for osteoporosis and fracture. Many of the drugs used to treat or control cancer contribute to bone loss, which may be further accelerated by inactivity during and following treatment.

Muscle atrophy from disuse can be slowly corrected with exercise. However, exercise may need to be modified to accommodate for loss of limb function, limited range of motion, peripheral

Take-Home Message

When a client is actively receiving chemotherapy with drugs such as paclitaxel, the fitness professional should be sure to ask whether she is experiencing any numbness in her fingers or toes. The longer the client is on chemotherapy with agents that cause peripheral neuropathy, the worse the condition is apt to get. The fitness professional should plan an exercise program that reduces the risk of dropping weights and works on balance.

neuropathy, and impaired balance. Core strength exercises should be used to help survivors with balance problems (fitness professionals should give examples and site the muscles to be used).

> ### Take-Home Message
> Cancer survivors may be debilitated with poor muscle strength and cardiopulmonary status. Fitness professionals need to assess what type and how much physical activity clients have been doing before they begin an exercise program. Many clients will say that they used to run and lift weights, but with further questioning, fitness professionals may discover that was 30 years ago! Exercise programs must be individualized to clients' abilities and where they are now, not where they were 30 years ago.

Patients with known bone metastasis or osteoporosis should be monitored closely. Weightlifting should be limited to weights they can manage using correct form throughout the full range of motion. Ideally, this would be determined through 1-repetition maximum testing, but rating of perceived exertion could also be used to determine appropriate weights. Balance and core strengthening are particularly important for people with these conditions to decrease their risk of falls and improve their balance.

Lymphedema is perhaps the most common and disabling side effect of surgery. Lymphedema causes swelling in the affected extremity, either from an abnormality in the production of lymph fluid or, more commonly, an obstruction of the circulating lymph fluid. Lymphedema can occur immediately following surgery or be triggered months or years after surgery as a result of radiation therapy or an infection. Common surgical sites related to lymphedema are dissection of the axillary nodes in the armpit and the inguinal nodes in the groin (less common). Lymphedema causes pain and shiny, swollen skin that feels full and tight. It can cause swelling in the fingers, hand, arm, or leg. Swelling may be intermittent, disappear entirely, or persist. Lymphedema impairs circulation and increases the risk of infection in the affected extremity.

Preventing lymphedema is difficult. Exercise, both aerobic and resistance, is safe.[11-13] However, resistance exercise must be done methodically. The exerciser should start a program without any additional resistance and slowly progress to adding resistance with weights. A recent study of women with lymphedema demonstrated that resistance exercise reduced the incidence and severity of lymphedema.[11] Many patients with lymphedema wear compression sleeves to control the swelling, and the National Lymphedema Network recommends that cancer survivors with lymphedema wear compression sleeves when they exercise.

Unilateral edema may be a sign of circulatory obstruction and should be considered a risk for exercise. Unless the cancer survivor can attribute the one-sided swelling to a specific recent injury, he should not be permitted to exercise. The cause of unilateral edema could be infection, a tumor compressing surrounding structures, or new-onset lymphedema. Survivors presenting with unilateral edema should be referred to their medical team for evaluation and treatment.

> ### Take-Home Message
> Clients at risk for lymphedema should be asked before every exercise session whether they feel any new or worsening swelling in their fingers, arm, or chest. The fitness professional should adjust the exercise session if the client reports new-onset or worsening of lymphedema and recommend that she talk with her medical team. The professional should make a note of this in the client's exercise chart and include details about when the lymphedema started, what the client is doing about it, and how the exercise program was modified.

Emergency Procedures

A facility should have written contingency plans in place to manage emergencies. The astute fitness professional can often prevent a serious emergency by carefully observing subtle changes in a cancer survivor and actively listening to the client. Most people either don't feel quite right or have unusual sensations or feelings prior to a significant event. Close attention to the onset of new symptoms and attenuation of the exercise program may be sufficient to thwart an emergency situation.

A fitness professional who recommends that a cancer survivor see a physician is responsible for documenting this and following up with the survivor, the medical team, or both. In an emergency, obtaining medical care promptly is critical. An emergency plan can be as simple as calling 911 and staying with the client. The fitness professional is not responsible for determining the cause of the illness, but is responsible for acting quickly and within the scope of practice, and for thoroughly documenting the event after the cancer survivor has been attended to by the appropriate medical personnel.

Documentation

Complete and accurate documentation is one of the most important skills for a fitness professional working with cancer survivors to develop. Accurate written documentation is an integral aspect of risk management and is critical when a client has new onset of symptoms, has a serious untoward event or emergency, or is returning to exercise after an illness. Fitness professionals can be held accountable for what they do or do not document about a client, so they need to think carefully about the sequence of events that occurred and document exactly what they did, and, if possible, cite any witnesses to the event.

All documentation should be written in ink and signed at the end of the note. If written on a computer, the document should be electronically signed or printed out and signed, and then added to the survivor's exercise record. (See figure 9.2 for a sample documentation form.) Fitness professionals need to maintain clear, accurate records of changes

in a client's health status, details of safety and emergency procedures, and records of referrals to medical care. Changes in health status should be documented including the date of onset, changes in medications, physical condition, and physical ability.

Following an emergency, documentation should include careful notation of the time and date of the incident, specifics of what happened to the client, and what was done to render aid. Documentation of where the client was sent for medical care and how the client was transported there should be recorded. All notes should be fully written out, in clear and concise statements. Before a cancer survivor returns to exercise, the fitness professional should ask for a medical release, or sign a release of responsibility if no medical consent for exercise is provided.

Take-Home Message
Clear, accurate documentation after every exercise session is important for planning the next exercise session and showing clients how they are progressing. Documentation is also important for risk management after an emergency.

Summary

Cancer-specific safety issues include susceptibility to infection, musculoskeletal and orthopedic changes, unilateral edema, fatigue, lymphedema, neurological changes, osteoporosis, and cognitive decline associated with treatment. Cancer-specific emergencies may be avoided by knowing the signs and symptoms of new-onset and major life-threatening complications of cancer. Any incident related to a cancer-specific adverse event should be well documented.

Figure 9.2 Incident Report Form

Date of incident: _____   Time of incident: _____

Client's primary complaint/problem: _____

_____

Details of Event

What was the client doing? _____

_____

When did it happen? _____

_____

How did it happen? _____

_____

Who else was present? _____

_____

Were there any witnesses present?_____

_____

What actions did you take? _____

_____

What medical attention was sought? _____

_____

Was client transported to:

Doctor?   ☐ Yes   ☐ No

Emergency department?   ☐ Yes   ☐ No

How was client transported?   ☐ Ambulance   ☐ Private car

Required before client can return to exercise:

☐ Medical release to exercise

☐ Review of any new exercise limitations with health care team

☐ Discussion and documentation of client's concerns and fears about returning to exercise

Sign: _____

Date: _____

From ACSM, 2012, *ACSM's guide to exercise and cancer survivorship* (Champaign, IL: Human Kinetics).

References

1. Rieger C, Herzog P, Eibel R, Fiegl M, Ostermann H. Pulmonary MRI—A new approach for the evaluation of febrile neutropenic patients with malignancies. *Support Care Cancer.* 2008; 16: 6, 599-606. Online publication date: July 1, 2008.

2. National Cancer Institute. Surveillance, Epidemiology, and End Results initiative (SEER). http://seer.cancer.gov. Accessed July 21, 2011.

3. Williams DM, Braun LA, Cooper LM, et al. Hospitalized cancer patients with severe sepsis: Analysis of incidence, mortality and associated costs of care. *Critical Care.* 2008, 8: R291-R298.

4. Regazzoni CJ, Irrazabal C, Luna CM, Poderoso JJ.Cancer patients with septic shock: Mortality predictors and neutopenia. *Support Care Cancer.* 2004; 12: 833-839.

5. Loblaw DA, Perry J, Chambers A, Laperriere NJ. Systematic review of the diagnosis and management of malignant extradural spinal cord compression: The Cancer Care Ontario Practice Guidelines Initiative's Neuro-Oncology Disease Site Group. *J Clin Oncol.* 2005: 9(20): 2028-2037.

6. Quasthoff S, Hartung PH. Chemotherapy-induced peripheral neuropathy. *J Neurol.* 2002; 249(1): 1432-1459.

7. Nunnelee J. Superior vena cava syndrome. *J Vasc Nurs.* 2007; 25(1): 2-5.

8. Wan JF, Bezjak A. Superior vena cava syndrome. *Emerg Med Clin North Am.* 2009; 27(2): 243-255.

9. Colen FN.Oncologic emergencies: Superior vena cava syndrome, tumor lysis syndrome, and spinal cord compression. *J Emerg Nurs.* 2008; 34(6): 535-7. Epub: September 5, 2008.

10. Walji N, Chan AK, Peake DR. Common acute oncological emergencies: Diagnosis, investigation and management. *Postgrad Med J.* 2008; 4(994): 418-427.

11. Schmitz KH, Troxel AB, Cheville A, et al. Physical activity and lymphedema (the PAL trial): Assessing the safety of progressive strength training in breast cancer survivors. *Contemp Clin Trials.* 2009; 30(3): 233-245. Epub: January 8, 2009.

12. Sagen A, Kåresen R, Risberg MA. Physical activity for the affected limb and arm lymphedema after breast cancer surgery. A prospective, randomized controlled trial with two years follow-up. *Acta Oncol.* 2009; 23: 1-9.

13. Harmer V. Breast cancer-related lymphoedema: Risk factors and treatment. *Br J Nurs.* 2009; 18(3): 166-172.

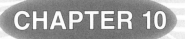

Program Administration

Carole M. Schneider, PhD

Content in this chapter covered in the CET exam outline includes the following:

- Knowledge of role in administration and program management within a cancer center, cancer treatment facility, and outpatient setting.

- Knowledge of the types of exercise programs available in the community and which of these programs cater specifically to the needs of cancer survivors.

- Knowledge of and ability to implement effective, professional business practices and ethical promotion of personal training services to the cancer care community (e.g., physicians, nurses, social workers, physical therapists, survivors and their families).

- Knowledge of the Health Insurance Portability and Accountability Act (HIPAA) and ability to implement systems to ensure confidentiality of cancer-related protected health information of participants.

- Knowledge and ability to obtain referral from physician and communicate with physician about adverse events, abilities and limitations of survivor, and outcomes of testing and training.

- Ability to recommend appropriate websites and refer to other health professionals.

- Knowledge of reimbursement programs as eligible/available.

- Knowledge and ability to recognize the limits in the scope of practice for exercise professionals in working with cancer survivors with complex medical issues.

- Knowledge of how to communicate effectively with the major medical specialties with whom cancer survivors may interact, including surgery, medical oncology, radiology, dietitians, and psychologists/psychiatrists.

Cancer exercise rehabilitation program development and administration requires that fitness professionals have the knowledge and skills to work with the medical community as well as the cancer survivor who may have multiple treatment-related complications. The goal of developing a cancer exercise rehabilitation program is to deliver quality care with appropriate exercise assessment, prescription, and intervention while also providing education and safe programs by certified and qualified personnel. This chapter presents information on the administration and management of cancer exercise rehabilitation programs with special emphasis on operational procedures, the roles and responsibilities of the rehabilitation team, reimbursement issues, and outcome evaluation.

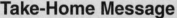

Take-Home Message

Because cancer survivors do not represent an "apparently healthy" population, cancer exercise rehabilitation should be conducted by trained and certified cancer exercise specialists, or trainers. These professionals need to be familiar with many types of cancer, the types of cancer treatments, and the side effects of the cancer and its treatments. Individualizing the program for each cancer survivor ensures the delivery of quality care.

The rehabilitation of cancer survivors and the amelioration of cancer treatment–related side effects originated with the National Cancer Act of 1971. The legislative objective directed funds to the development of training programs and research. In the same year, the National Cancer Institute sponsored the National Cancer Rehabilitation Planning Conference, which identified four objectives for the rehabilitation of cancer survivors: (1) psychosocial support, (2) optimization of physical functioning, (3) vocational counseling, and (4) optimization of social functioning.[1]

Cancer rehabilitation requires a multidisciplinary approach because of the many complications and toxicities of cancer and cancer treatments.[2] To meet the four objectives, the cancer care team included

physicians, case managers, oncology and rehabilitation nurses, social workers, psychologists, occupational therapists, dietitians, speech therapists, vocational counselors, and physical therapists. Physical therapists had the role of optimizing physical functioning. The difficulty with physical therapy is the limited time therapists have to evaluate and treat cancer survivors. As a result, Certified Cancer Exercise Trainers were needed in the field of exercise physiology and fitness.

Designing a Cancer Rehabilitation Program

Cancer exercise rehabilitation program development includes four steps: a needs assessment, program development, program implementation, and program evaluation.[3] The needs assessment involves surveying the needs of the cancer survivor population. This information, along with information about community needs (e.g., Is the local YMCA interested in offering exercise classes for cancer survivors? Are there any exercise classes in the cancer survivor's community?), can assist in the determination of programming and services.[4] The needs of survivors and their community can be determined using instruments and strategies such as market surveys, participant surveys, focus groups, current community program evaluations, and local organization databases (e.g., American Cancer Society).

Following the needs assessment and the determination of the community's needs, the next step is developing the program. Developing the program begins with creating a mission statement and then developing program goals that support that statement. Objectives, developed next, should support both the mission statement and the goals. Objectives form the basis for program decisions and help determine program success.[4] See the sidebar Mission Statement, Goals, and Objectives for a Cancer Rehabilitation Program.

Creating an organizational structure of program staff is the next step in program development. Figure 10.1 shows an example of an organizational structure. The board of director's role is leadership rather than management. The board provides oversight and direction to senior administration on

Mission Statement, Goals, and Objectives for a Cancer Rehabilitation Program

Mission Statement

Advance the quality of life of cancer survivors during and following cancer treatment through prescriptive exercise rehabilitation.

Goals

- To provide scientifically based individualized prescriptive exercise programs for cancer survivors.
- To increase the number of clients by 15% each quarter.
- To educate cancer survivors concerning the continuum of cancer care.

Objectives

- To gather research findings on exercise and cancer rehabilitation and design the exercise program based on these research findings.
- To prepare a brochure that defines the services of the cancer rehabilitation program.
- To provide cancer survivors with educational materials that enhance their understanding of the cancer care process.

issues such as financial oversight and governance. The director develops and implements policy and strategy, provides strategic leadership, works with the community, and manages staff and resources. The medical director oversees clinical care and works with the interdisciplinary team (nurses, physical therapists) to ensure quality patient care. The business manager may specialize in a specific area of the organizational operations. For example, a business manager may specialize in purchasing, personnel, or administrative services. In other cases, a business manager may be held accountable

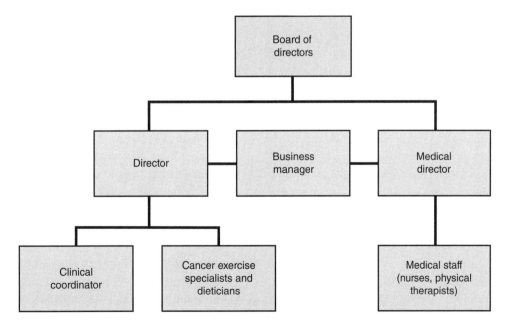

Figure 10.1 Organizational structure.

for the accuracy of the financial reporting for the organization. The clinical coordinator is responsible for the day-to-day operations of the clinic such as scheduling client appointments, managing the clinical staff (fitness professionals and dietitians), and developing the assessment and procedural manual for the clinic. The fitness professionals, dietitians, nurses, and physical therapists are responsible for the implementation of the program interventions.[4]

Program planning includes choosing the components of the cancer rehabilitation program. The Rocky Mountain Cancer Rehabilitation Institute has seven components: screening; physical examination; physiological and psychological assessment, reassessment, and prescription; dietary evaluation; individualized prescriptive exercise interventions; clinical and basic research; and advanced educational and professional development to promote high standards in cancer rehabilitation.[4,5] However, cancer rehabilitation program components will vary based on the results of the needs assessment and the program content.

Once program preparation is complete, budgeting, program pricing, and marketing plans should be established. Financial expenses may include employee salaries and benefits, equipment and materials, and marketing. Careful consideration must be given to the number of participants needed to at least break-even in regards to revenue and financial status. The financial statement should show the movement and availability of funds through and to the program over a given period of time. All financial revenues and expenses should be reviewed on a regular basis. Program implementation is based on the decisions made in the program planning phase regarding marketing strategies, staffing, and budget.

Program evaluation should begin during program implementation. Evaluation is essential to ascertain the effectiveness of the program and determine whether program and financial objectives are being met. Program evaluation is a systematic method for collecting, analyzing, and using information to answer basic questions about the program.

The types of program evaluation are process evaluation and outcome evaluation. Process evaluation assesses the effectiveness of the components of the program so that adjustments can be made, if necessary, to stay on track. Data are gathered from

Take-Home Message

A successful cancer rehabilitation program must have an evaluation process. Every program has to be justified to some type of higher administration. Program managers have to be able to show psychological and physiological progress in clients to merit continued funding.

staff and participants by asking survey questions such as the following: What are we doing? When? Where? How much? Are we delivering the program as planned? If not, why has it varied? Are we on track with time and resources? What is not working very well and why? Are we reaching the target audience? Questions should address the appropriateness of the facility, program delivery, staff performance, the schedule of activities, and the appropriateness of the screening process.[6]

Outcome evaluation looks at the program results. Questions to ask may include the following: What did we accomplish? Did we achieve our outcomes? Why or why not? What can we learn from the participants who dropped out of the program? What could we do differently next time to achieve better outcomes? Were there external influences that could have enhanced or hindered the achievement of expected outcomes? These questions address revenue versus expenditures, the number of new participants, and participant performance ascertained through pre- and postexercise assessments.

Evaluation can be performed at any time throughout the program.[6] Table 10.1 is a sample template of an outcome program evaluation plan.

Management of the program and personnel is necessary to provide physical, psychological, social, and professional conditions within the facility that will optimize the services offered. For cancer rehabilitation, this means responding to every aspect of the operation to ensure that exercise interventions are making a positive difference in the quality of life of cancer survivors. Successful management is based on leadership and vision. The director, or manager, should be able to empower others to act as needed to create an environment of trust, confidence, and pride.

TABLE 10.1   Template for Program Outcome Evaluation

Program goal	Target outcome	Steps to achieve the outcome	Results	Analysis and action plan	Person responsible
Provide a scientifically based, individualized prescriptive exercise intervention for cancer survivors	85% improvement in physical performance	Participants are offered a comprehensive, individualized three-month exercise intervention	Pre- and post-intervention fitness assessments that show that participants improved 75% on oxygen consumption and time on treadmill	Analyze program intervention to see where program can be strengthened	Clinical coordinator

Total quality management is a good theory to follow for cancer rehabilitation programs.[7] The scientific model that most closely fits the theory of quality management is the model of Grantham and colleagues[8]: the Theory of Quality Management. This model focuses on providing the best service in the most efficient way, which translates into high quality at low cost. If the management process is effective, every aspect of clinical service will be effective.

Cancer Rehabilitation Programs and Settings

A few factors to consider when developing a cancer rehabilitation program are the convenience of the facility location, scheduling that does not interfere with community programs, liability waivers and informed consent required in the area, the number of program participants in relation to the number of staff members, and the type of staff (e.g., cancer exercise specialists, physical therapists).

Cancer rehabilitation programs take place in a variety of settings. However, the majority of successful programs are clinical, occurring in hospital or physical therapy settings because of reimbursement issues and the access to cancer survivors. A limited number of cancer rehabilitation programs are located in community facilities such as YMCAs. Even fewer comprehensive cancer rehabilitation programs take place in commercial settings. These usually have programs for survivors following their cancer treatments.

Regardless of the setting, the target population determines the needs of the facility. In cancer rehabilitation, the needs of the target population usually are based on health goals or fitness goals. Clinical settings usually address health goals such as improving health and preventing the onset of recurrence while improving physical functioning. Programs address education, behavior modification, and exercise programming that emphasizes initial, improvement, and maintenance phases. The program begins with a gentle introduction to physical activity and emphasizes consistent participation and proper technique. The improvement phase provides gradual nonlinear progression based on the health status of the cancer survivor. Some days the person will not be able

Take-Home Message

The type of exercise program will depend on where the client is in the cancer continuum. If the client is in the treatment phase, then the exercise workout will be low to moderate in intensity with moderate-intensity workouts on good days and low-intensity workouts on bad days. Fitness professionals determine the good and bad days by asking clients how they feel that day. They should also take note of when the client had treatment; until more research is completed that may suggest otherwise, clients should not exercise the day of or the day following treatment.

to exercise as hard as on other days, especially if she is going through treatment. Therefore, progression will be gradual and nonlinear. The maintenance phase of the program encourages lifestyle changes in exercise habits and adherence to those changes.

A target population that consists of people who want to become more fit would receive programming based on the goal of getting stronger or losing weight. The programming would address looking better or feeling better, and the exercise prescription would concentrate more on the improvement phase of exercise programming. This type of programming would be for cancer survivors who are at least six months out from treatment.[3, 4]

Program Description and Operations

Although other cancer rehabilitation programs exist, this section provides an overview of a program that has been successful in meeting specific objectives such as improved psychological and physiological performance and high levels of participation. The cancer survivor chart should be developed first so as to assist in the collection of important information. Figure 10.2 displays what should be in the client's chart.

Every client should have a health screening prior to participation in the program. Screening forms can be sent to clients so they have time to complete them before coming to the facility. The health screening should include a cancer history, medical and family history, risk factor analysis, lifestyle evaluation, fatigue scale analysis, depression inventory, quality of life index, and dietary record. A physical examination is not always necessary, but if a physician is available to do one, the fitness professional should present the client to the physician (figure 10.3). A comprehensive fitness and nutritional assessment should be conducted because cancer treatment–related toxicities affect the entire body. Assessments should include cardiorespiratory endurance, pulmonary function, pulse oximetry, muscular strength and endurance, balance, body composition and circumference measurements, flexibility and range of motion, and dietary analysis and counseling.

Take-Home Message
Assessments should include possible toxicities clients may have experienced with cancer treatment (e.g., cardiovascular assessment because of cardiovascular toxicities with chemotherapy). Because no direct correlation exists between symptoms and toxicities, a variety of assessments should be done that include all systems of the body.

Individualized or personalized exercise prescriptions should be based on the client's assessment results, and exercise interventions or programs offered at the facility should be based on the exercise prescription. For example, if an intervention or program is to be offered for cancer survivors who are new to exercise, and their prescription recommends supervised exercise at a moderate-intensity, then the intervention or program should be just that. Following the program planned length of your exercise intervention, reassessments identical to the initial assessments should be completed to determine whether the objective of improving fitness has been met.[4, 5]

A well-designed operational plan should be established for the facility. Basic procedures such as opening and closing procedures, quality control within the facility, and emergency procedures need to be established and carefully implemented. Because clients will expect consistency in the opening and closing of the facility, an employee should be assigned this task and be given a checklist that outlines the opening procedures and closing procedures. The opening checklist may include checking the cleanliness of equipment (especially important for cancer survivors who are highly susceptible to infections), checking the availability of perishable supplies used for the program, and ensuring that safety equipment is functional. The closing checklist should include securing all doors and windows and turning on alarms. The sidebar Topics for Operating Procedures for Cancer Rehabilitation Facilities lists topics that need to be a part of the operational plan of the facility.

Figure 10.2 Chart Contents: Initial Assessment

Name: _____

Document	Date completed	Initials
Right side		
Charting sheet		
Exercise prescription		
Data collection sheet (assessment)		
Biodex printout		
Pulmonary printout		
Piper Fatigue Scale		
Beck Scale		
Quality of life index		
Informed consent		
Cardiovascular disease risk factors		
Lifestyle evaluation		
Dietary analysis		
Correspondence		
Left side		
Problem list		
Cancer history		
Medical history		
Physical exam		
Insurance information		

From ACSM, 2012, *ACSM's guide to exercise and cancer survivorship* (Champaign, IL: Human Kinetics). Reprinted from C.M. Schneider, C.A. Dennehy and S.D. Carter, 2003, *Exercise and cancer recovery* (Champaign, IL: Human Kinetics), 167. Used by permission of the Rocky Mountain Cancer Rehabilitation Institute.

Figure 10.3　Presenting the Cancer Survivor to the Physician

Name: _____　Age: _____

Referral source: _____　Primary care physician: _____

Last visit to cancer rehabilitation center was _____ years ago.

Diagnosis

Type of cancer (location): _____

Stage of cancer (if known): _____

History of Present Illness (HPI)

Date/s of diagnosis: _____

Surgeries (type and date): _____

Chemotherapy: _____

Radiation: _____

Cancer History

Since last visit to cancer rehabilitation center, cancer history (circle one):　Has changed　Has not changed

Changes include: _____

Recurrence: _____

New treatment: _____

Completed treatment: _____

Problem List

Other significant medical illnesses: _____

Current problems: _____

Medical History

Since last visit to cancer rehabilitation center, medical history (circle one):　Has changed　Has not changed

Changes include: _____

Medications (circle one):　　Has changed　　Has not changed

Medications and reasons for particular medications: _____

Changes include (new medication, discontinued medication, and change in prescribed amount):_____

_____

Family History

Other cancers: _____

Serious diseases: _____

Allergies

Medications: _____

Latex, tape, and so on: _____

Figure 10.3 Presenting the Cancer Survivor to the Physician *(continued)*

Current level of activity

Type of exercise: _____

Duration: _____

Frequency: _____

Length of time client has participated in this type of exercise: _____

Lab

Recent significant results, if known: _____

_____

Goals

Short and long term during the exercise program: _____

_____

Accessibility to exercise equipment, facilities, and transportation:_____

_____

From ACSM, 2012, *ACSM's guide to exercise and cancer survivorship* (Champaign, IL: Human Kinetics). Reprinted, by permission, from Rocky Mountain Cancer Rehabilitation Institute.

Quality control is essential for client safety and satisfaction. Regular inspections of the workout area, exam rooms, assessment rooms, and bathrooms are important. Inspections should include checking the cleanliness of air vents, workout equipment (treadmills, bikes, weight equipment, poles, bands, balls, spirometer), carpets, water fountains, and so forth, because of clients' susceptibility to infection. Additionally, emergency procedures are crucial (see chapter 9).

Personnel issues and equipment selection are important considerations in the operational plan. Job descriptions help define the responsibilities and expectations of employees in specific positions. Hiring qualified, personable personnel will keep clients returning to the program. Cancer survivors will come to the facility not only to seek enhanced physical functioning but also because they may feel, for the first time since their cancer diagnosis, that they have some control in their lives. They enjoy the

Topics for Operating Procedures for Cancer Rehabilitation Facilities

- Entry and dismissal of clients
- Client records and charts
- Billing and insurance
- Communication with health care professionals, clients, employees
- Facilities
- Opening and closing procedures

- Maintenance and quality control
- Cleaning
- Emergency plans
- Program assessments
- Prescription development and dissemination
- Exercise interventions
- Changing and adapting to clients' needs

normalcy of their time at the facility and working with healthy, happy personnel.

The most important personnel in the cancer rehabilitation facility are the fitness professionals. These people need to recognize, address, and manage cancer-related symptoms; ensure the safety of each client; promote a positive and supportive environment; promote adherence; help clients meet their program goals during and following treatment; adjust the exercise prescription and intervention to meet client needs; and monitor client progress and communicate with clients, physicians, and other service providers. Of most importance is that the fitness professional recognize the scope of practice when working with cancer survivors. Specifically, the fitness professional must know when and how to communicate effectively with the major medical specialties with whom cancer survivors may interact, including surgery, medical oncology, radiology, psychiatrists or psychologists, and dieticians. A fitness professional, for example, should not be consulting on dietary practices nor medications to be taken.

Equipment selection should be based on the clientele, be safe and dependable, offer variety, accommodate client volume and need, and be modifiable. Equipment selection will also be based on the facility space and budget. Clients can use equipment similar to those in other fitness facilities with some modifications. For example, weight equipment often has weights that are too heavy for cancer survivors; these clients need extensive balance equipment (balance poles, balance pads) because of potential neuropathies, lightweight bands, balls, and lightweight dumbbells. As mentioned, equipment should be cleaned after the workout of every cancer survivor. Also, if at all possible, only cancer survivors should be working in the workout area to avoid exposing them to colds, flu, and coughing that could compromise their already compromised immune systems.[4]

To be comprehensive, a cancer rehabilitation facility will need to rely on ancillary services for specialized expertise. These services may include massage therapy, occupational therapy, physical therapy, lymphatic massage, pain management, biofeedback, and psychological counseling.

Policies and Procedures

Policies and procedures for cancer rehabilitation programs should meet or exceed the standards set by local, state, regional, and national health care and exercise organizations. Programs should follow published guidelines (e.g., *Health/Fitness Facility Standards and Guidelines* from the American College of Sports Medicine) that set the gold standards for patient care. These guidelines use standards of care that address legal liability.[9]

The setting of the cancer rehabilitation facility will affect the type of standards employed. For example, if the program is located within a hospital, then the hospital's policies and procedure manual will dictate infection control, emergency management, and other policies. If the program is in a community-based setting, a policies and procedures manual should be developed that addresses the management of the environment in relationship to space use, acquisition of equipment, control of hazardous materials, prevention of injuries, safety training, and staff training for emergencies. The policies and procedures manual should contain measures to ensure quality programs and the attainment of outcomes. The manual should also have procedures for information management—handling patient records, patient confidentiality, data storage, and insurance billing.[4] Lastly, policies and procedures need to address assessment and care from the time clients enter the program until they leave.

The American College of Sports Medicine recommends standards for fitness facilities that should also be standards for cancer rehabilitation facilities.[1] These standards are listed in the sidebar American College of Sports Medicine Standards for Health/ Fitness Facilities.

Legal Issues and Documentation

Legal considerations should be a high priority in the field of cancer rehabilitation. Management and employees should recognize the legal responsibilities involved in rehabilitation. The fitness professional's involvement in legal issues is associated with the environment and the services rendered. A strong management, or operational, plan should include high standards of care within all services and consistency among those delivering the services.

Within the operational plan, the management of the cancer rehabilitation program along with designated lawyers should develop a legal issues

American College of Sports Medicine
Standards for Health/Fitness Facilities

1. Facility operators shall offer a general pre-activity screening tool (e.g., Par-Q) and/or specific pre-activity screening tool (e.g., health risk appraisal [HRA], health history questionnaire [HHQ]) to all new members and prospective users.

2. General pre-activity screening tools (e.g., PAR-Q) shall provide an authenticated means for new members, and/or users to identify whether a level of risk exists that indicates that they should seek consultation from a qualified healthcare professional prior to engaging in a program of physical activity.

3. All specific pre-activity screening tools (e.g., HRA, HHQ) shall be reviewed and interpreted by qualified staff (e.g., a qualified health/fitness professional or healthcare professional), and the results of the review and interpretation shall be retained on file by the facility for a period of at least one year from the time the tool was reviewed and interpreted.

4. If a facility operator becomes aware that a member, user, or prospective user has a known cardiovascular, metabolic, or pulmonary disease, or two or more major cardiovascular disease risk factors, or any other self-disclosed medical concern, that individual shall be advised to consult with a qualified healthcare provider before beginning a physical activity program.

5. Facilities shall provide a means for communicating to existing members (e.g., those who have been members for greater than 90 days) the value of completing a general and/or specific pre-activity screening tool on a regular basis (e.g., preferably once annually) during the course of their membership. Such communication can be done through a variety of mechanisms, including but not limited to a statement incorporated into the membership agreement of the facility, a statement on the new-member pre-activity screening form, and a statement on the website.

6. Once a new member or prospective user has completed a pre-activity screening process, facility operators shall then offer the new member or prospective user a general orientation to the facility.

7. Facilities shall provide a means by which members and users who are engaged in a physical activity program within the facility can obtain assistance and/or guidance with their physical activity program.

8. Facility operators must have written emergency response policies and procedures, which shall be reviewed regularly and physically rehearsed at least twice annually. These policies shall enable staff to respond to basic first-aid situations and emergency events in an appropriate and timely manner.

9. Facility operators shall ensure that a safety audit is conducted that routinely inspects all areas of the facility to reduce or eliminate unsafe hazards that may cause injury to employees and health/fitness facility members or health/fitness facility users.

10. Facility operators shall have a written system for sharing information with members and users, employees, and independent contractors regarding the handling of potentially hazardous materials, including the handling of bodily fluids by the facility staff in accordance with the guidelines of the U.S. Occupational Safety and Health Administration (OSHA).

11. In addition to complying with all applicable federal, state, and local requirements relating to automated external defibrillators (AEDs), all facilities (e.g., staffed or unstaffed) shall have as part of their written emergency response policies and procedures a public access defibrillation (PAD) program in accordance with generally accepted practice, as highlighted in this section.

12. AEDs in a facility shall be located within a 1.5-minute walk to any place an AED could be potentially needed.

(continued)

13. A skills review, practice sessions, and a practice drill with the AED shall be conducted a minimum of every six months, covering a variety of potential emergency situations (e.g., water, presence of a pacemaker, medications, children).

14. A staffed facility shall assign at least one staff member to be on duty during all facility operating hours who is currently trained and certified in the delivery of cardiopulmonary resuscitation and in the administration of an AED.

15. Unstaffed facilities must comply with all applicable federal, state, and local requirements relating to AEDs. Unstaffed facilities shall have as part of their written emergency response policies and procedures a PAD program as a means by which either members and users or an external emergency responder can respond from time of collapse to defibrillation in four minutes or less.

16. The health/fitness professionals who have supervisory responsibility and oversight responsibility for the physical activity programs and the staff who administer them shall have an appropriate level of professional education, work experience, and/or certification. Examples of health/fitness professionals who serve in a supervisory role include the fitness director, group exercise director, aquatics director, and program director.

17. The health/fitness and healthcare professionals who serve in counseling, instruction, and physical activity supervision roles for the facility shall have an appropriate level of professional education, work experience, and/or certification. The primary professional staff and independent contractors who serve in these roles are fitness instructors, group exercise instructors, lifestyle counselors, and personal trainers.

18. Health/fitness and healthcare professionals engaged in pre-activity screening or prescribing, instructing, monitoring, or supervising of physical activity programs for facility members and users shall have current automated external defibrillation and cardiopulmonary resuscitation (AED and CPR) certification from an organization qualified to provide such certification. A certification should include a practical examination.

19. Facilities shall have an operational system in place that monitors, either manually or technologically, the presence and identity of all individuals (e.g., members and users) who enter into and participate in the activities, programs, and services of the facility.

20. Facilities that offer a sauna, steam room, or whirlpool shall have a technical monitoring system in place to ensure that these areas are maintained at the proper temperature and humidity level and that the appropriate warning systems and signage are in place to notify members and users of any risks related to the use of these areas, including subsequent unsafe changes in temperature and humidity.

21. Facilities that offer members and users access to a pool or whirlpool shall provide evidence that they comply with all water-chemistry safety requirements mandated by state and local codes and regulations.

22. A facility that offers youth services or programs shall provide evidence that it complies with all applicable state and local laws and regulations pertaining to their supervision.

23. When a child is under direct staff supervision of a facility, as a participant in either an organized activity or in an ongoing facility program, or is just under temporary staff supervision while the parent or legal guardian is using the facility, the responsible staff person shall have ready access to the child's basic medical information, which has been previously collected from the parent as part of the child registration process.

24. The registration policy of a facility that provides child care shall require that parents or guardians of all children left in the facility's care complete a waiver, an authorization for emergency medical care, and a release for the children whom they leave under the temporary care of the facility.

25. The facility shall require that parents and guardians provide the facility with names of persons who are authorized by the parent or legal guardian to pick up each child. The facility shall not release children to any unauthorized person, and furthermore, the facility shall maintain records of the date and time each child checked out and was dropped off and the name of the person to whom the child was released.

26. Facilities shall have written policies regarding children's issues, such as requirements for staff providing supervision of children, age limits for children, restroom practices, food, and parental presence on site. Facilities shall inform parents and guardians of these policies and require that parents and guardians sign a form that acknowledges that they have received the policies, understand the policies, and will abide by the policies.

27. Facilities, to the extent required by law, must adhere to the standards of building design that relate to the designing, building, expanding, or renovating of space as detailed in the Americans with Disabilities Act (ADA).

28. Facilities must be in compliance with all federal, state, and local building codes (chapter 6).

29. The aquatic and pool facilities must provide the proper safety equipment according to state and local codes and regulations.

30. Facility operators shall post proper caution, danger, and warning signage in conspicuous locations where facility staff know, or should know, that existing conditions and situations warrant such signage.

31. Facility operators shall post the appropriate emergency and safety signage pertaining to fire and related emergency situations, as required by federal, state, and local codes.

32. Facility operators shall post signage indicating the location of any AED and first-aid kits, including directions on how to access those locations.

33. Facilities shall post all ADA and OSHA signage that is required by federal, state, and local laws and regulations.

34. All cautionary, danger, and warning signage shall have the required signal icon, signal word, signal color, and layout as specified in ASTM F1749.

Reprinted, by permission, from American College of Sports Medicine, 2012, *ACSM's health/fitness facility standards and guidelines*, 4th ed. (Champaign, IL: Human Kinetics), 74-76.

manual. Legal issues should be made known to all involved in the facility, and risk management principles should be applied to enhance the quality of service, improve client satisfaction, reduce the probability of injuries, and reduce the chance of legal litigation.

Although laws affecting the rehabilitation staff and the facility vary from country to country and state to state, fundamental legal principles apply to all. Two overreaching legal concepts, contract law and tort law, are involved in the exercise cancer rehabilitation setting. Contract law delineates activities among individuals. The basic contract addresses agreements with the facility, agreements with clients, and waivers and releases.

An example of breach of contract for failure to obtain adequate information would be not obtaining informed consent from the client, although this more readily falls under negligence. Informed consent obligates the facility and the fitness professional to present to clients the details, benefits, and potential risks of all proposed intervention strategies so they can make informed choices about participation. A proper informed consent that details the risks and benefits of the program may be used as legal defense to claims on either contract or tort principles. Defense counsel would use the informed consent as an assumption of risks of the plaintiff. This, however, does not excuse the fitness professional from acting in a competent and professional manner. An ethical component of informed consent is veracity, or the obligation to speak and act truthfully.

A tort occurs when a person fails to observe a duty of care or responsibility (negligence or malpractice) that results in personal injury or death. This could involve defective equipment, hazardous surroundings, or failure to properly supervise the client.[3, 4]

Currently no specific standards exist for cancer exercise rehabilitation. However, there are standards for rehabilitation facilities and centers, such as the Manual of Standards for Rehabilitation Centers and Facilities developed the U.S. Department of Health and Human Services. The board of directors of a cancer rehabilitation facility may want to seek legal advice about which standards to use as guidelines for clinical practice until standards are developed and accepted in the area of cancer exercise rehabilitation. The best way to avoid circumstances that could result in litigation is to operate according to practices that minimize the risk of injury or negligence and ensure the safety of clients.[4]

Confidentiality is important for all staff and employees of a cancer rehabilitation facility. The Health Information Portability and Accountability Act (HIPAA) is a U.S. federal law designed to protect the confidentiality of protected health information, whether it is oral, written, or electronic. A violation of HIPAA may have serious consequences including disciplinary action, fines, and imprisonment. Strategies to ensure confidentiality include assigning a number to the patient to be used in databases; placing patient files in a locked file cabinet; identifying patients by number when using communication media such as e-mail; requiring that all patient files remain at the facility; shredding all patient materials; and using HIPAA signature forms, which should be signed by all staff, employees, and interns and kept on file for proof that the facility is in compliance with the federal law.[4]

Reimbursement Concerns

Exercise cancer rehabilitation is not yet recognized by insurance companies as a category for reimbursement. However, physical therapy and oncologists can obtain reimbursement for their services (e.g., physical examinations, some assessments). Facilities that have a physician or physical therapist on staff need to obtain a provider number for billing. In a hospital setting, the billing can be completed through the hospital billing department. Outpatient

clinics that are not connected to a hospital but have the possibility of hiring a physician or physical therapists may be able to use the physician's or physical therapists' provider number for reimbursement. Diagnostic codes can be found online. Primarily, the facility should use the Medicare guidelines (section 2535) as the gold standard. Billing and documentation (e.g., SOAP notes: subjective, objective, assessment, and patient plan) requirements of third-party payers should be followed to receive reimbursement. Networking with cancer centers and cancer treatment facilities can also help with reimbursement.[4]

Local organizations such as a Susan G. Komen Race for the Cure affiliate represent another avenue of securing funds for a cancer rehabilitation facility. Self-pay can also be explored, although many cancer survivors have extensive medical bills and so are less likely to self-pay unless they can be convinced of the importance of exercise in their cancer recovery. Many U.S. state and federal agencies have grants for cancer survivorship (e.g., the American Cancer Society, the National Institutes of Health), which may be available to facilities involved in research.

Community-Based Support

Establishing a cancer rehabilitation facility requires both public relations and marketing outreach to the medical and lay communities. This outreach builds support, increases awareness, and creates positive attitudes. Once people in the community recognize the need for a cancer rehabilitation program, they are more likely to participate.[10]

Successful cancer rehabilitation programs are recognized and supported by physicians, especially oncologists, who often refer their clients. Establishing a rapport with the oncology community will increase patient awareness of the services provided, increase the chances of exercise intervention both during and following treatment, and improve cancer survivors' attitudes concerning recovery. Cancer rehabilitation services should be clearly defined and communicated stressing the program's features and benefits to the cancer community. Spokespeople for programs should emphasize that a majority of cancer survivors experience negative cancer treatment side effects and need help with their cancer recovery.

During the planning phase, program developers identify the objectives that would demonstrate program effectiveness. Once program managers have collected data on the effectiveness of the program, they should present their data to the oncology community in a short report that emphasizes specific psychological and physiological benefits, potential risks, research references supporting cancer rehabilitation, and the qualifications of the staff. The presentation should leave no doubt in the physicians' minds about the benefits of the program to their patients. Additionally, the support of cancer support group moderators, service organizations, and clinical providers will help with program promotion.

Program promotion strategies include creating brochures outlining the program and delivering them to community oncologists and other health care providers. Follow-up calls to oncologists who received the brochure could be fruitful. Programs should also advertise in local medical newsletters, make presentations at local hospitals, and offer a week of free exercise for cancer survivors following their treatment.

Programs can make patient referrals very simple and fast for oncologists and other physicians by developing a prescription pad (figure 10.4) that physicians can just sign after checking the services they want for their patients.[4] Communication with the physician after referral depends on the physician's preference. Some want to receive the results of the assessments and know how their patient is tolerating exercise, whereas others do not want any information about their patients. Regardless of what physicians want regarding information on patients, programs should develop a charting form that outlines the name of the cancer survivor, the date, and the time of exercise to document any adverse events that may have to be reported to the physician.

Summary

Cancer exercise rehabilitation program development includes four steps: a needs assessment, program development, program implementation, and program evaluation. A mission statement, goals, and objectives should be established to ensure quality care. Programs should be safe and administered by certified and qualified personnel; they should provide appropriate exercise assessment, prescription, and intervention protocols, as well as client education.

Figure 10.4 **Sample Prescription Pad**

Patient: _____   Date: _____

Diagnosis: _____

Rx

☐ Fitness assessment and exercise prescription

☐ Supervised cancer exercise rehabilitation program

☐ Cardiorespiratory endurance

☐ Muscular strength and endurance

☐ Other (please explain): _____

☐ Flexibility and range of motion

☐ Balance and agility

☐ Water treadmill

☐ Nutritional analysis

I deem this Rx medically necessary.

Physician or primary care: _____   MD/DO/PA/CNP

Printed name:_____

Telephone number: _____

From ACSM, 2012, *ACSM's guide to exercise and cancer survivorship* (Champaign, IL: Human Kinetics). Adapted, by permission, from Rocky Mountain Cancer Rehabilitation Institute.

Once program preparation is complete, developers should establish budgeting, program pricing, and marketing plans, followed by evaluation procedures. Evaluation is essential to ascertain the effectiveness of the program and whether the program and financial objectives are being met. Programs should include behavior modification and exercise programming that emphasizes initial, improvement, and maintenance phases. Quality control is essential to ensure client safety and satisfaction. Policies and procedures should meet or exceed the standards set by local, state, regional, and national health care and exercise organizations.

Finally, establishing a cancer rehabilitation facility requires both public relations and marketing outreach to the medical and lay communities. There are many strategies for effective administration; fitness professionals need to determine the best strategy for their clients and their communities. This chapter provides a starting place.

References

1. Kaplan RJ, Van Zandt JE. Cancer rehabilitation. eMedicine Physical Medicine and Rehabilitation. http://emedicine.medscape.com. Updated 2009. Accessed September 24, 2009.

2. DeVita VT, Lawrence TS, Rosenberg SA. *Cancer Principles & Practice of Oncology*. 8th ed. Philadelphia: Wolters Kluwer/Lippincott Williams & Wilkins; 2008.

3. American College of Sports Medicine. *ACSM's Resource Manual for Guidelines for Exercise Testing and Prescription*. 3rd ed. Baltimore: Williams & Wilkins; 1998.

4. Schneider CM, Dennehy CA, Carter SD. *Exercise and Cancer Recovery*. 1st ed. Champaign, IL: Human Kinetics; 2003.

5. Schneider CM, Dennehy CA, Roozeboom M, Carter SD. A model program: Exercise intervention for cancer rehabilitation. *Integr Cancer Ther*. 2002; 1(1): 76-82.

6. U.S. Department of Health and Human Services, Centers for Disease Control and Prevention. *Physical Activity Evaluation Handbook*. http://www.cdc.gov/nccdphp/dnpa. Updated 2002. Accessed September 25, 2009.

7. Deming WE. *Quality, Productivity, and Competitive Position*. Cambridge, MA: Massachusetts Institute of Technology, Facility for Advanced Engineering Study; 1982.

8. Grantham WC, Patton RW, York TD, Winick ML. *Health Fitness Management*. Champaign, IL: Human Kinetics; 1998.

9. American College of Sports Medicine. *ACSM's Health/Fitness Facility Standards and Guidelines*. 3rd ed. Champaign, IL: Human Kinetics; 2007.

10. Kotler P. *Marketing for Nonprofit Organizations*. Englewood Cliffs, NJ: Prentice Hall; 1975.

Appendix

ACSM/ACS Certified Cancer Exercise Trainer

Job Task Analysis

Exercise Physiology and Related Exercise Science

1.1.1 Knowledge of physiologic outcomes that may be improved by exercise training among cancer survivors.

1.1.2 Knowledge of symptoms and psychological attributes that may be improved by exercise training among cancer survivors.

1.1.3 Knowledge of lymph, immunologic, cardiac, neurologic, and hematologic systems as they pertain to cancer-specific exercise issues.

1.1.4 Knowledge of acute and chronic effects of exercise on temperature regulation and the adverse thermoregulatory/vasomotor symptoms (e.g., hot flashes) experienced by many cancer survivors.

1.1.5 Knowledge of cancer diagnosis and treatment effects on physiological response to acute and chronic exercise, particularly with regard to physical deconditioning, body composition changes, and range of motion.

Health Appraisal, Fitness, and Clinical Exercise Testing

1.3.1 Ability to obtain a basic history regarding cancer diagnosis (e.g., type, stage) and treatment (e.g., surgeries, systemic and targeted therapies).

1.3.2 Knowledge of and the ability to recognize the adverse acute, chronic, and late effects of cancer treatments.

1.3.3 Ability to obtain medical history for other health conditions (e.g., neurological, cardiovascular, musculoskeletal, pulmonary) that may cooccur and interact with adverse effects of cancer treatments.

1.3.4 Knowledge of and ability to discuss physiologic systems affected by cancer and treatment and how this would affect the major components of fitness, including balance, agility, speed, flexibility, endurance, and strength.

1.3.5 Knowledge of how cancer and its treatments may alter balance, agility, speed, flexibility, endurance, and strength in cancer survivors and ability to select/modify and interpret tests of these fitness elements.

1.3.6   Knowledge of how cancer and its treatments may affect body composition in cancer survivors and ability to select/modify and interpret tests of body composition in cancer survivors.

1.3.7   Knowledge of categories of patients that require medical clearance prior to testing or exercise prescription.

1.3.8   Knowledge of cancer-specific relative and absolute contraindications to exercise testing.

Exercise Prescription and Programming

1.7.1   Knowledge of current American Cancer Society guidelines for exercise in cancer survivors.

1.7.2   Ability to describe benefits and risks of exercise training in the cancer survivor.

1.7.3   Ability to recognize relative and absolute contraindications for starting or resuming an exercise program, and knowledge of when it is necessary to refer participant back to an appropriate care provider.

1.7.4   Knowledge, skill, and ability to modify exercise prescription/program based on:
   a. current medical condition
   b. time since diagnosis on or off adjuvant treatment
   c. type of current therapies (e.g., no swimming during radiation)
   d. type and recency of surgical procedures (e.g., curative or reconstructive)
   e. range of motion
   f. presence of implants
   g. amputations/fusions
   h. effects of treatment on all elements of fitness (agility, speed, coordination, flexibility, strength, and endurance)
   i. hematologic considerations (e.g., anemia, neutropenia)
   j. presence of a central line (PIC or Port)
   k. current adverse effects of treatment, both acute and chronic
   l. individuals that may be at increased risk for adverse late effects that could increase risks associated with exercise (e.g., heart failure)

1.7.5   Knowledge of potential for overtraining with the cancer survivor.

1.7.6   Knowledge of and ability to use appropriate sun protection for outdoor programming.

Nutrition and Weight Management

1.8.1   Knowledge of common effects of cancer treatment on energy balance and body composition for individuals with nonmetastatic disease.

1.8.2   Knowledge of effects of cancer cachexia on energy balance, intake, and activity level among individuals with metastatic disease.

1.8.3   Knowledge of relationship between body composition as a risk factor for the development of some cancers, and possibly as a risk factor for cancer recurrence.

1.8.4   Knowledge that many cancer survivors may use complementary and alternative medicine (CAM) approaches, and of the potential for these remedies to influence exercise testing and prescription parameters.

1.8.5   Ability to identify unintentional weight change that may relate to disease status, and recommend that the client seek appropriate medical attention.

1.8.6   Knowledge of effect of chemotherapy and radiation on the mouth and gastrointestinal system, and the result of these changes on appetite and food preferences and choices.

1.8.7   Ability to discern when a participant's nutritional questions or status would be best managed by referral to a registered dietitian.

1.8.8   Knowledge of current American Cancer Society nutrition guidelines during and after cancer treatment.

1.8.9   Knowledge of hydration needs specific to cancer patients and survivors.

1.8.10   Knowledge of safety of weight loss programs for cancer survivors.

Human Behavior and Counseling

1.9.1   Knowledge to identify a teachable moment for cancer survivors and ability to use that time to provide appropriate information and education about resuming or adopting an exercise program.

1.9.2   General knowledge of psycho-social problems common to cancer survivors, such as depression, anxiety, fear of recurrence, sleep disturbances, body image, sexual dysfunction, and work and marital difficulties.

1.9.3   Knowledge of behavioral strategies that can enhance motivation and adherence (e.g., goal setting, exercise logs, planning).

1.9.4   Knowledge of the impact of cancer diagnosis and treatment on quality of life (QOL), and the potential for exercise to enhance a range of QOL outcomes for survivors (e.g., sleep, fatigue, and other factors).

1.9.5 Knowledge of and ability to determine effectiveness of group exercise programming vs. individual exercise to meet client's needs.

1.9.6 Knowledge of how cancer and cancer treatment relate to ability and readiness to start an exercise program.

1.9.7 Ability to facilitate the social support needs that are cancer specific including connections to websites and local support groups.

Safety, Injury Prevention, and Emergency Procedures

1.10.1 Knowledge of and ability to recognize and respond to cancer-specific safety issues, such as susceptibility to infection, musculoskeletal and orthopedic changes, unilateral edema, fatigue, lymphedema, neurological changes, osteoporosis, cognitive decline associated with treatment.

1.10.2 Knowledge of and ability to respond to cancer specific emergencies, including: sudden loss of limb function, fever in immune-incompetent patient, and mental status changes.

1.10.3 Knowledge of and ability to respond to the signs and symptoms of new-onset and major life-threatening complications of cancer, such as superior vena cava syndrome (SVCS), sepsis or infection, and spinal cord compression.

1.10.4 Knowledge of and ability to write up incident documentation related to cancer specific adverse events.

Program Administration, Quality Assurance, and Outcome Assessment

1.11.1 Knowledge of role in administration and program management within a cancer center, cancer treatment facility, and outpatient setting.

1.11.2 Knowledge of the types of exercise programs available in the community and which of these programs cater specifically to the needs of cancer survivors.

1.11.3 Knowledge of and ability to implement effective, professional business practices and ethical promotion of personal training services to the cancer care community (e.g., physicians, nurses, social workers, physical therapists, survivors and their families).

1.11.4 Knowledge of the Health Insurance Portability and Accountability Act (HIPAA) and ability to implement systems to ensure confidentiality of

cancer-related protected health information of participants.

1.11.5 Knowledge and ability to obtain referral from physician and communicate with physician about adverse events, abilities and limitations of survivor, and outcomes of testing and training.

1.11.6 Ability to recommend appropriate websites and refer to other health professionals.

1.11.7 Knowledge of reimbursement programs as eligible/available.

Clinical and Medical Considerations

1.12.1 Knowledge of the major long-term effects of treatment among childhood cancer survivors that may require careful screening and program adaptation for these individuals.

1.12.2 Knowledge of the common side effects and symptoms of typical cancer treatments (surgeries, chemotherapy, radiation, hormone manipulations, other drugs).

1.12.3 Knowledge that cancer treatment may accelerate functional decline associated with aging, particularly in the elderly, and that exercise programming may need to be adjusted accordingly.

1.12.4 Knowledge of the combined effects of aging and cancer treatment on exercise capacity and selection of appropriate testing modalities and interpretation of results.

1.12.5 Knowledge of the common sites of metastases and ability to design and implement appropriate exercise programs consistent with this knowledge.

1.12.6 Knowledge of the signs and symptoms associated with new-onset lymphedema, and the major cancer types associated with increased lymphedema risk (e.g., breast, head, and neck cancer).

1.12.7 Knowledge of National Lymphedema Network (NLN) 18 risk reduction practices, and exercise guidelines.

1.12.8 Knowledge of how cancer treatment may alter cardiovascular risk factors, and inappropriate cardiovascular responses to exercise testing or training.

1.12.9 Knowledge of lymphatic, neurological, and immune system factors in cancer survivors that may require further evaluation by medical or allied health professionals before participation in physical activity.

1.12.10 Knowledge of how common cancer treatments affect the ability of cancer survivors to perform exercise, and how to adjust programs accordingly.

1.12.11 Knowledge of the effect of cancer treatment on balance and mobility and the ability to develop an appropriate exercise program that minimizes fall/injury risk.

1.12.12 Knowledge and ability to recognize the limits in the scope of practice for exercise professionals in working with cancer survivors with complex medical issues.

Physiology, Diagnosis, and Treatment

1.15.1 Knowledge of currently accepted screening practices for surveillance of recurrence for common cancers (e.g., mammography, colonoscopy, prostate specific antigen, pap smears).

1.15.2 Knowledge of the pathology tests used to diagnose common cancers (e.g., biopsy, imaging technologies, and blood tests for tumor markers).

1.15.3 Knowledge of how to communicate effectively with the major medical specialties with whom cancer survivors may interact, including surgery, medical oncology, radiology, dietitians, and psychologists/psychiatrists.

1.15.4 Knowledge of the most common warning signs of recurrence for common cancers, and when to recommend that clients seek additional medical evaluation.

1.15.5 Understand typical durations of cancer therapy for the major cancers (breast, prostate, melanoma, ovary, lung, colon), and that therapies are continually evolving/changing.

1.15.6 General knowledge of current cancer treatment strategies, including surgery, systemic therapies (e.g., chemotherapy) and targeted therapies (e.g., anti-angiogenesis inhibitors).

1.15.7 Knowledge of how lifestyle factors, including nutrition, physical activity, and heredity, influence hypothesized mechanisms of cancer etiology.

1.15.8 General knowledge of the descriptive epidemiology of cancer, including the prevalence, incidence, and survival statistics for the major cancer types.

1.15.9 General knowledge of cancer biology (e.g., initiation, promotion/progression, and metastases), particularly for the four most common cancers: lung, breast, colon, and prostate.

© American College of Sports Medicine 2008. All rights reserved. Available: www.acsm.org/AM/Template.cfm?Section=ACSM_ACS_Certified_Cancer_Exercise_Trainer&Template=/CM/ContentDisplay.cfm&ContentFileID=2173

Index

Note: The italicized *f* and *t* following page numbers refer to figures and tables, respectively.

About the Editor

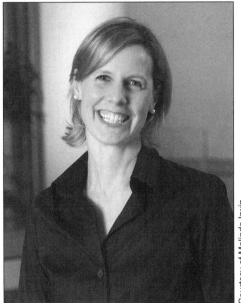

Courtesy of Melinda Irwin.

Melinda L. Irwin, PhD, MPH, is an associate professor in the Yale School of Public Health and codirector of the cancer prevention and control research program at Yale Cancer Center. Dr. Irwin's research focuses on how exercise and weight influence cancer risk and survivorship. Dr. Irwin is the principal investigator of a number of research studies at Yale University and collaborates on various national projects and initiatives focused on exercise and cancer survivorship. She has received funding from the National Cancer Institute, American Cancer Society, Komen for the Cure, Lance Armstrong Foundation, and American Institute for Cancer Research and has published her research findings in top medical journals. Dr. Irwin also serves on various national advisory committees to develop consensus statements on physical activity, diet, weight control, and cancer prevention and control.

About the ACSM

The **American College of Sports Medicine (ACSM)**, founded in 1954, is the world's largest sports medicine and exercise science organization with more than 45,000 national, regional, and international members and certified professionals in more than 90 countries. With professionals representing more than 70 occupations, ACSM offers a 360-degree view of sports medicine and exercise science. From academicians to students and from personal trainers to physicians, the association of sports medicine, exercise science, and health and fitness professionals is dedicated to helping people worldwide live longer, healthier lives through science, education, medicine, and policy. For more information, visit www.acsm.org.

You'll find
other outstanding
ACSM resources at

www.HumanKinetics.com

In the U.S. call

1-800-747-4457

Australia...08 8372 0999
Canada 1-800-465-7301
Europe..+44 (0) 113 255 5665
New Zealand..0800 222 062

HUMAN KINETICS
The Information Leader in Physical Activity & Health
P.O. Box 5076 • Champaign, IL 61825-5076 USA